CURRENT
SURGERY
OF THE HEART

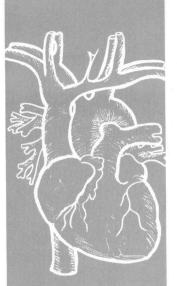

Editor
ARTHUR J. ROBERTS, M.D.

Professor and Chairman
Department of Cardiothoracic Surgery
University Hospital at Boston University Medical Center
Boston, Massachusetts

Associate Editor
C. RICHARD CONTI, M.D.

Professor of Medicine
Director, Cardiology Division
University of Florida College of Medicine
Gainesville, Florida

With 42 Contributors

CURRENT SURGERY OF THE HEART

J. B. LIPPINCOTT COMPANY
PHILADELPHIA
London   Mexico City   New York
St. Louis   São Paulo   Sydney

Acquisitions Editor: **Robert W. Reinhardt**
Sponsoring Editor: **Delois Patterson**
Manuscript Editor: **Margaret E. Maxwell**
Indexer: **Catherine Battaglia**
Art Director: **Tracy Baldwin**
Design Coordinator: **Don Shenkle**
Designer: **Maria S. Karkucinski**
Production Supervisor: **J. Corey Gray**
Production Coordinator: **Kathleen R. Diamond**
Compositor: **Progressive Typographers**
Printer/Binder: **R. R. Donnelley & Sons Company**

The authors and publisher have exerted every effort to ensure that drug selection and dosage set forth in this text are
in accord with current recommendations and practice at the
time of publication. However, in view of ongoing research,
changes in government regulations, and the constant flow
of information relating to drug therapy and drug reactions,
the reader is urged to check the package insert for each drug
for any change in indications and dosage and for added
warnings and precautions. This is particularly important
when the recommended agent is a new or infrequently employed drug.

1   3   5   6   4   2

Library of Congress Cataloging-in-Publication Data

Current surgery of the heart.

Includes bibliographies and index.
1. Heart—Surgery. I. Roberts, Arthur J. (Arthur
James) II. Conti, C. Richard (Charles Richard),
DATE.   [DNLM: 1. Heart Surgery—trends.
WG 169 C976]
RD598.C86   1987   617'.412   86-10259
ISBN 0-397-50724-0

CONTRIBUTORS

ROBERT A. BAUERNFEIND, M.D., F.A.C.C.
Division of Cardiology
Department of Medicine
Medical College of Virginia
Virginia Commonwealth University
Richmond, Virginia

WILLIAM F. BERNHARD, M.D.
Cardiovascular Surgeon
The Children's Hospital and Brigham and Women's
  Hospital;
Professor of Surgery
Harvard Medical School
Boston, Massachusetts

ALFRED E. BUXTON, M.D.
Director, Clinical Electrophysiology Laboratory
Department of Medicine
University of Pennsylvania School of Medicine
Philadelphia, Pennsylvania

JAMES G. CARR
Associate Director
Cardiovascular Surgical Research Laboratory
The Children's Hospital
Boston, Massachusetts

DANIEL S. J. CHOY, M.D., F.A.C.P.
Director of Laser Laboratory
St. Luke's Roosevelt Hospital Center;
Lenox Hill Hospital
New York, New York

WARREN CLAY, B.S.M.E.
Mechanical Engineer
Medical Products Division
Thermedics, Incorporated
Waltham, Massachusetts

C. RICHARD CONTI, M.D.
Professor of Medicine
Director, Cardiology Division
University of Florida College of Medicine
Gainesville, Florida

JOSEPH N. CUNNINGHAM, JR., M.D.
Director, Department of Surgery and Division of Thoracic
  and Cardiovascular Surgery
Maimonides Medical Center
Brooklyn, New York;
Professor of Surgery, Department of Cardiovascular
  Surgery
State University of New York
New York, New York

DAVID P. FAXON, M.D.
Associate Professor of Medicine
Section of Cardiology
Boston University Medical Center
Boston, Massachusetts

ROBERT W. M. FRATER, M.D.
Chief of Cardiothoracic Surgery
Montefiore Medical Center
Bronx, New York

ALEXANDER S. GEHA, M.D.
Professor and Chief
Section of Cardiothoracic Surgery
Department of Surgery
Yale University School of Medicine
New Haven, Connecticut

EUGENE A. GROSSI, M.D.
Department of Cardiovascular Surgery
New York University Medical Center
New York, New York;
Maimonides Medical Center
Brooklyn, New York

THOMAS HANKINS, C.C.P.
Department of Cardiothoracic Surgery
Boston University Medical Center
Boston, Massachusetts

JOHN M. HERRE, M.D., F.A.C.C.
Assistant Professor of Medicine
School of Medicine
University of California, San Francisco
San Francisco, California

THOMAS HOUGEN, M.D.
Cardiologist
The Children's Hospital;
Assistant Professor of Pediatrics
Harvard Medical School
Boston, Massachusetts

NANCY A. HOWELL
Research Associate
Cardiovascular Surgical Research Laboratory
The Children's Hospital
Boston, Massachusetts

EDUARDO JORGE, M.D.
Instructor in Surgery
Department of Surgery
The Milton S. Hershey Medical Center
The Pennsylvania State University College of Medicine
Hershey, Pennsylvania

AHMAD RAJAII KHORASANI, M.D.
Assistant Professor of Surgery
University Hospital
Boston, Massachusetts

JOHN C. LASCHINGER, M.D.
Department of Cardiovascular Surgery
New York University Medical Center
New York, New York;
Maimonides Medical Center
Brooklyn, New York

HAROLD L. LAZAR, M.D.
Assistant Professor of Surgery
Department of Cardiothoracic Surgery
Boston University Medical Center
Boston, Massachusetts

PAUL A. LEVINE, M.D.
Associate Professor of Medicine
Boston University School of Medicine;
Director of the Clinical Electrophysiology and
    Electrocardiology Laboratories
University Hospital
Boston, Massachusetts

JOHN R. MCCORMICK, M.D.
Associate Professor of Surgery
Department of Cardiothoracic Surgery
Boston University School of Medicine
Boston, Massachusetts

NOEL L. MILLS, M.D.
Department of Surgery
Ochsner Clinic and Alton Ochsner Medical Foundation
New Orleans, Louisiana

JOHN M. MORAN, M.D.
Surgeon-in-Chief
Division of Cardiothoracic Surgery
Rhode Island Hospital;
Professor of Surgery
Brown University
Providence, Rhode Island

JUDY O'YOUNG, M.D.
Assistant in Anesthesia
Cardiac Anesthesia Group
Department of Anesthesia
Harvard Medical School at Massachusetts General Hospital
Boston, Massachusetts

G. ARNAUD PAINVIN, M.D.
Associate Registrar
The College of Physicians and Surgeons of Ontario
Toronto, Ontario, Canada

WILLIAM E. PARKS, JR., M.D.
Clinical Instructor of Surgery
Humana Hospital
Loyola University
Louisville, Kentucky

DANIEL M. PHILBIN, M.D.
Associate Professor of Anesthesia
Director of Cardiac Anesthesia
Department of Anesthesia
Harvard Medical School at Massachusetts General Hospital
Boston, Massachusetts

STEVEN J. PHILLIPS, M.D.
Mercy Hospital Medical Center;
Clinical Assistant Professor
College of Osteopathic Medicine and Surgery;
Adjunct Associate Clinical Professor
College of Pharmacy
Drake University
Des Moines, Iowa

WILLIAM S. PIERCE, M.D.
Department of Surgery
The Milton S. Hershey Medical Center
The Pennsylvania State University College of Medicine
Hershey, Pennsylvania

BRUCE A. REITZ, M.D.
Cardiac Surgeon-in-Charge
Johns Hopkins Hospital
Baltimore, Maryland

ARTHUR J. ROBERTS, M.D.
Professor and Chairman
Department of Cardiothoracic Surgery
University Hospital at Boston University Medical Center
Boston, Massachusetts

TIMOTHY A. SANBORN, M.D.
Assistant Professor of Medicine
Boston University Medical Center
Boston, Massachusetts

FREDERICK J. SCHOEN, M.D., Ph.D.
Associate Professor of Pathology
Harvard Medical School;
Director, Cardiac Pathology Laboratory
Brigham and Women's Hospital
Boston, Massachusetts

WILL C. SEALY, M.D.
Professor of Surgery
Mercer University School of Medicine;
Chief of Surgery
Medical Center of Central Georgia
Macon, Georgia

JAY G. SELLE, M.D.
Sanger Clinic
Charlotte, North Carolina

NATHANIEL SIMS, M.D.
Assistant in Anesthesia
Cardiac Anesthesia Group
Department of Anesthesia
Harvard Medical School at Massachusetts General Hospital
Boston, Massachusetts

RONALD J. SOLAR, Ph.D.
Vice President
Versaflex Delivery Systems, Inc.
San Diego, California

THOMAS L. SPRAY, M.D.
Assistant Professor of Cardiothoracic Surgery
Washington University
St. Louis, Missouri

WILLIAM J. WELCH, M.D., F.A.C.C.
Division of Cardiology
Department of Medicine
Medical College of Virginia
Virginia Commonwealth University
Richmond, Virginia

BENJAMIN M. WESTBROOK, M.D.
Department of Cardiothoracic Surgery
University Hospital at Boston University Medical Center
Boston, Massachusetts

LEWIS WETSTEIN, M.D., F.A.C.C., F.C.C.P.
Associate Professor of Surgery
Division of Thoracic and Cardiac Surgery
Department of Surgery
Medical College of Virginia
Virginia Commonwealth University
Richmond, Virginia

PREFACE

It is probable that the number of open-heart surgical procedures will continue to decline over the next several years. The main reason for this change is the relative decrease in the number of coronary bypass procedures performed on an annual basis. The factors that have influenced this modification include results of the coronary artery surgery study (CASS), success in percutaneous transluminal coronary angioplasty (PTCA), socioeconomic pressures to control medical expenses, progress in coronary risk-factor modification, long-term inadequacy of the saphenous vein conduit, and improved medical therapy for coronary artery disease. Nevertheless, there are exciting developments in cardiac surgery that continue to stimulate those involved in the field of cardiovascular diseases. The purpose of *Current Surgery of the Heart* is to identify and describe selected major advances related to the surgical treatment of heart disease.

In the field of pediatric open-heart surgery, there has been greater reliance on primary corrective repair of congenital heart defects early in life. Such an approach has been associated with excellent 20-year survival for lesions such as tetralogy of Fallot. Importantly, postoperative growth and mental development for many children with such defects have been rewarding. Nevertheless, difficult clinical anomalies such as interrupted aortic arch and hypoplastic left-sided heart syndrome are still associated with high mortality rates. Dr. Thomas Spray describes these and other conditions in Chapter 17, Pediatric Cardiac Surgery.

Interest in electrophysiologic phenomena has stimulated the development of mapping techniques to chart the course of certain electrical patterns in the heart. Such procedures are performed in the cardiac catheterization laboratory and in the surgical operating room. Atrial arrhythmias, in particular Wolff-Parkinson-White syndrome, have been managed successfully with either surgical or medical treatment. In Chapter 9, Surgical Treatment of Supraventricular Arrhythmias, Dr. Will Sealy, a pioneer in this field, outlines the historical and current clinical results in this area. Ventricular arrhythmias, especially those associated with discrete ventricular aneurysms, can be successfully eradicated by electrophysiologically guided surgery. Presently, the endocardial resection procedure has gained popularity because it usually eliminates the site of arrhythmogenic foci in the myocardium. The various surgical techniques and clinical results in this field are described by Dr. Lewis Wetstein in Chapter 11, Surgery for Ventricular Tachyarrhythmias. Electrophysiologic information has also been harnessed for use during surgery on the thoracic aorta. In these situations, spinal cord ischemia with resulting paraplegia is a dreaded complication. By monitoring evoked potentials, the operating room team can identify early spinal cord ischemia. In some cases, by modifying the surgical procedure, surgeons can prevent serious injury to the nervous system. Dr. Joseph Cunningham has been active clinically and experimentally in this area. He relates his experience with this technique in Chapter 12, Use of Somatosensory Evoked Potentials During Thoracic Aneurysm Surgery. The conduction system of the heart remains a vital electrical system that has received increased attention in recent years. A new generation of complicated, programmable pacemakers has been associated with a high level of sophistication in cardiac pacing. Consequently, patients who receive the newer cardiac pacing systems require careful follow-up and regular intra- and postoperative evaluations. In Chapter 20, Cardiac Pacing: Past, Present, and Future, Dr. Paul Levine characterizes his experience with the various challenges presented by modern cardiac pacemakers.

At present, the selection of patients for myocardial revascularization involves several therapeutic choices. In addition to coronary artery bypass graft (CABG) surgery, PTCA, intravenous and intracoronary streptokinase as well as tissue plasminogen activator (TPA) offer relatively noninvasive alternative methods of affording myocardial revascularization. Further studies are necessary to clarify the relative efficacy of each of these three procedures and their influence on myocardial perfusion and patient survival. In Chapter 14, Selection of Patients for Myocardial Revascularization, Dr. David Faxon describes the current status of patient selection for procedures that potentially improve coronary blood supply.

In the field of coronary artery disease, many other interesting developments can also be identified. The laser has been used to vaporize atherosclerotic obstructions in the coronary arteries both in the catheterization laboratory and in the operating room. Dr. Daniel Choy has been influential in the initial clinical applications of this exciting development and describes his experience with this technology in Chapter 1, Lasers in Cardiovascular Disease. The application of laser technology to the treatment of coronary disease has far-reaching implications. In fact, the Boston University group has adopted laser technology over the relatively noninvasive intravascular cardiac catheter. They have lased the first several diseased human coronary arteries *in vivo* in the United States. Evaluation of surgical treatment with the laser can be assessed by the newer generation of fiberoptic angioscopes. Dr. Timothy Sanborn presents his experience with vascular angioscopy in Chapter 2, Angioscopy in Cardiac Surgery. He and his associates have also used the angioscope intraoperatively to evaluate native coronary arteries and saphenous vein bypass grafts. As the impetus to perform more complete myocardial revascularization becomes established, adjunctive intraoperative measures that help to accomplish this goal are being evaluated. Borrowing from the experience gained from PTCA, intraoperative balloon-tipped catheter dilatation of coronary artery lesions has been successfully employed. Dr. Noel Mills outlines his experience with this technique in Chapter 3, Intraoperative Coronary Artery Balloon-Catheter Dilatation.

The optimal performance of cardiac surgery requires the support of an experienced cardiac anesthesiologist. Recent advances in perioperative patient monitoring and pharmacologic manipulations to decrease myocardial ischemia have been associated with clinical stability during the induction and pre–cardiopulmonary bypass phases of cardiac surgery. Dr. Daniel Philbin describes the major advances in this area of cardiac physiology in Chapter 22, Cardiac Anesthesia.

Surgical treatment of patients with unstable angina syndromes remains a challenging clinical problem. Patients with unstable angina frequently may be stabilized with the use of mechanical or pharmacologic therapy prior to surgery. Dr. C. Richard Conti utilizes his previous experience, including his involvement with a national cooperative study of unstable angina patients, to outline current management of this patient group, as described in Chapter 23, Pre- and Postinfarction Unstable Angina: Thoughts on Pathogenesis and Therapeutic Strategies. The patient subgroup with refractory postinfarction angina pectoris continues to be a most difficult group of patients to manage surgically. In Chapter 18, Myocardial Revascularization in Patients with Post–Myocardial Infarction Unstable Angina, Dr. John McCormick describes his experience with surgical intervention for this patient category. Operative mortality for this group of patients, especially those with moderate to severely depressed left ventricular function following a recent myocardial infarction, continues to be high (5% to 10%). On the other hand, patients with an acute evolving myocardial infarction may be successfully treated by urgent myocardial revascularization. Dr. Steven Phillips reports his success with an aggressive surgical approach in Chapter 19, Surgery in Evolving Acute Myocardial Infarction. However, it remains uncertain whether surgery for this acute clinical syndrome is superior to nonoperative or less invasive, catheterization-based revascularization therapy. In both stable and unstable coronary artery syndromes, perioperative coronary artery spasm, on occasion, may be a serious contributor to perioperative morbidity and mortality. Fortunately, the widespread use of calcium channel blockers and intravenous nitroglycerin has limited the clinical impact of perioperative coronary artery spasm. Dr. Alfred Buxton presents his experience with perioperative coronary spasm in Chapter 10, Perioperative Coronary Artery Spasm.

Progress in the art and science of perfusion technology has led to important advances in recent years. In addition to newer equipment developed for use in conjunction with the heart-lung machine, the computer has recently been shown to be applicable to the management of cardiopulmonary bypass. In Chapter 21, Perfusion Technology, Mr. Thomas Hankins relates his innovative investigations in this field. The area of myocardial protection continues to evolve, despite relatively few important changes in recent years. However, the use of oxygen free-radical scavengers and coronary sinus interventions are among the newer techniques that have had a positive impact in this important area. In Chapter 16, Myocardial Protection, Dr. William Parks reviews this topic. The use of noninvasive techniques such as radionuclide ventriculography and two-dimensional echocardiography to objectively evaluate the results of cardiac surgery is outlined by Dr. Harold Lazar. He discusses the available data relating to the efficacy of these and other newer techniques for describing cardiac surgical results in Chapter 13, Noninvasive Techniques to Evaluate Results in Cardiac Surgery.

Innovative types of artificial heart valves continue to be introduced into the clinical arena. Improved preservation techniques for tissue valves and more favorable hemodynamic performance in some recent-generation mechanical heart valves have influenced both early and late clinical results associated with heart valve replacement. Dr. Alexander Geha describes his experience in choosing the appropriate heart valve in Chapter 7, Evaluation of Newer Heart Valve Prostheses. Simultaneously, the repair of native heart valves, especially in the mitral position, has finally begun to gain increasing application in the United States. Dr. Robert Frater has been active in valvular reconstruction. He discusses the surgical techniques available in this dynamic area in Chapter 6, Mitral Valvuloplasty. It appears that the mitral valve may be repaired more frequently than anticipated, and left ventricular performance following repair of the mitral valve may be better than that observed following replacement of the mitral valve.

Despite many advances in the performance of cardiac surgery, there is still a small number of open-heart cases that require mechanical assist devices to support the circulation postoperatively. Left ventricular mechanical assist devices have been available for approximately 15 years, but newer generation technology has resulted in greater biocompatibility and less destruction of formed blood elements. In Chapter 8, Assist Devices for Left- and Right-Sided Heart Support, Dr. William Bernhard reviews the current status of this evolving field. In addition, right ventricular support, including the use of pulmonary artery counterpulsation, has been advocated in several centers active in the performance of cardiac surgery. Dr. John Moran has been vitally involved in this area. He describes recent developments in right ventricular assistance for right ventricular failure and/or refractory pulmonary hypertension in Chapter 15, Right Ventricular Support by Pulmonary Artery Counterpulsation. The mechanical heart continues to capture the imagination of many investigators. Although mechanical performance is improving in the newer versions of the mechanical heart, thrombus formation and stroke-related problems continue to be a major source of morbidity and mortality in artificial-heart recipients. In certain centers, the mechanical heart is being used as a temporary device during procurement of a suitable donor for cardiac transplantation. Dr. William Pierce relates his experience after years of fundamental research in this area in Chapter 4, Development of a Clinical Artificial Heart. Interest in cardiac transplantation has been renewed in recent years because of improvements in perioperative patient selection and management as well as newer immunosuppressive treatment, specifically the use of cyclosporine. In Chapter 24, Heart Transplantation: Current Status and Prospects, Dr. Arnaud Painvin relates the current experience in this field. More recently, the application of combined heart and lung transplantation has been attempted in a smaller group of selected patients with some initial clinical success. Dr. Bruce Reitz has been a pioneer in this area. He describes his experience with this complicated procedure in Chapter 5, Heart-Lung Transplantation. Undoubtedly, further investigations and developments in the field of transplantation and cardiac replacement will continue to occupy an important part of the treatment of cardiac diseases in the foreseeable future.

If the authors are successful in conveying the excitement associated with the present advances in the management and treatment of cardiovascular diseases, the time and effort involved in producing *Current Surgery of the Heart* will have been worthwhile. It appears to us that this period is an important and perhaps transitional one in the history and development of cardiac surgery. The relative importance of the various developments identified in this present work remain to be proven by future evaluations. Regardless of the eventual place of the therapeutic modalities described herein, it has been enjoyable and rewarding for us to be involved in the evolution of new treatments for cardiovascular diseases in an exciting period of adjustment.

Arthur J. Roberts, M.D.

C. Richard Conti, M.D.

CONTENTS

CURRENT
SURGERY
OF THE HEART

1

LASERS IN CARDIOVASCULAR DISEASE

Daniel S. J. Choy

HISTORY

The maser (microwave amplification by stimulated emission of radiation) was invented by C. H. Townes of Columbia University in 1951. In 1958, in collaboration with A. Schawlow of Bell Telephone Laboratories, Townes proposed the term "laser" (light amplification by stimulated emission of radiation). The first working laser, based on the Ruby crystal, was constructed by T. H. Maiman in 1960. Since then, numerous types of lasers based on liquid, gas, and crystal gain media, with wavelengths from x-ray to infrared, have been demonstrated. Of these, only the lasers with relevance to medicine will be discussed.

PHYSICS

LASERS

A typical laser is represented in Figure 1–1. The resonator chamber containing the gas, liquid, or crystal medium is terminated at one end by a mirror and at the other end by a semitransparent mirror. In gas lasers, an electric discharge generated by the electrodes at the sides of the chamber "pumps" or raises the atoms of the medium to an excited quantum level. When each atom falls back to its ground level, a photon is emitted. In steady-state operation, photons are reflected back and forth between the end mirrors and stimulate the emission of just enough additional photons to provide the optical output power from the semitransparent mirror. The photon wavelength is determined by the energy difference between the ground and the excited quantum levels. The laser thus converts electrical power into highly monochromatic optical power. The laser output takes the form of a well-collimated pencil beam (Fig. 1–2). The laser energy may be emitted as single pulses, with a duration expressed in nanoseconds (10^{-9}) or microseconds (10^{-6}), or as a continuous wave (CW). The power of a laser beam is expressed in watts; the total energy, or watts × time (seconds), as joules. Power density is expressed as watts/cm², and incident energy density as joules/cm². "Q" switching is a method of generating short energetic pulses by means of an optical switch inside the resonator that prevents laser action until a large number of excited atoms are stored. Opening the switch then produces a sudden burst of stimulated emission. The term "Q" is derived from standard radio and microwave terminology and refers to the quality factor of a resonating system. Peak laser power ranges from milliwatts to megawatts over pulse lengths in the microsecond range.

The lasers with relevance to medicine are listed with their wavelengths (1 nm $= 10^{-9}$M $= 10$ angstroms) below.

Helium-neon	632.3 nm
Ruby	694.3 nm
Argon	488 nm and
	514.5 nm

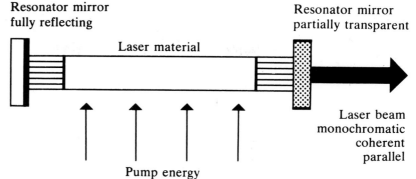

FIG. 1–1. Basic elements of a laser. (Hofstetter A, Frank J: The Neodymium-YAG Laser in Urology. Basel, Switzerland, Editiones "Roche," 1980)

Resonator mirror fully reflecting

Laser material

Resonator mirror partially transparent

Laser beam monochromatic coherent parallel

Pump energy

Neodymium:YAG (yttrium aluminum garnet)	1060 nm and 1318 nm
Carbon dioxide (CO_2)	10,600 nm
Dye	Various, 630 nm
Excimer (ultraviolet [UV])	193 nm, 248 nm, 330 nm, 350 nm

WAVEGUIDES

A low transmission loss, flexible optical fiber can serve as a waveguide for a laser beam and thereby greatly expand the applicability of the laser to endoscopic use in the body. The usual optical fiber (Fig. 1–3) consists of a silica glass core with a glass cladding of a slightly lower-refractive index surrounding it. The higher-refractive index of the core causes a light beam entering one end of an optical fiber to be internally reflected within the core until it emerges from the distal end. If the fiber is bent beyond a critical radius (± 1 cm), the angle of incidence of a light beam at the curve can exceed a critical angle beyond which total reflection will no longer occur, and some light will be refracted through the cladding. Optical-fiber waveguides used in medical applications typically have core diameters ranging from 80 μm to 600 μm (10^{-6}M). Allowable power density and fiber flexibility decrease with increasing core diameter. Power density outside the fiber is also a function of beam divergence and distance from the fiber tip (Table 1–1).

Certain laser wavelengths are difficult to transmit through optical fibers and must be delivered along line-of-sight optical paths with articulating mirrors. Each mirror interface results in energy loss. In practice, delivery systems for the CO_2 laser are designed with the minimum number of mirrors that will allow sufficient maneuverability of the hand-held applicator for surgical use. In spite of recent reports, there is as yet no practical optical fiber for the CO_2 laser.[1,2] The excimer (from excited dimer) laser suffers from the same drawback. The 193-nm wavelength cannot be transmitted through a silica fiber, although fibers are transparent to somewhat longer wavelengths.[3]

DIFFERENT LASERS AND INTERACTION WITH TISSUE

In general, lasers produce a thermal and a nonthermal effect on tissues.

The nonthermal effects associated with pulsed

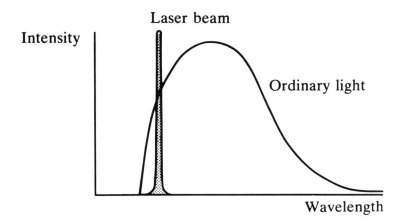

Intensity

Laser beam

Ordinary light

Wavelength

FIG. 1–2. Ordinary light is noncoherent. A laser beam consists of light waves that are coherent. (Hofstetter A, Frank J: The Neodymium-YAG Laser in Urology. Basel, Switzerland, Editiones "Roche," 1980)

laser systems, with the exception of photo dissociation, which is discussed further below, are chiefly of interest to physicists.[4]

Thermal effects are a function of the wavelength of the laser; the color and color-related energy-absorption coefficient of the target tissue; the power delivered; the local cooling factors, such as capillary blood flow, infused saline, and so forth; and the thermal relaxation time, in the case of pulsed laser energy delivery. Destruction of tissue by laser, with the exception of the excimer laser, is achieved by almost instantaneous heating of the target tissue to a temperature in excess of 100°C, with vaporization of all tissue components.

We will now consider the tissue interaction characteristics of the specific lasers of importance in clinical medicine.

The CO_2 laser emits at the infrared portion of the spectrum and acts by vaporizing water. Cellular water is boiled off and the tissue evaporates. The visible color of the tissue is relatively unimportant with respect to energy absorption at this wavelength. Because CO_2 laser energy is strongly absorbed by water, tissue penetration is low. Cutting effect is pronounced.

The Nd:YAG laser at 1060 nm exhibits greater tissue penetration and produces greater forward scatter than the CO_2 and argon lasers (Fig. 1–4). There is more protein coagulation than with the argon laser. Darker-colored tissues absorb Nd:YAG laser energy more strongly than tissues that are lighter colored.

The Nd:YAG line at 1318 nm, in comparison with the more common line at 1060 nm, is associated with lower coagulative and higher cutting and evaporative tissue effects.[4]

In the "Q"-switched form, with extremely short pulse duration and high peak power, the

TABLE 1–1
POWER DENSITY AS A FUNCTION OF
DISTANCE FROM FIBER TIP, ASSUMING
A POWER OUTPUT OF 10 WATTS

Distance from Tip (mm)	Power Density (w/cm²)
0	3536
1	372
2	132
3	67
4	41
5	27

(Choy DSJ et al: Embolization and wall perforation in argon laser recanalization. Lasers Surg Med 5:297–308, 1985)

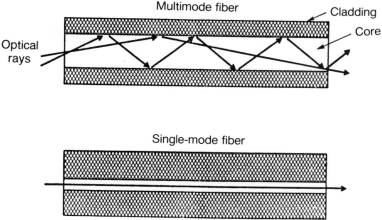

Nd : YAG laser will produce vaporization of thin cell layers. This effect is utilized in posterior capsulotomy.

The argon laser emits a blue-green light that is freely transmitted through water and preferentially absorbed by tissues of complementary colors (*i.e.*, red). It is completely absorbed even by dilute blood.[5] It produces greater evaporative effects and less forward scatter than the Nd : YAG laser. For equal power, it results in a zone of coagulation narrower than that associated with the Nd : YAG laser.

The excimer laser at shorter wavelengths (193 nm) produces disruption of molecular bonds (photo dissociation) with exquisite precision (Fig. 1–5). With longer wavelengths, there is increasing thermal effect. It is absorbed by water and has not at present been used *in vivo*. Its potential in medicine lies in its nonthermal effect and great precision.

The dye laser at 630 nm is a red light. This laser is useful for maximal tissue penetration in photodynamic therapy, which is discussed in greater detail later in this chapter. Dye lasers of other wavelengths are produced by varying the dye.

The copper vapor and frequency-doubled Nd : YAG lasers are considered together because the generated wavelength of 530 nm is essentially similar to that of the argon laser. The tissue interactions of these two lasers are therefore similar to those of the argon laser. These lasers may assume greater importance in the future because of greater power output.

LASERS IN MEDICINE

It was appropriate that lasers found their first application in clinical medicine in the field of ophthalmology, because the lens of the eye is a natural window for the transmission of laser light into the body. Argon laser photocoagulation for diabetic retinopathy has been established therapy for over a decade. Posterior capsulotomy has already been mentioned. Newer applications include gastroenterology: upper gastrointestinal bleeding, esophageal tumors, and condyloma acuminata; neurosurgery: meningiomas and arteriovenous malformation; gynecology: endometriosis, fallopian tube reconstruction, and cervical dysplasia; dermatology: hemangiomas, tattoo removal, and malignant tumors; urology:

FIG. 1–4. Tissue interaction with CO_2, argon, and ND:YAG lasers. CO_2 laser has low penetration; argon laser has higher, but still low, penetration; Nd:YAG laser has the highest penetration. (Hofstetter A, Frank J: The Neodymium-YAG Laser in Urology. Basel, Switzerland, Editiones "Roche," 1980)

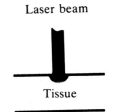

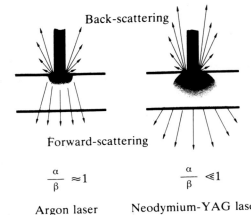

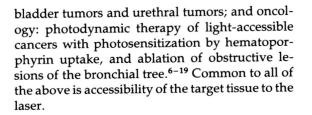

bladder tumors and urethral tumors; and oncology: photodynamic therapy of light-accessible cancers with photosensitization by hematoporphyrin uptake, and ablation of obstructive lesions of the bronchial tree.[6-19] Common to all of the above is accessibility of the target tissue to the laser.

LASERS IN CARDIOVASCULAR DISEASE

Against the background cited above, and with the increasing sophistication of the optical-fiber industry, it was only a question of time before lasers found an application in the cardiovascular area. In a discussion of this rapidly expanding field, the following outline of the use of lasers in cardiovascular disease may be helpful for purposes of perspective:

1. Ablation of pathologic tissue
   A. Conductive tissue
   B. Valves
   C. Myocardium
   D. Septum
2. Vessel anastomosis
3. Arterial recanalization
   A. History
   B. *In vitro* data
   C. *In vivo* animal data
   D. *In vivo* human data
      (1) Peripheral arteries
      (2) Coronary arteries
   E. Current problems
   F. Future considerations

ABLATION OF CONDUCTIVE TISSUES

Several groups have succeeded in ablating the canine bundle of His *in vivo* by utilizing standard endocardial mapping techniques to locate the target tissue, maneuvering a catheter with an optical fiber coupled with an argon or an Nd:YAG laser until the tip is against the tissue, then applying laser energy until atrioventricular dissociation is achieved.[20,21] A potential use that would

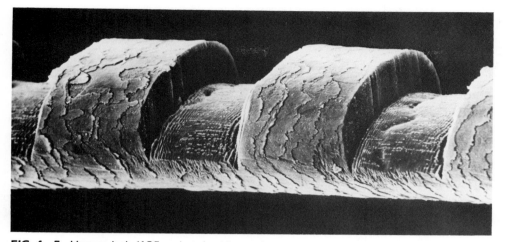

FIG. 1–5. Human hair (125 μm) etched by excimer laser. (Work by R. Srinivasan, IBM Thomas J. Watson Research Center, and Professor W. M. Hess, Brigham Young University)

be of great value is percutaneous ablation of accessory bundles in Wolff–Parkinson–White (WPW) syndrome.

Valves. Macruz and colleagues induced pulmonic stenosis in dogs and subsequently perforated the stenotic valves with argon laser energy conducted by an optical fiber.[22] Isner and associates ablated the calcific deposits from human aortic valves obtained during valve replacement surgery and at necropsy using a CO_2 laser coupled with a dissecting microscope.[23] This particular approach would be difficult to adapt for use *in vivo* because there are at present no practical optical fibers for the CO_2 laser and a dry field would have to be achieved.

Myocardium. Myotomy for hypertrophic cardiomyopathy is complicated by the difficulty of visualizing the myocardium deep in the ventri-

cle. Morrow states that myotomy incisions "must extend to the apical termination of the muscular ridge," and "for this to be accomplished, the knife must be plunged into the septum until it is out of sight, completely."[24] Isner's group, after canine experimentation, performed the first argon laser myotomy in a patient with hypertrophic cardiomyopathy in 1984.[25] The chief advantages of using an argon laser are twofold: the laser light illuminates the ventricular wall, and the argon laser wavelengths of 488 nm and 514 nm are ideally suited to the absorption spectra of myoglobin, which range from 400 nm to 650 nm.

Septum. Our group has proposed use of the Nd:YAG laser catheter to produce interatrial septal defects percutaneously for the treatment of intractable left ventricular failure. This is based on the work of Case and colleagues, who were able to relieve ischemic left ventricular failure in dogs by creating atrial septal defects.[26–29]

VESSEL ANASTOMOSIS

The CO_2, argon, and Nd:YAG lasers at low power all have been used in pioneering efforts by Neblett, Gomes, Jain, and Dew.[30–33] Arteries as small as 0.5 mm in outside diameter (OD) can be anastomosed by laser "welding." The advantages of using a laser for vessel anastomosis are applicability to vessels deep in the operative field, relative lack of the foreign-body reaction that is always seen with suture anastomosis, rare reocclusions by thrombi, and a time-saving as high as fivefold compared with that of anastomosis by suture.

ARTERIAL RECANALIZATION WITH THE LASER CATHETER

In 1980 two investigators independently proposed the use of an optical fiber incorporated in a catheter to conduct external laser energy to the site of an atherosclerotic plaque to ablate the lesion and thus create a new lumen.[34,35] In 1978, our group, using a Coherent Model 900 argon laser, tunneled through a fresh human thrombus (Fig. 1-6). Abela reported *in vitro* data comparing the effects of the CO_2, argon, and Nd:YAG lasers on atherosclerotic plaque.[36] Our group performed successful *in vivo* recanalizations of an experimentally thrombosed rabbit aorta and a canine femoral artery in 1981.[37] Gerrity and associates reported complete endothelial repair in

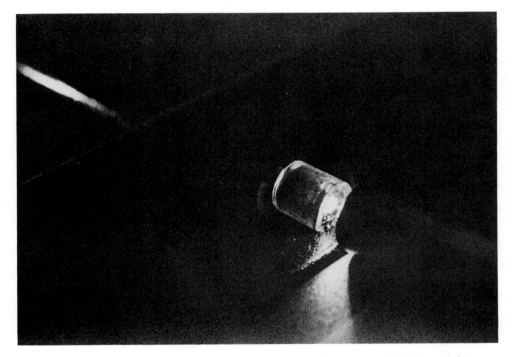

FIG. 1–6. Fresh human thrombus in PVC tubing that has been tunneled through by argon laser. Note the beam distal to the thrombus.

swine arteries irradiated with laser energy.[38] Lee and colleagues confirmed the feasibility of vaporizing atherosclerotic plaque and thrombi with the argon and Nd:YAG lasers.[39] In 1983 Ginsburg's group at Stanford successfully recanalized the femoral artery of a patient about to undergo amputation using an argon laser system under fluoroscopic control.[40] In 1984 Geschwind reported on three femoral arteries recanalized with an Nd:YAG laser.[41] Choy and associates performed intraoperative coronary recanalization in humans at the University of Toulouse, France on September 17, 1983.[42] Subsequent *in vivo* human clinical trials by Ginsburg, Geschwind, and Choy will be described later in this chapter.

In Vitro **Data.** Gas chromatography and absorbance spectroscopy and mass spectroscopy of gases generated by vaporization of plaque and thrombi indicate the chief constituents to be water vapor, nitrogen, carbon dioxide, hydrogen, and trace amounts of short-chain carbon molecules (Table 1–2).[43,44] Case and associates demonstrated a lack of particulate matter in the effluent of arterial thrombi and plaque vaporized by an argon laser.[45] Absence of particulate matter and distal embolization was confirmed by other studies.[46–48] Perforations of vessels reported by a number of investigators were probably the result of early inexperience, use of the Nd:YAG laser, absence of a coaxial relationship between the fiber and vessel, and direct mechanical perforation by the hard, unprotected fiber itself.[49–51] Histologic changes induced by absorption of laser energy by tissue consist of, in order of occurrence, a superficial zone of carbonization, a zone of lacunae that probably represents pockets of trapped water vapor, and lastly a zone of thermal coagulation of protein material (Fig. 1–7). These changes are produced by the CO_2, argon, and Nd:YAG lasers used in the CW mode. Recent work suggests that the Nd:YAG laser used in a pulsed mode, with extremely short pulses (in the nanosecond range), will allow relatively long thermal relaxation times.[52] This may totally eliminate the thermal component of tissue damage and result in smooth-cut surfaces resembling those produced by the excimer laser.

In spite of recent publicity on the excimer laser, use of this laser is at present impractical because

TABLE 1–2

COMPOSITION OF VAPOR GENERATED BY LASING OF THROMBUS AND PLAQUE CONCENTRATION, PERCENT BY VOLUME

	Thrombus	Plaque
Nitrogen	17.3	24
Oxygen	1.16	3.6
Argon	0	0.1
Carbon dioxide	50+	29.6
Hydrogen	14.9	15.3
Methane	2.9	13.5
Ethane	1.54	2.3
Ethylene	5.7	4.8
Propane	1.35	1.81
Propylene	3.5	3.9
C4+ hydrocarbons	0.67	1.21
Aromatic hydrocarbons	0.1	0

(Kaminow IP, Wiesenfeld JM, Choy DSJ: Argon laser disintegration of thrombus and atherosclerotic plaque. Applied Optics 23(9):1301–1302, 1984)

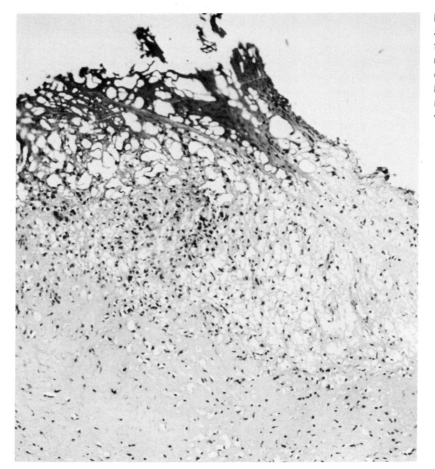

FIG. 1–7. Histologic appearance of a lasered surface. Note the thin carbonized layer and underlying zones of protein coagulation and multiple lacunae. The latter may represent pockets of water vapor.

of low power per pulse, difficulty of coupling the beam to a fiber, lack of suitable fibers for transmission of UV at the shorter wavelengths (193 nm), and concerns about possible carcinogenicity. If these problems can be solved, the excimer laser could prove to be the laser of choice.

The dye laser has been used in conjunction with hematoporphyrin derivative (HPD) by Spears.[53] HPD is taken up by dividing cells in the perinuclear region and is selectively eliminated at rates that differ with varying tissues. The shortest rate of elimination is seen in normal cells, and the longest in neoplastic tissue. When exposed to light energy, photoactivation analogous to that seen in porphyria occurs with the formation of singlet oxygen. Necrosis of cells then takes place. Arteriosclerotic plaque consists of collagen, lipids, and smooth muscle cells. The latter absorb HPD, which is then activated by exposure to light from a rhodamine dye laser (630 nm). The choice of 630 nm is dictated by the high penetration of light through tissue at this wavelength. Suggestive but not entirely convincing results have been obtained in experimentally induced atherosclerotic plaques in rabbit aortas.

Angiograms of a human coronary artery and a femoral artery recanalized by laser are shown in Figures 1 – 8 and 1 – 9, respectively. Of note is the smooth surface of the laser-irradiated femoral artery contrasted with the irregular plaque-beaded surface of the distal, untreated artery.

In Vivo **Animal Data.** Sanborn, Lee, Abela, and our group have all successfully recanalized thrombus- and plaque-occluded arteries in the rabbit and canine models (Fig. 1-10).[37,49,50,54,55] The highest incidence of perforations was associated with the Nd : YAG laser, for the reasons previously discussed, and the lowest incidence of perforations occurred with the argon laser. Atherosclerosis induced in the rabbit model with high-lipid diets is not comparable to the process in humans; the rabbit plaques are considerably softer, contain less collagen, and are not calcified. Macruz proposed engrafting atherosclerotic human arteries onto canine femoral arteries as an experimental model. At least one group in the United States has attempted this procedure.[56] Our group found graft rejection with this system, and we do not consider it to be a good model of human atherosclerosis.

In Vivo **Human Data.** Peripheral Arteries. The largest clinical experience has been that of Ginsburg. His group at Stanford, using an argon laser with maximum power output at the resonator of 16 watts, has treated 20 patients with stenotic lesions of the femoral artery with severe distal ischemia, recommended amputation, and medical contraindication to surgery.* Successful recanalization was accomplished in 50%. Only a small lumen was achieved in most cases (1 mm in

* Ginsburg R: Personal communication, 1985.

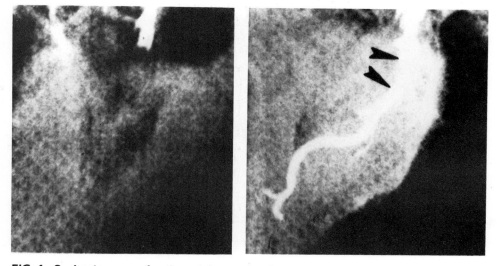

FIG. 1 – 8. Angiograms of cadaver left anterior descending coronary artery showing total occlusion by thrombus and patency after laser recanalization. Arrows indicate site of thrombus.

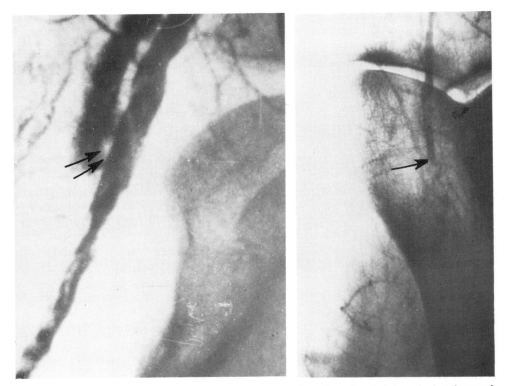

FIG. 1–9. Angiograms of femoral and popliteal arteries, showing total occlusion **(arrow)** preoperatively and patency after laser recanalization. The anastomotic site between the popliteal artery and the Gortex graft **(double arrow)** has also been opened. Note the smooth wall of the laser-irradiated artery compared with the plaque-beaded wall of the untreated distal artery.

6-mm vessels); in these cases, the procedure was supplemented by balloon dilatation. There were two perforations. These procedures were all performed under fluoroscopic guidance, with introduction of the catheter accomplished with the Seldinger technique. Of interest is Ginsburg's "pullback" technique. Whenever possible, a fiber is passed beyond the lesion (in those that were not 100% obstructions), and the laser is fired as the fiber is pulled in a retrograde direction. This approach minimizes the hazard of mechanical perforation by the fiber and tends to keep the fiber coaxial to the vessel. Long-term follow-up data are unavailable.

Geschwind reported on 14 human femoral arteries recanalized with an Nd:YAG laser.[57] The last ten laser recanalizations were supplemented with balloon dilatation. There were four late reocclusions.

Carotid Arteries. Choy, Ascher, and colleagues recanalized nine of ten cadaver carotid arteries using a percutaneously inserted and fluoroscopically guided laser catheter, and they partially ab-

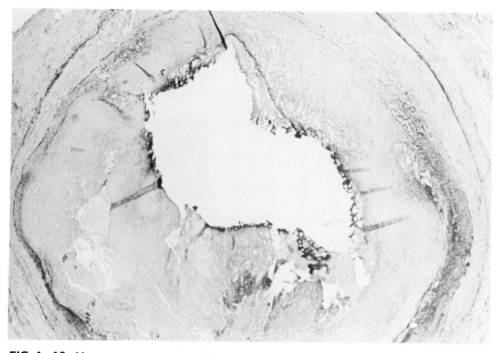

FIG. 1–10. Human coronary artery immediately after argon laser recanalization. The lumen, formerly 10% of normal, is now 70% of normal in the cross-sectional area.

lated a common carotid arteriosclerotic plaque in one human patient in June 1985.[58]

Coronary Arteries. Our group performed intraoperative argon laser recanalization in high-grade stenoses in three left anterior descending and two right coronary arteries during coronary artery bypass graft surgery in France in September 1983.[42] One artery was mechanically perforated and immediately repaired. Four arteries were successfully recanalized. For ethical reasons, all were bypassed with saphenous vein grafts. One laser-irradiated artery was immediately excised for histologic examination (Fig. 1–10). This revealed a new lumen approximately 70% of normal. One laser-treated artery was pat-

ent at 25 days (Fig. 1–11). At 3 months, all laser-recanalized arteries were reoccluded.

In January 1984, during cardioplegic arrest employed for coronary artery bypass graft surgery of stenotic left anterior descending (LAD) and circumflex arteries, we successfully recanalized three totally occluded right coronary arteries with the argon laser catheter.[59] All three patients had complete transmural infarcts distal to the right coronary lesions. One of the three lesions was heavily calcified. There were no perforations. At 3 months, two of the three arteries were reoccluded. The third patient refused postoperative angiography, and the fate of his right coronary artery is unknown.

As of this writing, 27 and 24 months after the

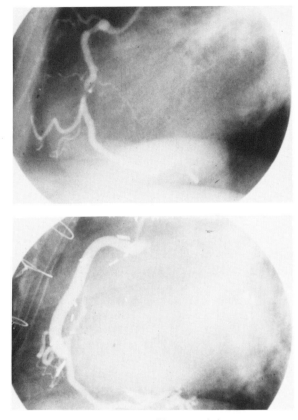

FIG. 1–11. Angiograms of human right coronary artery preoperatively showing 95% stenosis **(top)**, and 25 days after laser recanalization and bypass grafting showing continued patency of the lasered segment **(bottom)**.

procedures, all eight patients are alive and well after intraoperative coronary laser treatment.

Current Problems. The question of distal embolization has been discussed above. We do not consider distal embolization to be a problem.

Vessel perforation is the chief concern of all investigators in the field. The danger of perforation can be minimized by exercising care in maintaining a strict coaxial relationship between the laser catheter and the vessel, use of Ginsburg's pullback technique, and use of the argon laser. During intraoperative use, when direct visual control is exercised, the vessel being recanalized should be dissected free to facilitate visual monitoring of the entire circumference. A plaque adds to the vessel-wall thickness, thus reducing transmission of laser light; such areas appear dark in comparison with a normal vessel wall. Laser recanalization is then accomplished by "sculpting" the interior of the vessel until light transmission is uniform throughout. Protective amber goggles that are 50% of the optical density of the standard goggles should be used; these permit visual monitoring of the transmitted laser light while protecting one's eyes. In the final analysis, of course, successful laser recanalization depends largely on operator experience.

Laser recanalization under fluoroscopic guidance is more difficult because the visual means of assessing vessel-wall thickness are absent. In our opinion, the angioscope, which is a coherent bundle of optical fibers with a light source, is of little value because it adds to the diameter of the catheter; it provides a somewhat distorted, essentially two-dimensional image of a three-dimensional situation; and it is expensive and not cost effective. We use a combination of the pullback technique when treating incomplete occlusive lesions, and a short-exposure, short-advance technique in treating total obstructions. This consists of three steps performed repetitively:

1. Angiogram
2. A flush with saline
3. A 1- to 2-second exposure of the argon laser

The saline flush is essential because the interaction of an argon laser with radiocontrast material produces precipitates of unknown chemical composition.

A more sophisticated approach to the problem of vessel perforation lies in the creation of conditions to enhance energy absorption by target tissue rather than the vessel wall, in effect enlarging the therapeutic index. Studies of nontoxic dyes with high affinity for plaque are under way at several institutions. The ideal dye would have a color complementary to the blue-green of the argon laser (*i.e.*, red) and would adsorb strongly to a plaque on the first pass of the circulation and not at all to intact intima.

Another problem is that of "burnback." When the fiber tip is in direct contact with a lesion, if dissipation of the heat generated is insufficient, the fiber-tip temperature can increase to ignition level and cause a literal burnback of the fiber. Various protective methods, such as shields and a tip with a high flash point, are being studied.

Catheter guidance or steerability is important to the laser angiographer. Present methods of preformed tips and guidewires are usable, but not ideal. The ideal laser catheter should have a built-in method of tip guidance that does not unduly increase the diameter of the catheter. The catheter tip should be highly flexible, for ease of following the complex curves of the arterial tree. Forty percent of Ginsburg's, 29% of Geschwind's, and all of our cases were reoccluded at varying durations after laser recanalization. We believe this to be the most serious problem of all. At this point, we can only speculate that the reocclusions were chiefly due to endothelial disruption with possible increased thrombogenicity and reduced blood flow through the laser-treated segments. In Ginsburg's and Geschwind's cases reocclusions probably occurred because of the small lumens created, and in our cases because of competitive flow in the first five cases and the known reduction of flow to infarcted myocardial tissue.[60] Using an *ex vivo* system and [111]indium-labeled platelets, we are working with Fuster and colleagues to study platelet aggregation on a lasered vessel surface and with Weksler and associates to study prostacyclin production by a laser-irradiated intimal surface. We also plan to institute a more aggressive antithrombosis regimen in the next group of patients treated.

The Future. The general enthusiasm with which the new field of laser recanalization has been received by the cardiology community augurs well for the future. Since its inception in the late 1970s and early 1980s, laser recanalization has attracted increasing numbers of highly competent investigators to its study and development. Regulatory agencies have not been far behind in recognizing its potential. The Food and Drug Administration has currently approved human clinical trials in peripheral arteries, albeit with the constraint of immediately removing the lasered vessel for histologic examination, in three institutions: Seton Medical Center, Cedars–Sinai (Los Angeles), and University of Florida; in intraoperative use of a CO_2 laser for endarterectomy in coronary arteries at the Texas Heart Institute; and for both peripheral and coronary arteries with the argon laser catheter, without the requirement to remove the vessels, at our institution, St. Luke's–Roosevelt Hospital Center.

We believe that cooperative studies eventually will take place, a central registry will be established at the National Institutes of Health (NIH), and the chief problems will be solved to a point at which laser recanalization as a relatively noninvasive method of revascularization for peripheral, renal, cerebral, and coronary arteries will become established, routine therapy. It should, in the meantime, serve as an increasingly useful means to assist the peripheral vascular surgeon and the cardiac surgeon in achieving a more complete revascularization of ischemic tissues.

REFERENCES

1. Eldar M, Battler A, Neufeld H et al: Transluminal carbon dioxide laser catheter angioplasty for dissolution of atherosclerotic plaques. J Am Coll Cardiol 3:135–137, 1984

2. Takahishi K, Yoshida N, Yakota M: Optical fibers for transmitting high powered carbon dioxide laser beam. Sumitomo Electronics Technical Review 23:203–210, 1984

3. Grundfest WS, Litvack F, Forrester JS et al: Laser ablation of human atherosclerotic plaque without adjacent tissue injury. J Am Coll Cardiol 5:929–933, 1985

4. Goldman L: The Biomedical Laser: Technology and Clinical Applications. Heidelberg, Springer–Verlag, 1981

5. Kaplan MD, Case RB, Choy DSJ: Vascular recanalization with the Argon laser: The role of blood in the transmission of laser energy. Lasers Surg Med 5:275–279, 1985

6. Dwyer RM, Bass M: Laser phototherapy in man using Argon and Nd : YAG lasers. Gastrointest Endosc 24:195–196, 1978

7. Mellow MH, Pinkas H: Endoscopic therapy for esophageal carcinoma with Nd : YAG laser: Prospective evaluation of efficacy, complications and survival. Gastrointest Endosc 6:334–339, 1984

8. Scott RS, Castro DJ: Treatment of condyloma acuminata with carbon dioxide laser: A prospective study. Lasers Surg Med 4(2):157–162, 1984

9. Cerullo LJ: Laser neurosurgery: Past, present, and future. IEEE J Quant Elect QE-20, 12:1397–1400, 1984

10. Fasano VA: The treatment of vascular malformation of the brain with laser surgery. Presented at Congress of Laser Neurosurgery II, Chicago, IL, September 1982

11. Bellina JH, Voros JI, Fick AC, Jackson JD: Surgical management of endometriosis with the carbon dioxide laser. Microsurgery 5:4, 1984

12. Bellina JH: Microsurgery of the fallopian tube with the carbon dioxide laser: Analysis of 230 cases with a 2 year follow up. Lasers Surg Med 3:255, 1983

13. Anderson MC: Treatment of cervical intraepithelial neoplasia with the carbon dioxide laser: Report of 543 patients. Obstet Gynecol 59:720, 1982

14. Apfelberg DB, Moser MR, Lasl H: Progress report on extended clinical use of the Argon laser for cutaneous lesions. Lasers Surg Med 1:71–83, 1980

15. Bailin DS, Katz JL, Levine AL: Removal of tattoos by carbon dioxide laser. J Dermatol Surg Oncol 6:997–1001, 1980

16. Koslov AP, Moskalik KG: Pulsed laser radiation therapy of skin tumors. Cancer 46:2172–2178, 1980

17. Hofstetter A, Frank F, Keiditsch E, Bowering R: Endoscopic Nd : YAG laser application for destroying bladder tumors: Clinical papers. Eur Urol 7:278–282, 1981

18. Hofstetter A: Laser application for destroying ureter tumors (abstr). Lasers Surg Med 3:152, 1983

19. Dougherty TJ, Kaufman JE, Goldfarb A et al: Photoradiation therapy for treatment of malignant tumors. Cancer Res 38:2628–2635, 1978

20. Lee BI, Fletcher RD, Cohen AI et al: Transcatheter endocardial ablation — comparison of laser photo ablation and electrode shock ablation (abstr). J Am Coll Cardiol 3(2):536, 1984

21. Narula OS, Bharati S, Chan MC et al: Laser micro transection of the His bundle: A pervenous catheter technique (abstr). J Am Coll Cardiol 3(2):537, 1984

22. Macruz R, Armelin E, Gomes OM et al: Aplicacao do laser no sistema cardiovascular. Arq Bras Cardiol 39(1):5–10, 1982

23. Isner JM, Michlewitz H, Clarke RH et al: Laser photo ablation of aortic valve calcium: Evaluation of Argon versus carbon dioxide laser using excised surgical and postmortem specimens (abstr). J Am Coll Cardiol 3:558, 1984

24. Morrow AG: Hypertrophic subaortic stenosis: Operative methods utilized to relieve left ventricular outflow obstruction. J Thorac Cardiovasc Surg 76:423–430, 1978

25. Isner JM, Clarke RH, Pardian NG et al: Laser myoplasty for hypertrophic cardiomyopathy: In vitro experience in human postmortem hearts and in vivo experience in a canine model (transarterial) and human patient (intraoperative). Am J Cardiol 53:1620–1626, 1984

26. Case RB, Roven RB, Crampton RS: Relief of high left atrial pressure in left ventricular failure. Lancet, pp 841–842, (Part II), 1964

27. Roven RB, Crampton RS, Case RB: Influence of venous shunts on left atrial pressure in left ventricular failure. Clin Res 12(2):56, 1964

28. Roven RB, Crampton RS, Case RB: Surgical approach to the relief of left ventricular failure. Circulation (Suppl III) 29(30):55, 1964

29. Roven RB, Crampton RS, Case RB: Effect of compromising right ventricular function in left ventricular failure by means of interatrial and other shunts. Am J Cardiol 24:209–219, 1969

30. Neblett CR: Reconstructive vascular surgery with use of the carbon dioxide laser. Presented at Congress of Laser Neurosurg II, Chicago, 1982

31. Gomes OM, Macruz R, Armelin E et al: Vascular anastomosis by Argon laser beam. Texas Heart Institute Journal 10:145–150, 1983

32. Jain KK: Sutureless microvascular extracranial anastomosis with Nd : YAG laser. Lasers Surg Med 3:311, 1984

33. Dew DK: Laser microsurgical repair of soft tissue: A demonstration of surgical techniques. Lasers Surg Med 3:351, 1984

34. Choy DSJ: Fiberoptic laser tunneling device: The laser

catheter. Beijing/Shanghai Proceedings of an International Conference on Lasers, pp 685–690. New York, Wiley–Interscience, 1980

35. Macruz R, Martins JRM, Tupinamba AS et al: Possibilidades terapeuticas do raio laser em ateromas. Arq Bras Cardiol 34(1):9–12, 1980

36. Abela GS, Normann S, Cohen D et al: Effects of carbon dioxide, Nd : YAG, and Argon laser radiation on coronary atheromatous plaques. Am J Cardiol 50(6):1199–1205, 1982

37. Choy DSJ, Stertzer SH, Rotterdam HZ et al: Transluminal laser catheter angioplasty. Am J Cardiol 50(6):1206–1208, 1982

38. Gerrity RG, Loop FD, Golding LAR et al: Arterial response to laser operation for removal of atherosclerotic plaques. J Thorac Cardiovasc Surg 85:409–421, 1983

39. Lee G, Ikeda RM, Kozina J, Mason DT: Laser dissolution of coronary atherosclerotic obstruction. Am Heart J 102:1074–1075, 1981

40. Ginsburg R, Kim DS, Cuthener D et al: Salvage of an ischemic limb by laser angioplasty: Description of a new technique. Clin Cardiol 7:54–58, 1984

41. Geschwind H, Boussignac G, Teisseire B et al: Percutaneous transluminal laser angioplasty in man (letter). Lancet 1:844, 1984

42. Choy DSJ, Stertzer SH, Myler RK et al: Human coronary laser recanalization. Clin Cardiol 7:377–381, 1984

43. Clarke RH, Donaldson RF, Isner JM: Identification of photoproducts liberated by in vitro laser irradiation of atherosclerotic plaques, calcified valves, and myocardium (abstr). Lasers Surg Med 3(4):358, 1984

44. Kaminow IP, Wiesenfeld JM, Choy DSJ: Argon laser disintegration of thrombus and atherosclerotic plaque. Applied Optics 23(9):1301–1302, 1984

45. Case RB, Choy DSJ, Dwyer EM, Jr, Silvernail PJ: Absence of emboli during in vivo laser recanalization. Laser Surg Med 5:281–289, 1985

46. Choy DSJ, Stertzer SH, Myler RK et al: Argon laser coronary angioplasty: Mass spectrometer evaluation, technetium 99 scintigraphy, human intraoperative evaluation (abstr). J Am Coll Cardiol 3(2):489, 1984

47. Abela GS, Pepine CJ, Conti RC: Effects of laser irradiation on human blood: Relation between exposure and debris formation (abstr). J Am Coll Cardiol 3(2):489, 1984

48. Isner JM, Clarke RH: The current status of lasers in the treatment of cardiovascular disease. IEEE J Quant Elect QE-20, 12:1406–1419, 1984

49. Abela GS, Cohen D, Feldman RL et al: Use of laser radiation to recanalize stenosed arteries in a live animal model. Circulation 66(II):366, 1982

50. Sanborn TA, Faxon DP, Haudenschild CC et al: Angiographic and histopathologic consequences of in vivo laser radiation of atherosclerotic lesions. AHA 56th Scientific Sessions. Abstract 577. Circulation, 1983

51. Jain A, Dedhia H, Savrin R, Withers A: Laser angioplasty in chronic occlusion of canine arteries (abstr). Eur Heart J 5:64, 1984

52. Deckelbaum L, Donaldson RF, Isner JM et al: Elimination of pathologic injury associated with laser induced tissue ablation using pulsed energy delivery at low repetition rates. J Am Coll Cardiol 5(2):408, 1985

53. Spears JR, Serur J, Shropshire D, Paulin S: Fluorescence of experimental atheromatous plaques with hematoporphyrin derivative. J Clin Invest 71:395–399, 1983

54. Lee G, Ikeda RM, Stobbe D et al: Intraoperative use of dual fiberoptic catheter for simultaneous in vivo visualization and laser vaporization of peripheral atherosclerotic obstructive disease. Cathet Cardiovasc Diagn 10:11–16, 1984

55. Marco J, Silvernail PJ, Fournial G et al: Complete patency in thrombus-occluded arteries two weeks after laser recanalization. Lasers Surg Med (in press)

56. Abela GS, Normann S, Feldman RL et al: A new model for evaluation of transluminal recanalization: Human atherosclerotic coronary artery heterografts. Circulation 66(III):5, 1982

57. Geschwind H, Boussignac G, Teisseire B: Transluminal laser angioplasty in man (abstr). Circulation 70:298, 1984

58. Choy DSJ, Ascher P, Lammer J et al: Percutaneous laser recanalization of carotid arteries in seven cadavers and one human patient. Am J Neuroradiol (in press)

59. Choy DSJ, Marco J, Fournial G, Stertzer SH: Argon laser recanalization of three totally occluded human right coronary arteries. Clinical Cardiology 9:296–298, 1986

60. Prioleau WH, Clark S, Gross A et al: Flow in coronary artery bypass grafts to totally and partially occluded left anterior descending coronary arteries. Ann Thorac Surg 34:490–492, 1982

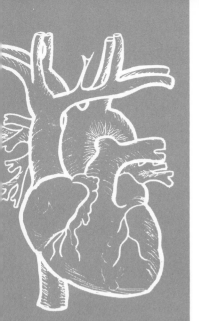

2

ANGIOSCOPY IN CARDIAC SURGERY

Timothy A. Sanborn
Benjamin M. Westbrook
Arthur J. Roberts

Before recent developments in fiberoptic technology, attempts to visualize intracardiac structures or the interior of blood vessels had only modest success over the past 70 years.[1-14] Now, with small, flexible fiberoptic catheters that are 1.5 mm to 3.7 mm in diameter, several groups have demonstrated the feasibility of vascular endoscopy or angioscopy.[18-21] Although additional technical developments are still required for better documentation, better directional control of the catheter, and clearing of blood from the field of vision, considerations should also be addressed to determining the clinical indications of this emerging technology and the circumstances under which it adds useful information that is unavailable through current techniques of cardiac catheterization, cineangiography, echocardiography, or direct inspection.

HISTORICAL PERSPECTIVE

THE RIGID CARDIOSCOPE

Intracardiac endoscopy was first attempted in 1913 by Rhea and Walker, who designed a cardioscope that consisted of a rigid cylindric tube carrying electric light in a sheath and a cutting knife for cutting the mitral valve in mitral stenosis. Because the lens was recessed in a sheath, direct contact between the lens and the object was impossible and circulating blood interfered with vision. This pioneering work in dogs was deemed unsatisfactory and, therefore, was never published. It was referred to, however, in a review by Cutler.[1]

In 1922 Allen and Graham improved on the cardioscope by placing a rounded glass cap at the end of the device.[2] This modification allowed them to visualize intracardiac structures of dogs when direct contact was established. Although a transventricular approach resulted in a 50% mortality, the transauricular approach was very successful and allowed them to perform mitral valvulotomy under direct vision. In 1923 the first clinical attempt in a patient with mitral stenosis was unsuccessful, however, because of the difficulty of fixing the auricle close against the cardioscope. Before inspection or any other measure could be carried out, the patient died.[1] Cutler and associates continued experimental investigations in dogs with a similar device that was combined with a valvulotome, but they never convinced themselves of the benefit to be derived from such limited visualization.[1] Vision was hindered by the intermittent contact of the cardioscope with the structures of the pulsating heart, as well as by the small field of vision. Later, in 1948, Brock attempted to use a rigid cardioscope to visualize the pulmonic valve in three patients with pulmonic stenoses but found the approach through the left pulmonary artery to be generally unsuccessful. Direct inspection was believed to be more reliable.[3]

The interference of blood with visualization of intracardiac structures continued to be the main problem in vascular endoscopy until 1943 when Harken and Glidden attached a transparent balloon to the distal end of a cardioscope to displace blood from the field of vision.[4] With this scope in position, the balloon could be inflated with 8 ml to 15 ml of clear saline solution and the opaque blood displaced to allow visualization of the intracardiac structures of the left atrium and ventricle of surgically exposed dog hearts. Because balloon inflation caused temporary circulatory obstruction, it was necessary to deflate the balloon and allow circulation to recover for 10 to 15 seconds between each observation period of 20 to 30 seconds.

Another method for improving visualization was to disperse the blood with clear saline irrigation. In 1950 Bloomberg described a method by which a stream of clear saline was injected under pressure to displace blood and allow visualization of a relatively large field of vision inside all four chambers of the dog heart.[5] Despite the large area of inspection available, the cardiac valves moved so rapidly that they had to be caught and held by a hook attached to the end of the cardioscope for good visualization. In addition, a large amount of fluid was needed to maintain clear vision; this volume load put too much strain on the dog heart.

In 1958 Sakakibara summarized the clinical results of studies in which a curved cardioscope with a rubber balloon-tip and saline irrigation of the heart were used to successfully visualize valvular pathology in seven patients with aortic stenosis, as well as additional references to prior successful studies in patients with mitral and pulmonic stenosis.[6]

Additional improvements of the cardioscope were made in the early 1950s when plastic materials that had light-transmission properties were used. Butterworth reported on a cardioscope that retained the contact vision principle but utilized a unique light-transmitting property of solid Perspex (methyl methacrylate).[7] The major advantages of this scope were claimed to be the following: a wide, brilliantly illuminated field that extended to the extreme edge without obstruction by light source or metal casing; absence of lens aberration; and removal of the light source to a position outside the instrument where it could be altered or interchanged while keeping the instrument in position. When a cutting knife was attached to this scope, both could be passed through the left auricular appendage or the left ventricle to cut the mitral valve cusp in animals and blood-filled cadaver hearts with good results. Bolton designed a similar cardioscope, which utilized the light-carrying properties of a Lucite rod and an ordinary room light entering the scope for illumination.[8] Thus, the need for an additional light source was eliminated entirely. This device was of particular value in estimating the size and location of intra-atrial septal defects. With a large-bore shaft along the side of the scope, instruments could be passed for a valvulotomy procedure.

Despite all of these experimental studies, the fact that the investigators failed to pursue significant clinical application of these rigid cardioscopes indicates the inadequacies of these devices. Furthermore, as open-heart surgery developed with the advent of the heart bypass machine, direct visualization of intracardiac structures became available and the need for an intraoperative endoscopic approach disappeared. What remained to be determined was whether cardiac or vascular endoscopy could be performed for diagnostic or therapeutic indications without an open surgical procedure.

TOWARD A TRANSLUMINAL APPROACH

In 1961 Carlens and Silander made the first step toward the transluminal application of a cardioscope by inserting a 7-mm right-angled telescope through the right external jugular vein of anesthetized dogs to visualize structures in the right side of the heart.[9] With a thin rubber bladder inflated with 5 ml of saline over the distal end of the scope, the instrument could be pressed lightly against vascular and cardiac walls for good visualization of structures such as the orifice of the azygous vein in the superior vena cava, the coronary sinus, the atrial septum, and the base and commissures of the tricuspid valve.

Clear visualization of an artificially induced atrial septal perforation was also possible. The instrument could also be inserted into the right ventricle for short periods to visualize valves, papillary muscles, and chordae tendineae. Overall, the procedure was well tolerated with no evidence of stasis or circulatory compromise. Extrasystoles and atrial tachycardias occurred during passage through the valves and occlusion of the inferior vena cava, but these were transient and were relieved by repositioning the instrument. Although the instrument had adequate illumination for the purpose of inspection, photography required an exposure time of approximately 1 minute and therefore could only be obtained in blood-filled hearts at a standstill. This rigid device was subsequently used clinically by Silander in 1964 to visualize and document the presence and anatomical location of atrial septal defects in seven patients.[10] However, the rigidity of the instrument probably precluded further clinical application.

THE EMERGENCE OF FLEXIBLE FIBEROPTIC DEVICES

Using a 7-mm flexible choledochoscope with optical, lighting, and irrigation systems all enclosed in a single latex and vinyl copolymer sheath, Greenstone and colleagues first demonstrated the feasibility of intravascular endoscopy with a flexible fiberoptic device in large vessels such as the aortic, iliac, and femoral arteries of anesthetized dogs and human cadavers.[11] With the segments of the vessels occluded at both ends and side branches controlled to eliminate backflow of blood into the lumen, the endoscope could be introduced through a small arteriotomy and retained blood could be rapidly cleared with the high-flow irrigating system. A high degree of intimal detail was obtained. In the dog, normal

anatomy as well as the arteriotomy and patch closure sites were readily visualized, whereas in the cadaver studies, varying degrees of atheromatous changes and thrombi were easily recognized. Optical visualization did require that the instrument be aligned with the axis of the arterial lumen. This required external manipulation of the artery around the viewing end of the instrument.

Gamble and Innis advanced the technique of cardiac endoscopy further by introducing a 4.1-mm flexible fiberoptic device through femoral arteries or veins, carotid arteries, or jugular veins of anesthetized dogs to visualize intravascular and intracardiac structures of the right and left sides of the heart.[12] By inflating an air-filled balloon at the tip of the scope, the details of normal aortic valves, mitral valve chordae, and papillary muscles as well as the apex endocardium were all visualized; however, the single-frame photographic reproductions were of only fair quality and merely suggestive of the anatomical detail visualized. Interestingly, in these studies with the balloon inflated with 4 cc to 7 cc of air, there were some extrasystoles but no compromises, as evidenced by a less than 5 mm Hg drop in systolic arterial pressure. Tanabe and associates have now reported on the clinical intracardiac application of a 4-mm fiberoptic endoscope used during preoperative cardiac catheterization for various right-sided cardiac diseases (primarily atrial septal defects).[13]

Although several additional reports documented the usefulness of intraoperative vascular peripheral endoscopy as a means of following and documenting the completeness of the semiclosed thromboendarterectomy in peripheral vascular surgery, and intracardiac endoscopy is now technically feasible using standard techniques of cardiac catheterization, clinical application is again hindered by the lack of additional useful diagnostic information that is over and above that currently available by cardiac catheterization, angiocardiography, or noninvasive echocardiography.[14-16]

CORONARY ANGIOSCOPY

Clinical coronary angioscopy was first performed in 1983 when Spears and associates used a 1.8-mm ultrathin fiberscope (Olympus) for intraluminal visualization of the coronary artery in dogs using catheterization techniques, and in four patients during the course of coronary artery bypass surgery.[17] To reduce the outer diameter of this device to 1.8 mm, only two fiberoptic bundles for illumination and visualization were included. The angulation system and the channels usually provided in standard endoscopes had to be eliminated. Using a 10F guiding catheter inserted from a carotid arteriotomy in anesthetized dogs, this fiberscope could be directed into the left main coronary artery for visualization of the left main bifurcation using an infusion of either oxygenated Krebs – Ringer's solution or perfluorocarbon emulsion. *In vivo* human coronary angioscopy was performed in four patients during coronary artery bypass surgery while the hearts were arrested. The catheter could be placed through either a side branch of a saphenous vein graft after completion of the distal anastomosis or directly into the native left anterior descending arteriotomy prior to completion of the anastomosis. Intraluminal visualization of atherosclerotic plaque within the lumen of the coronary artery was achieved in all four patients by perfusing a crystalloid cardioplegic solution.

In a discussion of the potential clinical applications of this device, Spears and associates note that, during diagnostic catheterization or cardiac surgery, coronary angioscopy may provide useful information on the nature of vascular pathology (atheroma or thombus), which appears as a defect on standard coronary angiography only. It was suggested that this diagnostic advantage over angiography may have clinical application during thrombolytic therapy to distinguish atheroma from residual thrombus or in understanding the nature of abrupt reclosure after balloon angioplasty.

Additional experience with intraoperative coronary angioscopy was reported by two other groups.[18,19] Litvack and colleagues performed saphenous vein and native coronary artery angioscopy in eight patients by placing either a 1.5-mm (American Edwards) or 1.8-mm (Olympus) angioscope through the proximal end of a saphenous vein graft after completion of the distal anastomosis but prior to the aortic anastomosis.[18] Images of the vein graft were obtained in all eight patients, with photography demonstrating a characteristic fish-mouth anastomosis and individual black sutures. Images of the native coronary arteries were obtained in four patients. Interestingly, inspection of a right coronary artery revealed a small plaque that was not demonstrated at angiography.

In our studies, intraoperative saphenous vein graft and native coronary artery angioscopy were performed in 17 patients during coronary artery bypass surgery using a 1.7-mm fiberoptic catheter (Trimedyne).[19] Good to excellent visualization and video recording of 10 of 11 proximal and 10 of 10 distal coronary anastomoses were obtained promptly and consistently (Fig. 2 – 1). The one failure in visualizing a proximal anastomosis was due to inadequate clearing of blood away from the anastomosis. Visualization of three native coronary arteries through complete anastomosis was possible but was limited to the area immediately distal to the anastomotic site because of the large catheter size relative to the small size of the distal coronary vessel. Lack of an angulation system did preclude examination of a large posterior descending artery through a distal right coronary artery anastomosis. Visualization of native coronary arteries directly through an arteriotomy was adequate in only three of eight

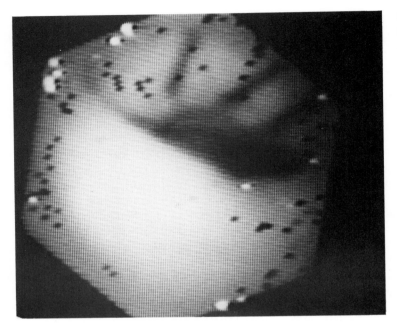

FIG. 2–1. Visualization of a proximal coronary anastomosis.

patients because of the persistence of intraluminal blood. Perfusion with 3 ml to 5 ml of clear cold saline flushes was required to obtain useful images in three patients.

LIMITATIONS OF CURRENT CORONARY ANGIOSCOPY

In all of these clinical studies, the feasibility of performing intraoperative coronary angioscopy has been demonstrated without significant consequences.[17-19] The latter two studies do make the point that the quality of the images improved with operator experience. However, several limitations still exist with the current state-of-the-art coronary angioscopic catheters. First, as has been a problem throughout the history of angioscopy, blood interference with the visual field remains a potential problem. Even the smallest amount of intraluminal blood can produce a hazy red image that can only be cleared with good irrigation. Second, the coaxial advancement of these flexible catheters was not a problem in vein grafts or straight native coronary arteries, but the lack of an angulation system did limit the extent of the coronary vasculature that could be visualized. Finally, despite the smaller size of these angioscopic catheters, they still may be too large because only the larger nondiseased portions of the coronary arteries could be visualized.

INDICATIONS FOR ANGIOSCOPY IN CARDIAC SURGERY

As has been reported for peripheral vascular angioscopy, coronary angioscopy must be able to provide clinically relevant information over and above that currently available with angiography or direct inspection.[14-16] The greatest potential value of this technique could lie in its ability to provide immediate qualitative and quantitative information during intraoperative coronary procedures. Potentially, this could be as simple as inspection of the anastomotic site as either an instructional aid or for answering questions about the quality of the anastomosis. Indeed, in a more recent analysis of their angioscopic series, Grundfest and associates reported three cases of misplaced sutures documented by angioscopy that led to revision of the anastomosis.[20]

Potential indications for intraoperative coronary angioscopy include the ability to evaluate the results of balloon or laser angioplasty. With the current emphasis on complete myocardial revascularization, intraoperative balloon-catheter dilation and laser vaporization of distal diseased vessels or sequential lesions are attractive adjunctive procedures to coronary artery bypass surgery when intraoperative angiography is either unavailable or impractical because of limitations of space and time.[21]

CONCLUSION

In summary, cardiac endoscopy or angioscopy has developed considerably over the past 70 years, with fiberoptic technology making significant advancement possible over the past 20 years. Current technological limitations of size, irrigation, and angulation could undoubtedly be resolved. Widespread clinical application of this procedure, however, requires a definite indication and advantage over existing diagnostic methods.

REFERENCES

1. Rhea L, Walker IC, cited in Cutler EC, Levine SA, Beck CS: The surgical treatment of mitral stenosis: Experimental and clinical studies. Arch Surg 9:689–690, 1924
2. Allen DS, Graham EA: Intracardiac surgery: A new method. JAMA 79:1028–1030, 1922
3. Brock RC: Pulmonary valvulotomy for relief of congenital pulmonary stenosis. Br Med J 1:1121, 1948
4. Harken DE, Glidden EM: Experiments in intracardiac surgery. II. Intercardiac visualization. J Thorac Surg 12:566–572, 1943
5. Bloomberg AE, in discussion in Bailey CP, Glover RP, O'Neil TJE, Ramirez HPR: Experiences with the experimental surgical relief of aortic stenosis. J Thorac Surg 20:516, 1950
6. Sakakibara S, Ilkawa T, Hattori J, Inomata K: Direct visual operation for aortic stenosis: Cardioscopic studies. J Int Coll Surg 29:548, 1958
7. Butterworth RF: A new operating cardioscope. J Thorac Surg 22:319–322, 1951
8. Bolton HE, Bailey CP, Costas–Durieux J, Gemeinhardt W: Cardioscopy—simple and practical. J Thorac Surg 27:323–329, 1954
9. Carlens E, Silander T: Method for direct inspection of the right atrium: Experimental investigation in the dog. Surgery 49:622, 1961
10. Silander T: Cardioscopy without thoracotomy. Acta Chir Scand 127:67–84, 1961
11. Greenstone SM, Shore JM, Heringman EC, Massell TB: Arterial endoscopy (arterioscopy). Arch Surg 93:811–813, 1966
12. Gamble HA, Innis RE: Experimental intracardiac visualization. N Engl J Med 276:1397–1403, 1967
13. Tanabe T, Yokotu A, Sugie S: Cardiovascular fiberoptic endoscopy: Development and clinical application. Surgery 87:375–379, 1980
14. Crispin HA, Van Baarle AF: Intravascular observation and surgery using the flexible fiberscope. Lancet 1:750–751, 1973
15. Vollman JF, Storz LW: Vascular endoscopy. Possibilities and limits of its clinical application. Surg Clin North Am 54:111–122, 1974
16. Towne JB, Bernard VM: Vascular endoscopy: Useful tool or interesting toy. Surgery 82:415–419, 1977
17. Spears JR, Marais HJ, Serur JM et al: In vivo coronary angioscopy. J Am Coll Cardiol 1:1311–1314, 1983
18. Litvack F, Grundfest WS, Lee ME et al: Angioscopic visualization of blood vessel interiors in animals and humans. Clin Cardiol 8:65–70, 1985
19. Sanborn TA, Rygaard JA, Westbrook BM et al: Interoperative saphenous vein and coronary artery angioscopy. J Thorac Cardiovasc Surg 91:339–343, 1986
20. Grundfest WS, Litvack F, Sherman T et al: Delineation of peripheral and coronary detail by intraoperative angioscopy. Ann Surg 202:394–400, 1985
21. Roberts AJ, Faro RS, Feldman RL et al: Comparison of early and long term results with intraoperative transluminal balloon catheter dilatation and coronary artery bypass grafting. J Thorac Cardiovasc Surg 83:435–440, 1983

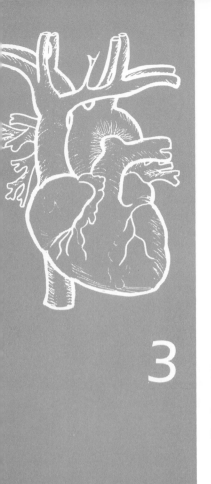

3

INTRAOPERATIVE CORONARY ARTERY BALLOON-CATHETER DILATATION

Noel L. Mills
Ronald J. Solar

To achieve long-term anginal relief and improved longevity, a variety of strategies to approach total myocardial revascularization at the time of coronary artery bypass operation have been endorsed.[1-6] Grafts are placed in an increasing number of branches in the coronary arterial tree, and endarterectomies are more commonly employed. However, certain pathologic and anatomical conditions continue to limit the ability to achieve total revascularization. For example, diffuse distal disease often occurs in vessels that are too small or inaccessible for grafting. These lesions may limit runoff of a proximally placed bypass graft and also may obstruct flow to potentially important but relatively small arteries. In these circumstances, intraoperative balloon-catheter dilatation is an important adjunct to bypass grafting, offering a chance for more complete myocardial revascularization. In this chapter, the pathophysiology of balloon angioplasty is reviewed, indications and the intraoperaive technique are discussed, and the various types of dilatation catheters available for intraoperative use are compared. Our clinical experience with intraoperative coronary artery balloon-catheter dilatation is presented.

PATHOPHYSIOLOGY OF BALLOON ANGIOPLASTY

When Dotter and Judkins first suggested in 1964 that atherosclerotic lesions could be permanently dilated, it was believed that the increase in lumen diameter was due to compression and remodeling of the plaque against the arterial wall, along with the simultaneous release of fluid components of the plaque.[7,8] More recent studies[9-13] have disproved this early theory, finding no evidence of significant plaque compression, remodeling, or fluid extrusion. The dominant mechanisms by which atherosclerotic lesions are dilated include plaque disruption (such as splitting and separation from the arterial wall), intimal fracture, and stretching of the media and adventitia (sometimes with tearing). Generally, the orientation of the disruption and tearing is longitudinal (*i.e.*, parallel to the blood flow). This may account for the relative scarcity of postdilatation complications, such as intimal flaps and dissecting aneurysms; unlike a transverse tear, longitudinal tears would not be subjected to the lifting force of the blood flow. Despite the traumatic nature of dilatation, there is a relatively low incidence of embolization or thrombosis after this procedure. As discussed by Fogarty and associates, this may be explained by the lack of atheroma fragmentation, the continued attachment of the plaque to the arterial wall, the increased laminar flow across the dilated area, and the increased usage of antiplatelet agents.[10,14]

Just as certain types of coronary lesions are more amenable to endarterectomy, certain coronary lesions are more amenable to balloon angioplasty. Atherosclerotic disease in the coronary artery may range from soft, semisolid plaque material, to areas of fibrosis with a paucity of cholesterol, or to lesions with varying degrees of calcification and solidification. In studying the effects of balloon dilatation in human postmortem coronary arteries, ten lesion variations and possible results from dilatation were identified.[13] These are shown in Figure 3–1. Often, the surgeon may get a "feel" for the type of disease at hand, and this may influence the decision as to whether or not angioplasty should be performed. For example, if the atherosclerotic disease appears to contain much liquid cholesterol and debris, antegrade angioplasty may be avoided because there may be an increased risk of embolization of this debris into distal coronary branches, thereby jeopardizing the bypass graft.

INDICATIONS AND CONTRAINDICATIONS

In general, intraoperative coronary angioplasty is indicated in patients presenting with multiple segmental coronary artery lesions that are difficult to approach by standard bypass techniques (*i.e.,* lesions in vessels too small to accept a graft and anatomical locations inaccessible to normal bypass techniques). Calcification is not a contraindication to operative angioplasty and has been revoked as a contraindication to percutaneous coronary angioplasty. Specific examples include the following: left anterior descending

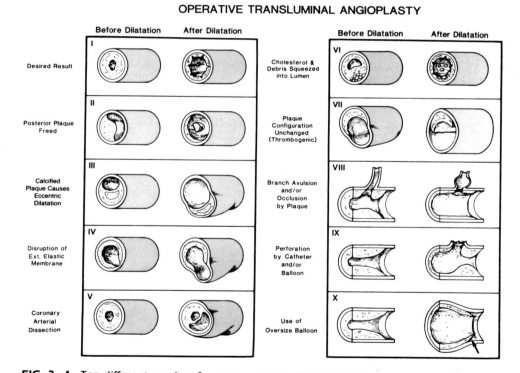

OPERATIVE TRANSLUMINAL ANGIOPLASTY

FIG. 3–1. Ten different results of coronary artery dilatation in freshly autopsied hearts. (After Mills NL, Doyle DP: Does operative transluminal angioplasty extend the limits of coronary artery bypass surgery? A preliminary report. Circulation (Suppl I) 6:I–26, 1982; by permission of the American Heart Association, Inc)

(LAD) coronary artery with a proximal lesion that has a second significant lesion at the apex (intraoperative dilatation has been shown to offer collateral circulation by way of the distal vessel); lesions obstructing flow to a branch (*e.g.,* diagonal, secondary circumflex marginal branches, and distal right coronary artery (RCA) branches too small to accept a graft); proximal LAD artery with tandem lesions (dilating the more distal lesion may offer flow to the trapped branches and increase runoff); proximal or mid-RCA stenosis in conjunction with a proximal posterior descending artery (PDA) lesion in which sequential grafting is not feasible; and the main left coronary artery, which may be dilated by way of the aorta to offer more blood flow to proximal branches that cannot be bypassed (Fig. 3–2).[15] Although other researchers have suggested that angioplasty is feasible for heavily calcified or fibrotic arteries that may be difficult to enter safely for performance of grafting, we would treat such lesions with endarterectomy.[14,16] There are several specific settings in which intraoperative angioplasty is contraindicated.

> It is not used to dilate arterial anastomoses that have been somewhat narrowed secondary to technical reasons. The anastomosis should be redone.
>
> Angioplasty is not used to dilate a diseased coronary artery for the purpose of enlarging it to more easily accept a bypass graft. An endarterectomy is indicated in this case.
>
> Antegrade dilatation of proximal lesions that could embolize debris to the distal coronary bed should be avoided.
>
> Dilatation of proximal lesions that may allow competition with the bypass graft from the native circulation should be avoided.

In general, whenever an endarterectomy or sequential grafting can be used within reason, in-

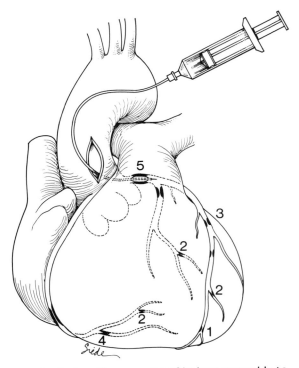

FIG. 3–2. Specific examples of lesions amenable to intraoperative coronary dilatation. **(1)** The most common site is in the distal LAD. **(2)** Lesions obstructing the flow to branches that are too small to accept a bypass graft. **(3)** Tandem LAD lesions with interim vessels. **(4)** Posterior descending stenosis in conjunction with a right coronary artery stenosis for which bypass to the distal right coronary system is not feasible. **(5)** Main left coronary artery by way of the aorta to offer more blood flow to proximal branches that cannot be bypassed.

traoperative angioplasty should be avoided. Other researchers have suggested that dilatation of secondary lesions should be used instead of sequential grafting and endarterectomy.[14,17] Because the angioplasty procedure requires much less time, the aortic cross-clamp time may be reduced. In addition, endarterectomy may be associated with side-branch shearing, a high incidence of reocclusion, and a higher incidence of perioperative infarction. However, observations of percutaneous coronary angioplasty suggest that the restenosis rate within the first 6 to 12 months is 17% to 30%, and thus intraoperative angioplasty may not be as satisfactory as endarterectomy or, when possible, additional grafting procedures.[16,18] Therefore, until long-term results of intraoperative balloon angioplasty can be evaluated, we recommend endarterectomy or sequential grafting over angioplasty whenever practical. This recommendation is widely shared.[16,19,20]

TECHNIQUE

A hand drawing of the coronary artery tree with its lesions is used in the operating room as a guide to identify the correct anatomy, to localize lesions, and to plan the operative course (Fig. 3–3). Whenever possible, the epicardium over the lesion is opened, and the lesion is visualized and palpated. A coronary arteriotomy is made at the site of the proposed bypass grafting. The diameters of the lesion and the normal vessel adjacent to the lesion are measured (calibrated) with graduated probes; these measurements are compared with those taken from the preoperative arteriogram. If cardiac fat or the depth of the artery prevents direct visualization, the location of the lesion is determined by measuring the length of the calibrated probe from the lesion to the arteriotomy. The balloon size is selected on the basis of the diameter of the coronary artery adjacent to the lesion, as measured with the calibrated probe. The balloon diameter should be equal to or slightly larger (0.5 mm) than that of the coronary artery (*i.e.*, a 2-mm or a 2.5-mm diameter balloon is chosen for an artery that accepts a 2-mm probe but not a 2.5-mm probe). In the majority of our cases, a coaxial balloon catheter with a fixed guidewire tip (USCI, Billerica, MA; SciMed Life Systems, Inc., Minneapolis, MN) was employed. With this design, the balloon is

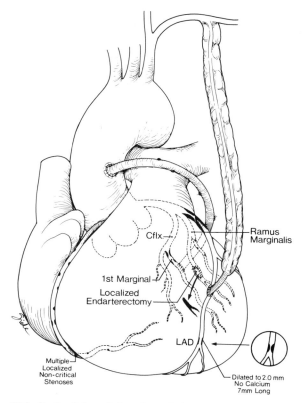

FIG. 3–3. *A hand drawing of the coronary artery tree with its lesions that is used in the operating room as a guide to identify the correct anatomy, to localize lesions, and to plan the operative dilatation.*

passed across the lesion and (whenever possible) situated such that the lesion is centered within the midportion of the balloon. These catheters have black markings, which are usually visible from within the artery, that facilitate balloon placement.

Prior to passage within the artery, the balloon catheter is first prepared. A stopcock and syringe (5 ml to 10 ml), partially filled with saline, are attached to the Luer fitting of the catheter. The catheter is then purged with normal saline to remove most of the trapped air (repeated inflation/deflation cycles using a saline-filled syringe provide for adequate purging), and then the balloon is held in the deflated state by creating a vacuum with the syringe and closing the stopcock. The balloon is then passed through the arteriotomy and across the lesion. By passing the catheter with the balloon held in the deflated condition (under vacuum), the smallest profile or diameter is attained, which facilitates crossing the lesion and minimizes the risk of damage to the normal endothelium of the adjacent arterial segment. Once the balloon is in position across the lesion, a 2.5-ml saline-filled syringe is connected to a pressure manometer, which is then connected to the catheter/stopcock assembly. The stopcock is opened and the syringe is compressed to inflate the balloon to 7 to 10 atmospheres of pressure. This pressure is held for 30 seconds and then the balloon is deflated by creating a vacuum with the syringe. This inflation/deflation is repeated for three successive cycles. The balloon is deflated and the catheter is

withdrawn, and the appropriate-size calibrated probe is passed across the dilated lesion to measure the dilated diameter. The site of the lesion is marked with a radiopaque clip for future angiographic reference. A commercial hand dilatation syringe-manometer system used for percutaneous transluminal coronary angioplasty (PTCA) may be used for operative angioplasty (Fig. 3–4).

The procedure is considered successful if the probe that calibrated the size of the normal artery proximal to the lesion can now be passed through the dilated segment. An "unsuccessful" procedure is one in which the lesion cannot be crossed with the catheter or cannot be dilated once crossed. In the case in which the lesion does not dilate, a larger diameter balloon (+0.5 mm) catheter may be tried, but with great caution. Care must be taken to dilate only the area of the lesion and not the normal coronary artery. Once the angioplasty procedure is completed, the bypass graft is anastomosed to the coronary artery

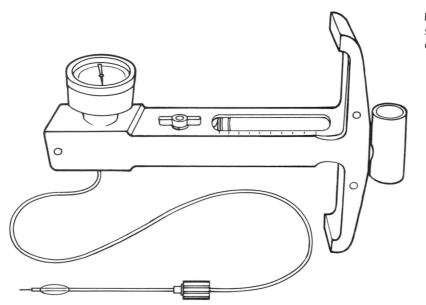

FIG. 3–4. Commercial syringe-manometer used for operative dilatation.

by routine technique. Generally, the intraoperative angioplasty procedure requires 5 to 10 minutes per lesion.

Although operative arteriography is available, it has not been used because of the added cross-clamp and cardiopulmonary bypass times, the increased risk of infection, and the fact that the information obtained would not influence the treatment (*i.e.*, an angiographically determined failure would not warrant any further manipulation of the area). Again, it is emphasized that only arteries that would otherwise be left unbypassed are selected for operative angioplasty. Postoperatively, aspirin (600 mg/day) and dipyridamole (75 mg/day) are given orally and continued indefinitely.

INTRAOPERATIVE ANGIOPLASTY CATHETER SYSTEMS

Since its beginning, the primary interest in angioplasty has been percutaneous applications. Consequently, the first intraoperative angioplasty catheters were simply modified versions of the percutaneous devices, and applications in adjunctive coronary angioplasty were limited. More recently, devices specifically designed for

FIG. 3–5. Four types of catheters used for intraoperative coronary angioplasty. **(A)** Balloon extruded from within catheter. **(B)** Standard catheter with balloon. **(C)** Balloon over guidewire. **(D)** Catheter advanced over guidewire.

OPERATIVE ANGIOPLASTY CATHETERS

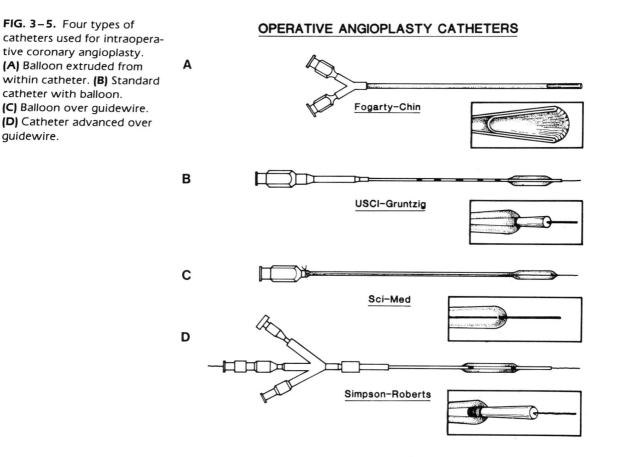

A — Fogarty–Chin

B — USCI–Gruntzig

C — Sci–Med

D — Simpson–Roberts

intraoperative coronary use have become available. At present, four types of catheters have been used for intraoperative coronary artery balloon angioplasty: fixed guidewire coaxial systems, fixed guidewire coaxial systems with a threaded tip, movable guidewire coaxial systems, and a linear extrusion system (Fig. 3–5). Each has advantages and disadvantages, and occasionally during the course of a procedure, two different systems may be used to complement each other. Balloon sizes range from 1.5 mm to 3 mm in diameter and are generally 20 mm in length.

FIXED GUIDEWIRE COAXIAL SYSTEMS

Fixed guidewire coaxial systems are the most commonly used catheters for intraoperative coronary applications. Two companies, USCI (Billerica, MA) and SciMed Life Systems, Inc. (Minneapolis, MN), presently manufacture these devices. Although materials and construction differ, the primary clinically observed differences between these two devices are dimensional. The SciMed catheter has a smaller deflated balloon profile, enabling balloon passage through tighter lesions. Its balloon is located closer to the tip of the guidewire (3 mm versus 10 mm for the USCI catheter). In the case of an immediate branching distal to the lesion, the size of the coronary artery decreases distally, and the long tip of the USCI catheter becomes a significant disadvantage; the catheter tip may traverse the lesion, but the balloon may not. Unlike the SciMed catheter, the USCI device lacks a smooth transition from the guidewire to the tip of the catheter; this may hang up on firm coronary lesions, preventing catheter passage or resulting in plaque dislodgement (Fig. 3–6).

FIXED GUIDEWIRE WITH THREADED TIP

The fixed guidewire with threaded tip device is similar to the SciMed catheter described above with the exception that the catheter tip (proximal

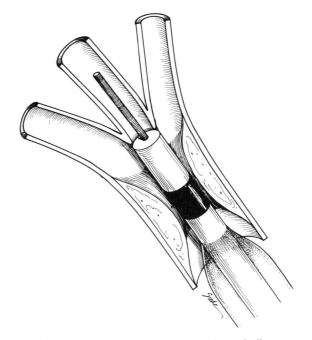

FIG. 3–6. Angioplasty device showing a balloon that cannot be advanced across the lesion because it is too remote from the catheter tip. Further advancement of the catheter is prevented by distal branching of the coronary arterial tree. Note the lack of taper from the guidewire to the catheter, which may result in artery damage or plaque dislodgement.

to the leading guidewire) has a threaded configuration (Fig. 3–7). It is useful in tight lesions where it is not desirable to force the catheter tip and balloon across the lesion. After the guidewire crosses the lesion, the catheter is gently rotated in a clockwise direction; the plastic threads engage the plaque and pull the balloon tip through the lesion. Although present experience with this device has been limited, the results are most promising; in eight of ten attempts, the threaded catheter safely crossed lesions that prohibited passage of nonthreaded-tip catheters.

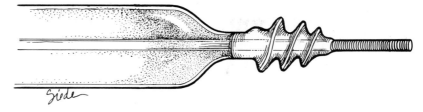

FIG. 3–7. Close-up of the threaded configuration of the catheter tip used for tight lesions in which it is not possible to advance the usual type of catheter device across the lesion.

MOVABLE GUIDEWIRE COAXIAL SYSTEMS

With movable guidewire coaxial systems (manufactured by Advanced Cardiovascular Systems, Inc., Mountain View, CA, and Meditech, Watertown, MA), a guidewire is first placed across the stenosis, and then the catheter is advanced over the guidewire. Although our experience with this catheter is limited, the system was found to have many of the same technical disadvantages described above (*i.e.*, large size, long tip, lack of smooth guidewire-to-tip transition).

LINEAR EXTRUSION SYSTEM (FOGARTY–CHIN)

In the linear extrusion system (manufactured by American Edwards Laboratories, Irvine, CA), the balloon is housed within the catheter. The catheter tip is positioned just proximal to the lesion. Fluid injection into the catheter with a syringe causes the balloon to "extrude" or unroll from inside the catheter and traverse the lesion as it unrolls. Continued fluid injection results in radial expansion of the balloon to its fixed diameter. Some compliance of the lesion and arterial wall is necessary for balloon extrusion. Unlike coaxial catheters, this system has the disadvantage of only a single use in patients with multiple lesions, because reinsertion of the balloon within the catheter is difficult and is discouraged.

In coronary applications, we have not shared the same clinical success with this system as that reported by Dr. Fogarty and colleagues.[10,14] We found that the 5F catheter size was often too large for distal coronary artery dilatation and that the catheter tip, having no taper, had a tendency to hang up on noncritical lesions as it was ad-vanced down the coronary artery to the site of the dilatation. In addition, the sudden uncontrolled extrusion of the balloon from within the catheter resulted in three complications. At the time of this writing, further modifications of this system are in progress by the manufacturer to avoid such problems. Wire and/or suture attachments to the balloon hopefully will allow a controlled extrusion of the balloon.

CLINICAL EXPERIENCE

The results of our clinical experience with intraoperative coronary balloon angioplasty are presented with respect to two study groups and are summarized in Table 3–1. Group 1 contains the first 81 operative coronary angioplasty patients (November 1980 to February 1983), and group 2 contains a later group of patients (June 1984 to April 1985). The patient population in both groups was similar with respect to age, sex, number of grafts, and location of lesion (approximately half of the lesions treated in each group were located in the distal LAD artery). In group 1, the fixed guidewire coaxial catheter (USCI) was used most often for reasons of availability and better clinical results; four movable guidewire coaxial catheters (ACS and Meditech) and ten linear extrusion catheters (American Edwards Laboratories) were also employed. In group 2, the newer low-profile fixed guidewire coaxial catheter (SciMed) was used most frequently. In addition, 10 catheters with threaded tips (SciMed) and 12 USCI catheters were also used in group 2.

TABLE 3–1
SUMMARY OF CLINICAL RESULTS

	Group 1 (11/80–2/83)	Group 2 (6/84–4/85)	Total Groups 1 and 2
No. of Patients	81	33	114
Male	72 (89%)	30 (91%)	102 (89%)
Female	9 (11%)	3 (9%)	12 (11%)
Age	34–73	36–77	34–77
Mean number of grafts	4.2	3.9	4.1
No. of Lesions	93	38	131
No. of calcified lesions	27 (29%)	3 (8%)	30 (23%)
Mean lesion length (cm) — successful	0.98	3.3	1.7
Mean lesion length (cm) — nonsuccessful	1.96	4	2.35
% of Lesions Crossed	78/93 (84%)	35/38 (92%)	113/131 (86%)
Operative Success Rate	75/93 (81%)	34/38 (90%)	109/131 83%)
Defective Catheters	23/91 (25%)	7/38 (18%)	30/129 (23%)
Balloon rupture	17 (19%)	4 (10%)	21 (16%)
Leaks	6 (6%)	3 (8%)	9 (7%)
Complications	5/93 (5.4%)	1/38 (2.6%)	6/131 (4.6%)
Perforations	2	—	2
Plaque dislodgement	1	—	1
MI	1	—	1
Vessel rupture	1	1	2

In both groups, the primary reason for failure of the procedure was the inability to cross the lesion. In group 1, the "crossing failure rate" was 16%, which was twice as high as that in group 2, suggesting a clear advantage of the low-profile catheter. Although calcification was encountered much less frequently in group 2, its lesions were two to three times as long as those found in group 1. These data and the literature suggest that longer lesions are associated with a higher failure rate.[10-20] Moreover, in group 2, there were seven instances in which the USCI catheter would not cross the lesion, whereas the low-profile catheter, which was used subsequently, crossed and dilated these lesions. The threaded-tip catheter was used successfully in eight cases and was unsuccessful in two; in these two lesions, no catheter was able to cross the lesion. The operative success rates for groups 1 and 2 were 81% and 90%, respectively, and 83% for both groups combined.

POSTOPERATIVE STUDIES

In group 1, 29 patients allowed postoperative coronary angiography to study 31 lesions for up to 1 year. Of 28 lesions that had a successful operative angioplasty, a good result was observed in 20, or 71%. This continued success rate curiously corresponds to the 30% restenosis rate reported by a number of centers performing percutaneous coronary angioplasty.[16,18] In group 2, only eight patients have been restudied to date, and six are enjoying continued success (75%).

COMPLICATIONS

By far the most common complication associated with operative angioplasty was balloon rupture or catheter leak. Although some improvements have been made (reduction of malfunctions from 25% to 18% from groups 1 to 2), this failure rate is much too high. In most cases, balloon rupture or catheter leak offers simply a "nuisance factor." However, in two cases, balloon rupture was associated with a tear of the coronary artery, with extrusion of fluid into the subepicardial area adjacent to the vessel. The problem was repaired by performing a manual core endarterectomy and suturing the tear with 8–0 proline over a 1-mm catheter. No untoward sequelae followed. Of the ten cases in which the linear extrusion catheter was employed, complications occurred in three. In one patient, the balloon, rather than traversing the plaque, dislodged it and pushed in distally. In the other two, the balloon extruded rapidly from the catheter and perforated the coronary artery near the proximal origin of the lesion; in one of these patients, an extensive distal endarterectomy with closure of the small coronary artery was required to repair the damaged artery.

In all patients, a search for perioperative myocardial infarction (MI) was carried out using serial electrocardiograms (ECGs) and creatine phosphokinase-MB (CPK-MB) isoenzymes. If the CPK measurement or ECG indicated perioperative MI, an isotope scan of the myocardium was performed. Two patients in group 1 had overt MIs, but only one was in the area of the operative dilatation. Congestive heart failure, prolonged cardiac drug support, or an intra-aortic balloon pump was not present in either series. There were no early or late deaths in group 1, and in group 2, one patient died 1 month postoperatively of noncardiac causes. Postmortem angiogram revealed a successful dilatation, and histology of the lesion showed "remodeling" of the dilated artery. Other than the perforations associated with the use of the linear extrusion system, known complications have been nil; spasm, arrhythmia, or late hemorrhage has not occurred.

DISCUSSION

Intraoperative coronary artery angioplasty was first performed in 1978.[21] The technique and indications are still evolving, and the long-term outlook depends on the late clinical results. Unfortunately, angiographic studies for a later follow-up are difficult to obtain. Because of the widespread interest in PTCA, catheter development for intraoperative angioplasty applications has lagged. Early attempts at intraoperative dilatation of potentially correctable lesions were often unsuccessful because of poor design of the intraoperative balloon catheters. However, as evidenced by comparisons of our early and late results, the recent development of the low-profile systems for intraoperative coronary use has contributed to a marked improvement in the operative success rate. Failures due to the inability to cross the lesion have been cut in half, from 16% to 8%. In addition, improvements in balloon technology have resulted in fewer balloon ruptures.

The single most obvious difference between percutaneous and intraoperative angioplasty is the use of angiography. Because angiography is not used in intraoperative angioplasty, it has been suggested that this is a blind procedure. On the contrary, during intraoperative angioplasty, the target artery is most often exposed under the direct vision of the operating surgeon. The surgeon can place the balloon catheter across the lesion using direct visual control, palpation, and measurements of catheter length from the arteriotomy. The use of probes to calibrate the artery and lesion has proved to be a simple, inexpensive, and safe procedure, and, in our studies and those of others, the correlation to measurements determined angiographically was extremely high.[17] Moreover, considering the varying nature of the atherosclerotic lesion, the surgeon may be in a better position to determine, by direct observation, which lesions can be dilated safely and effectively.

Recurrence, or restenosis of arteries that have been dilated, remains the "Achilles' heel" of any coronary angioplasty technique. Restenosis rates on the order of 30% may not be all that objectionable in PTCA if one considers the fact that these stenoses respond very well to a repeat PTCA and that the morbidity associated with the procedure is low. The restenosis rate of arteries subjected to intraoperative angioplasty to date is unknown. It may be higher than that for PTCA because the arteries treated are smaller and more distal. On the other hand, however, intraoperative angioplasty may have a restenosis rate lower than PTCA because of the precise control afforded by direct visualization at operation and the ability to repeatedly calibrate lesions until the stenosis is completely relieved.

The criterion for a "successful" PTCA has been stated as a 20% increase in lumen diameter at the stenosis as opposed to complete relief of the stenosis, which is the criterion used for operative angioplasty. The importance of precise balloon positioning such that only the lesion — and not the normal artery — is dilated is well established. Investigators who initially advocated extensive dilation into areas of normal coronary arteries have now reversed that philosophy.[22]

CONCLUSIONS

Intraoperative coronary balloon-catheter dilatation is a safe and effective technique that offers a chance for more complete myocardial revascularization, particularly in patients presenting with severe distal coronary artery disease. Recent improvements in catheter design have extended the application by allowing passage through smaller, more distal arteries. Because long-term results of intraoperative angioplasty are not known, it is strongly emphasized that coronary arteries that can be bypassed or safely endarterectomized should be treated with these techniques; angioplasty should be reserved for coronary arteries generally not amenable to the usual bypass techniques.

REFERENCES

1. Buda AJ, MacDonald IL, Anderson MJ et al: Long-term results following coronary bypass operation: Importance of preoperative factors and complete renovascularization. J Thorac Cardiovasc Surg 82:383, 1981
2. Lawrie GM, Morris GC, Silvers A et al: Influence of residual disease after coronary bypass on the 5-year survival rate of 1274 men with coronary artery disease. Circulation 66:717, 1982
3. Jones EL, Craver JM, Guyton RA et al: Importance of complete revascularization in performance of the coronary bypass operation. Am J Cardiol 51:7, 1983
4. Hossack KF, Bruce RA, Ivey TD, Kusumi F: Changes in cardiac functional capacity after coronary bypass surgery in relation to adequacy of revascularization. J Am Coll Cardiol 3:47, 1984
5. Iskandrian AS, Hakki AH, Nestico PF et al: Effects of residual coronary artery disease on results of coronary artery bypass grafting. Int J Cardiol 6:537, 1984
6. Cosgrove DM, Loop FD, Lytle BW et al: Primary myocardial revascularization. Trends in surgical mortality. J Thorac Cardiovasc Surg 88:673, 1984
7. Dotter CT, Judkins MP: Transluminal treatment of arteriosclerotic obstruction: Description of a new technique and a preliminary report of its application. Circulation 30:654, 1964
8. Dotter CT: Transluminal angioplasty — Pathologic basis. In Zeitler E, Gruntzig A, Schoop W (eds): Percutaneous Vascular Recanalization, p. 3. Berlin, Springer – Verlag, 1978
9. Castaneda – Zuniga WR, Formanek A, Tadavavarthy M et al: The mechanism of balloon angioplasty. Radiology 135:565, 1980
10. Fogarty TJ, Chin AK, Shoor PM et al: Adjunctive intraoperative arterial dilatation: Simplified instrumentation technique. Arch Surg 116:1391, 1981
11. Chin AK, Fogarty TJ, Kinney TB et al: Pathophysiologic bases for transluminal angioplasty. Surg Forum 32:323, 1981
12. Lyon RT, Zarins CK, Lu CT et al: Arterial wall disruption by balloon dilatation: Quantitative comparison of normal, stenotic, and occluded vessels. Surg Forum 32:326, 1981
13. Mills NL, Doyle DP: Does operative transluminal angioplasty extend the limits of coronary artery bypass surgery? A preliminary report. Circulation (Suppl I) 66:I–26, 1982
14. Fogarty TJ, Kinney TB: Intraoperative coronary artery balloon-catheter dilatation. Am Heart J 107:845, 1984
15. Mills NL, Ochsner JL, Doyle DP, Kalchoff WP: Technique

and results of operative transluminal angioplasty in 81 consecutive patients. J Thorac Cardiovasc Surg 86:689, 1983

16. Jones EL, King SB: Intraoperative balloon-catheter dilatation in the treatment of coronary artery disease. Am Heart J 107:836, 1984

17. Ross AM, Leiboff RH, Aaron BL et al: Intraoperative retrograde balloon-catheter dilatation to augment myocardial revascularization. Am Heart J 107:851, 1984

18. Kent KM, Bentivoglio LG, Black PC et al: Percutaneous transluminal coronary angioplasty: Report from the registry of the National Heart, Lung, and Blood Institute. Am J Cardiol 49:2011, 1982

19. Faro RS, Alexander JA, Feldman RL et al: Intraoperative balloon-catheter dilatation: University of Florida experience. Am Heart J 107:841, 1984

20. Wallsh E, Weinstein GS, Frazone AJ et al: Adjunctive operative coronary artery balloon-catheter dilatation: Review of Lenox Hill experience. Am Heart J 107:856, 1984

21. Turina M, Gruntzig AR, Krayenbuhl CH, Senning A: The role of the surgeon in percutaneous transluminal dilatation of coronary stenosis. Ann Thorac Surg 28:103, 1979

22. Roberts AJ, Alexander JA, Knauf DG et al: Clinical and angiographic experience with intraoperative transluminal balloon-catheter dilatation and coronary artery bypass surgery. J Cardiovasc Surg 26(3):207–211, 1985

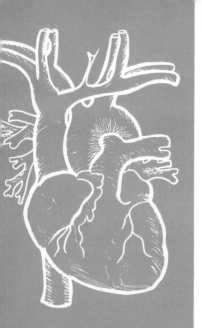

4

DEVELOPMENT OF A CLINICAL ARTIFICIAL HEART

Eduardo Jorge

William S. Pierce

Cardiovascular diseases continue to be the leading cause of death in the United States, with nearly one million deaths attributed to them yearly.[1] Myocardial infarctions represent over one half of these deaths. It has been estimated that approximately 14,000 people between the ages of 15 and 54 could have benefited from cardiac transplantation in 1980, but only 1932 would have met the selection criteria.[2] In addition, one of seven patients dies while waiting for a donor heart to become available. These figures illustrate the large patient population with end-stage heart disease for whom there are presently no further medical alternatives for improved cardiac function. A panel from the National Heart, Lung, and Blood Institute (NHLBI) estimated that 17,000 to 50,000 people per year could benefit from an artificial heart.[3]

During the 19th and early 20th centuries, numerous investigators developed blood pumps designed to be used for perfusion of isolated organs or to eventually replace the heart.[4] This led to the clinical use of a heart-lung machine by Gibbon in 1953.[5] In 1957 Akutsu and Kolff first replaced the heart of a dog with an intrathoracically located artificial heart.[6] The device was constructed of polyvinylchloride and was powered by an extracorporeal air pump. They were able to support the dog's circulation for 90 minutes. After a brief period of experimentation with electrically driven artificial hearts, Kolff's group "became restless with this slow progress" and continued their work on the pneumatically driven heart. In 1965 Nosé and colleagues reported over 24 hours' survival of a calf with a sac-type ventricular chamber constructed of Silastic.[7] A diaphragm pump designed by Kwann–Gett achieved a survival of 2 weeks in 1972.[8] Improvements in biomaterials and design allowed for further prolongation of animal survival. The use of segmented polyurethane as the blood-contacting surface provided an extremely smooth inner surface with excellent flex life in one of the most biocompatible materials available today.[9] In addition, evaluation of blood flow in these devices has allowed design modification to minimize regions of stasis within the artificial ventricles.[10] This has resulted in prolonging the functional lives of these pumps as well as minimizing thromboembolic complications. Animal survival up to 10 months has been achieved with currently available devices. Finally, in 1969 Cooley implanted the first temporary pneumatic artificial heart in a human while an allograft was located for transplantation.[11]

PNEUMATIC ARTIFICIAL HEART

DESIGN

There are many varieties of the air-powered artificial heart. The Pennsylvania State University heart is typical of those used worldwide. Two separate prosthetic ventricles are used to pump blood into the pulmonary and systemic circulations (Fig. 4–1). Unidirectional flow through the blood pumps is achieved by the use of one-

FIG. 4–1. Separate right and left ventricles of the pneumatic artificial heart. The individual grafts and atrial cuffs are attached to the natural aorta, pulmonary artery, and atrial remnants before being connected to the inlet and outlet ports of the prosthetic ventricles. (Pennock JL, Wisman CB, Pierce WS: Mechanical support of the circulation prior to cardiac transplantation. Heart Transplantation 1:299–305, 1982)

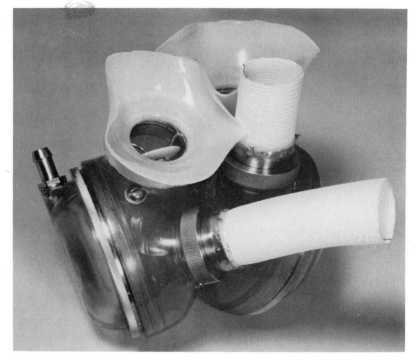

way valves at the inflow and outflow ports. Bjork–Shiley 60-degree concavo-convex tilting acetal disk valves are used instead of pyrolitic carbon disk or planodisk valves, which have been shown to undergo fractures of the disk or welded major strut, respectively, in mock loop and animal studies. The increased stress applied to these valves by an artificial heart may result in the earlier breakdown of these other valve models. Twenty-nine–mm and 25-mm valves are used for the inlet and outlet ports, respectively.

The outer case of the blood pumps is constructed of rigid polysulfone in the shape of an oblate spheroid with an elliptic cross section and a circular frontal section.[12,13] It is covered with a velour fabric prior to implantation to promote tissue ingrowth and, therefore, to allow for better fixation within the chest. The most crucial component of the pump is the flexible inner sac, which is the blood-contacting surface. The sacs are manufactured by dip casting segmented polyurethane on hollow wax forms to provide a seam-free and extremely smooth inner surface. Sac shape and valve orientation have been designed with the aid of flow visualization techniques, laser Doppler anemometry, and pulsed Doppler ultrasound to avoid areas of stasis, to provide good washout of blood, and, therefore, to minimize the tendency for thrombus formation. A polyurethane diaphragm separates the pneumatic portion of the pump from the blood sac. It also serves to limit pump stroke, preventing apposition of opposite sac walls, thereby reducing hemolysis.

The pneumatic power and control console is

located extracorporeally. It consists of four power units and a backup DC storage battery and air compressor. Two power units are used to drive the ventricles while the others serve as auxiliary units. Air pulses are delivered from the power console to the blood pumps through 10-mm internal diameter flexible hoses. These two hoses are tunneled under the skin and chest wall for approximately 20 cm and are brought through the skin by way of velour-covered telescoping sleeves to allow tissue ingrowth and to minimize infection.[14] The air pulses result in compression of the blood sacs against the rigid outer casing, causing the blood to be expelled into the aorta or pulmonary artery. During normal operation, the left systolic pressure is set between 200 mm Hg and 250 mm Hg, with a vacuum of 25 mm Hg to 50 mm Hg to aid diastolic filling. The right pump's pressures are set at 75 mm Hg to 125 mm Hg during systole, with a vacuum of 35 mm Hg to 40 mm Hg.

The pressure tracing derived from a transducer located on the left drive line (extracorporeally)

allows monitoring of left-pump function. Deflections of the baseline indicate complete pump filling, systolic phase, and complete pump emptying (Fig. 4–2). The fill time also provides an estimate of left atrial pressure.[15] Each pump's stroke volume is determined prior to implantation (approximately 70 ml). Therefore, provided that the pump is filling and emptying appropriately, the cardiac output may be calculated from the stroke volume and pump rate.

The output of the prosthetic ventricles must be regulated to allow for augmentation of cardiac output during exercise while avoiding excessive pulmonary flow and the development of pulmonary edema. The automatic control system developed by Landis and associates at The Pennsylvania State University uses the left ventricular air line pressure wave shape to derive aortic and left atrial pressures.[16] Because both pumps are always run in a full-to-empty mode, pump rate determines cardiac output. The automatic control system uses negative feedback loops to decrease left or right pump rates in response to ele-

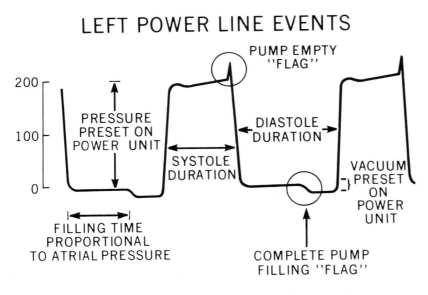

LEFT POWER LINE EVENTS

PUMP EMPTY "FLAG"

PRESSURE PRESET ON POWER UNIT

DIASTOLE DURATION

SYSTOLE DURATION

VACUUM PRESET ON POWER UNIT

FILLING TIME PROPORTIONAL TO ATRIAL PRESSURE

COMPLETE PUMP FILLING "FLAG"

FIG. 4–2. Left air line pressure tracing allows monitoring of pump function. Indications of left atrial and aortic pressures as well as pump filling and emptying can be derived from these tracings. (Pierce WS, Meyers JL, Donachy JH et al: Approaches to the artificial heart. Surgery 90:137–148, 1981)

vated aortic or left atrial pressures, respectively. Conversely, left or right pump rate is increased when aortic or left atrial pressures decrease. Therefore, variations of systemic vascular resistance will have an inverse effect on the left pump rate and consequently on cardiac output. Control of each pump by a separate feedback loop allows each to run at different rates. The right ventricle usually beats at a slower rate because passive flow-through accounts for a portion of the right-sided output. We try to achieve a cardiac output of approximately 90 ml/kg/minute at rest. This control system has several features that make it desirable. No invasive monitoring is required, preventing portals of entry for infectious agents and the thrombotic complications of long-term indwelling catheters. The wide range of cardiac outputs attainable with this system has allowed calves to go from the resting state to treadmill exercise without manual pump adjustments.

The groups at Salt Lake City and Cleveland have a control system based on Starling's law.[17,18] The system used in Salt Lake City is referred to as a "fill limited mode." In this system, systolic pressure and duration are preset to achieve complete emptying. At normal atrial pressures, the short diastolic duration prevents complete filling of the pumps. An increase in atrial pressures (*e.g.*, with exercise) results in increased pump filling and a corresponding increase in cardiac output. This system is simple and is capable of functioning without invasive monitoring. However, because the pump fails to fill with each beat, cardiac output control is achieved at the expense of economy of space. Additionally, pumping parameters may need to be adjusted during exercise to achieve the full range of pump output.

The Berlin group, on the other hand, uses the right atrial pressure to control pump frequency and pressure and, therefore, output.[19] Pressures in their device are monitored by way of air capsules incorporated into the pump connectors.

Elevation of the right atrial pressure in this system results in an increase in both pump rates. A safety negative feedback control is also used to decrease right systolic driving pressure if the left atrial pressure is significantly elevated. This group feels that much higher pump flows are required (*i.e.*, 130 ml/kg/minute) to achieve normal hemodynamics in calves.

ANIMAL IMPLANTATION

All of the prosthetic ventricles used at The Pennsylvania State University are manufactured by our group. Each ventricle is initially tested on a mock circulatory loop prior to implantation to screen for any mechanical defects as well as to determine each pump's stroke volume.

Calves weighing 85 kg to 100 kg are used for total artificial heart implantation because of their docile nature, adequate chest cavity size, and excellent tolerance of cardiopulmonary bypass. The implantation is performed through a right fifth intercostal space thoracotomy and requires approximately 2 hours of cardiopulmonary bypass. The ventricles are excised at the atrioventricular groove in a fashion similar to that used to prepare a recipient for cardiac transplantation. The aorta and pulmonary arteries are transected immediately cephalad to the semilunar valves. Vascular grafts with attached metal connectors are sutured to the great vessels. The atrial cuffs, made of a stretch fabric (14% polyurethane, 86% polyester) coated with filler-free silicone rubber with a metal connector, are attached to the respective atrial remnants. The right and left pumps are attached to the appropriate connectors and air is removed with a catheter introduced through the atrial suture lines. Pumping with the artificial heart is gradually increased as cardiopulmonary bypass is gradually removed. The calves can be extubated and can eat, drink, and stand on the day of surgery. They gain weight at a rate very similar to a normal calf and are able to exercise on a treadmill several times each week without difficulty.

Between 1980 and early 1985, pneumatic total artificial hearts were implanted in 27 calves with a mean survival of 80 days (range 1 to 269 days). The causes of death have included infection, pannus obstruction of inflow valves, hemorrhage, and mechanical failures (holes in blood sac or diaphragm, valve fractures, and so forth).

Some major problems limiting prolonged survival in these animals have been resolved or significantly ameliorated. Calcification of the blood sacs became apparent after animal survival was extended beyond 3 months. This is believed to be analogous to the calcification of xenograft valves in children and may be a finding that is limited to the growing animal.[20] These calcium deposits result in stiffening, flexion failures, and perforations of the blood sac. The use of warfarin sodium and etidronate disodium has nearly eliminated this problem.[21] Pannus formation on the atrial cuffs has often resulted in inflow obstruction when it extends over the valve orifice. The resulting decrease in cardiac output has led to the death of some animals. The precise cause of pannus growth is not clear. It may represent an organized thrombus that becomes secondarily infected. Design and biomaterial changes in the atrial connectors instituted in 1982 have resulted in the resolution of this difficult problem.[22]

Aside from weight gain and exercise tolerance, organ function and laboratory parameters appear to be minimally affected in these animals. It has been noted that with prolonged survival, the calves developed a "right heart syndrome" with elevated central venous pressure and ascites. This may represent the inability of these pumps to maintain an adequate cardiac output in these rapidly growing animals. Hematocrits of calves with artificial hearts are generally in the mid 20s (normal hematocrit 30%).[12] After the immediate postoperative period, plasma hemoglobin stays in the range of 10 mg/dl or less, indicating a low degree of hemolysis. This may be partially attributed to the four mechanical prosthetic valves. Other laboratory parameters (white blood cells, platelets, blood urea nitrogen [BUN], creatinine, and liver function) remain essentially unchanged.[12,23] Serum lactic acid dehydrogenase does remain elevated at appoximately twice the normal level, which may again reflect the level of hemolysis.

CLINICAL EXPERIENCE

To date, 20 patients have received a pneumatic total artificial heart. Fifteen patients have had the device implanted for circulatory support while awaiting a donor heart for transplantation.[11,24] In the remainder, it was implanted as a permanent cardiac replacement; these patients were not transplantation candidates.[25] Some of the same problems seen in the calf experiments (bleeding and prosthetic-valve failure) have been experienced clinically.

At The Pennsylvania State University, we have used the pneumatic total artificial heart as a "bridge" to tranplantation. Patients who are candidates for cardiac transplantation and who have completed the required testing may be candidates for the artificial heart. Should the clinical conditions of these patients deteriorate to the point where all other forms of therapy (inotropic agents, intra-aortic balloon pump, ventricular assist device) are not capable of adequate support, a pneumatic artificial heart would be implanted, utilizing a technique very similar to that described for the calves. Once a donor organ became available, the device would be removed and the allograft transplanted. The required period of support for the artificial heart may be as short as several days or as long as several months. One of the most crucial concerns in these immunosuppressed patients will be the risk of lethal infections. It is speculated that with the use of cyclosporine A, adequate immunosuppression can be achieved without unduly depressing the recipient's resistance to infection.[26]

ELECTRIC MOTOR–POWERED ARTIFICIAL HEART

The ultimate goal of artificial heart research is to devise a totally implantable system without a need for any portion of the system to traverse the skin. Pneumatically powered hearts require a bulky power-and-control console, which is located extracorporeally. Prior attempts at developing a nuclear-powered artificial heart were abandoned because of cost and safety considerations.[27] Several groups are currently involved in developing and testing electrically powered artificial hearts.[28,29]

Our group is currently using two different types of motor-driven hearts experimentally. In the cam-driven system, a brushless DC motor turns a drum cam that is positioned between two sac-type blood pumps. The blood sacs and their polysulfone outer casing are very similar to those employed in the pneumatically powered artificial heart. As the cam rotates, the cam followers and pusher plates are advanced in one direction. Pumping results from the pusher plates at each end of the cam follower, which alternately compress the two blood sacs (Fig. 4–3). This system has kept a calf alive for 222 days.[28]

The roller-screw system is similar in that pusher plates are also advanced alternately, compressing the two blood sacs.[30] However, the central portion consists of a screw that moves in a rectilinear fashion in response to the roller-screw nut, which is rotated by the motor. This system has had promising results in *in vitro* testing. Additionally, roller-screw ventricular assist devices have functioned well *in vivo*.

Control of the electrically driven hearts presents a different challenge because a single motor is used to power the right and left prosthetic ventricles. As in the pneumatic hearts, car-

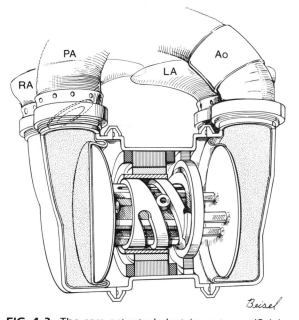

FIG. 4-3. The cam-actuated electric-motor artificial heart. Pusher plates alternately compress the right and left blood sacs. Unlike the pneumatically driven heart, a single, centrally located motor supplies the power for both left and right prosthetic ventricles. (**PA,** pulmonary artery graft; **RA,** right atrial cuff; **Ao,** aortic graft; **LA,** left atrial cuff). (Rosenberg G, Snyder AJ, Landis DL et al: An electric motor-driven total artificial heart: Seven months survival in the calf. Trans Am Soc Artif Intern Organs 30:69–74, 1984)

diac output is indirectly related to systemic vascular resistance, and balance between the right and left ventricles is adjusted according to the left atrial pressure. Aortic pressure is indirectly sensed by monitoring the motor current during left ventricular systole. Higher aortic pressures require an increase in motor current to maintain stroke speed. Left atrial pressure is inversely proportional to left pump fill time, as sensed by a Hall-effect switch. The left pump runs in a full-to-empty mode. As with the pneumatic heart,

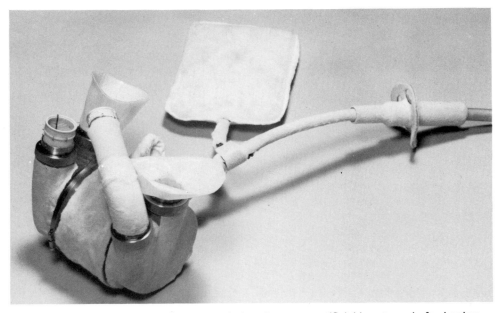

FIG. 4–4. Velour-covered cam-actuated electric-motor artificial heart ready for implantation. The attached compliance chamber serves as a reservoir for gas displaced from the centrally located motor.

pumping rate is increased in response to a decrease in aortic pressure, thereby increasing cardiac output. Because both pumps must run at the same rate, balance between the two must be achieved by varying the stroke volume of the ventricles. This can be accomplished by decreasing the filling period of the pump, whose output must be decreased. A shortened filling period prevents complete pump filling and decreases stroke volume. Because the motor is hermetically sealed, air is displaced into a compliance chamber to make up the volume differences between the two sacs. Without a compliance chamber, the trapped gas would increase the power requirements of the motor (Fig. 4–4).

Jarvik has developed an electrohydraulic-powered artificial heart that is similar to the Jarvik-7 pneumatic artificial heart.[3] The two ventricles are identical to those of the Jarvik-7. A high-speed (10,000 rpm) reversing brushless motor-driven turbine pumps silicone oil into the pumps to displace the diaphragms and to compress the blood sacs, as compressed air does in the pneumatic hearts. Reversal of pump rotation causes the silicone oil to flow out of one ventricle and into the other, thus alternating systole and diastole between the pumps. An effective control system still needs to be developed for this device. Only short-term animal studies have been performed thus far.

CONCLUSIONS

Great strides have been made in developing more reliable artificial heart systems in the past 28 years. Portable drive units for the pneumatic heart have enhanced patient mobility.[31] However, the need for percutaneous tubes with the air-powered ventricles will preclude their use as permanently implanted systems. The use of inductive coupling techniques may allow energy transmission to implanted coils in a totally implanted system. This latter system is expected to be used for permanent heart replacement in those patients who are unable to meet the selection criteria for cardiac transplantation.

REFERENCES

1. American Heart Association: Heart Facts, 1985. Dallas, American Heart Association National Center, 1985
2. Evans RG, Manninen DL, Gersh BJ et al: The need for and supply of donor hearts for transplantation. Heart Transplantation 4:57–62, 1984
3. Jarvik RK: The total artificial heart. Sci Am 244:74–80, 1981
4. Dale HH, Schuster EHJ: A double perfusion-pump. J Physiol 64:356–364, 1928
5. Gibbon JH, Jr: Application of a mechanical heart and lung apparatus to cardiac surgery. Minn Med 37:171–180, 1954
6. Akutsu T, Kolff WJ: Permanent substitutes for valves and hearts. Trans Am Soc Artif Intern Organs 4:230–235, 1958
7. Nosé Y, Topaz S, SenGupta A et al: Artificial hearts inside the pericardial sac in calves. Trans Am Soc Artif Intern Organs 11:255–262, 1965
8. Hershgold EJ, Kwann–Gett CS, Kawai J, Rowley K: Hemostasis, coagulation and the total artificial heart. Trans Am Soc Artif Intern Organs 18:181–185, 1972
9. Boretos JW, Pierce WS: Segmented polyurethane: A new elastomer for biomedical application. Science 158:1481–1482, 1967
10. Phillips WM, Brighton JA, Pierce WS: Artificial heart evaluation using flow visualization techniques. Trans Am Soc Artif Intern Organs 18:194–199, 1972
11. Cooley DA, Liotta D, Hallman GL et al: First human implantation of cardiac prosthesis for staged total replacement of the heart. Trans Am Soc Artif Intern Organs 15:252–263, 1969
12. Shaffer LJ, Donachy JH, Rosenberg G et al: Total artificial heart implantation in calves with pump of an angle port design. Trans Am Soc Artif Intern Organs 25:254–258, 1979
13. Pierce WS, Myers JL, Donachy JH et al: Approaches to the artificial heart. Surgery 90:137–148, 1981
14. Hastings WL, Aaron JL, Deneris J et al: A retrospective study of nine calves surviving five months on the pneumatic total artificial heart. Trans Am Soc Artif Intern Organs 27:71–76, 1981
15. Rosenberg G, Landis DL, Phillips WM et al: Determining arterial pressure, left atrial pressure, and cardiac output from the left pneumatic drive line of the total artificial heart. Trans Am Soc Artif Intern Organs 24:341–344, 1978
16. Landis DL, Pierce WS, Rosenberg G et al: Long-term in vivo automatic electronic control of the artificial heart. Trans Am Soc Artif Intern Organs 23:519–525, 1977
17. Mochizuki T, Hastings WL, Olsen DB et al: Postoperative hemodynamic changes in calves implanted with total artificial hearts designed for human application. Trans Am Soc Artif Intern Organs 26:55–59, 1980
18. Kasai S, Koshino I, Washyu T et al: Survival for 145 days with total artificial heart. J Thorac Cardiovasc Surg 73:637–646, 1977
19. Hennig E, Grobe–Seistrup C, Krautzberger W et al: The relationship of cardiac output and venous pressure in long surviving calves with total artificial heart. Trans Am Soc Artif Intern Organs 24:616–624, 1978
20. Kutsche LM, Oyer P, Shumway N, Baum D: An important complication of Hancock mitral valve replacement in children. Circulation (Suppl I) 60:98–103, 1979
21. Pierce WS, Donachy JH, Rosenberg G, Baier RE: Calcification inside artificial hearts: Inhibition by warfarin-sodium. Science 208:601–603, 1980
22. Pae WE, Rosenberg G, Donachy J et al: A solution to inlet pannus formation in the pneumatic artificial heart. Trans Am Soc Artif Intern Organs 31:12–16, 1985
23. Bürcherl ES, Henning E, Baer P et al: The artificial heart program in Berlin—Past, present, future. Heart Transplantation 1:306–317, 1982
24. Cooley DA, Akutsu T, Norman JC et al: Total artificial heart in two-staged cardiac transplantation. Cardiovascular Diseases Bulletin of the Texas Heart Institute 8:305–319, 1981
25. Joyce LD, DeVries WC, Hastings WL et al: Response of the human body to the first permanent implant of the Jarvik-7 total artificial heart. Trans Am Soc Artif Intern Organs 29:81–87, 1983
26. Pennock JL, Wisman CB, Pierce WS: Mechanical support of the circulation prior to cardiac transplantation. Heart Transplantation 1:299–305, 1982
27. Cole DW, Holman WS, Mott WE: Status of the USAEC's nuclear-powered artificial heart. Trans Am Soc Artif Intern Organs 19:537–541, 1973

28. Rosenberg G, Snyder AJ, Landis DL et al: An electric motor-driven total artificial heart: Seven month survival in the calf. Trans Am Soc Artif Intern Organs 30:69–74, 1984

29. Jarvik RK, Smith LM, Lawson JH et al: Comparison of pneumatic and electrically powered total artificial hearts in vivo. Trans Am Soc Artif Intern Organs 24:593–599, 1978

30. Rosenberg G, Snyder AJ, Weiss W et al: A roller-screw drive for implantable blood pumps. Trans Am Soc Artif Intern Organs 28:123–126, 1982

31. Frank J, Affeld K, Baer P et al: First experience with a mobile total artificial heart system. Trans Am Soc Artif Intern Organs 26:72–73, 1980

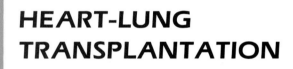

5

HEART-LUNG TRANSPLANTATION

Bruce A. Reitz

In the last 5 years, combined heart-lung transplantation has become a clinical reality for certain patients with end-stage pulmonary vascular disease.[1] This has resulted from general advances in heart transplantation, improved immunosuppression, and a growing clinical experience with heart-lung transplantation.

The technical ability to perform heart-lung transplantation has existed since the introduction of techniques for cardiopulmonary bypass.[2] Early efforts were unsuccessful because of the inability to detect and adequately treat allograft rejection and because toxic immunosuppression resulted in poor tracheal or bronchial healing. These results were similar to those of early attempts at single lung transplantation.[3] Subsequently, better laboratory animal models allowed the study of heart-lung transplantation, and cyclosporine improved immunosuppression.[4]

Clinical heart-lung transplantation was first performed in March 1981 at Stanford University Medical Center. Since that time, more than 60 patients in the United States and a similar number abroad have undergone the procedure with results approaching those of heart transplantation alone. The longest surviving patients are now alive more than 4 years following their transplant. This chapter will review the types of patients who can benefit from the procedure, their management, and the long-term results to be anticipated.

RECIPIENTS

Patients presently being considered for heart-lung transplantation are those with either primary pulmonary vascular disease or pulmonary vascular disease secondary to congenital heart disease. There are also other patients with diffuse lung disease who might be considered appropriate candidates if they have also developed secondary cardiac failure. Patients with primary pulmonary hypertension or Eisenmenger's syndrome have constituted approximately 90% of the heart-lung transplantations performed to date, and the early results are better in these patients.

The criteria are similar to those used to select heart transplant patients.[5] Age may vary between 10 and 50 years, and only those who are believed to have less than a year of anticipated survival without transplantation are considered. They must have no other significant systemic disease and must be medically compliant with good family support. A relative contraindication is a history of previous cardiac surgery. Dense adhesions present technical problems at the time of the transplant, with excessive collateral blood supply in the posterior mediastinum and difficulty in preserving the phrenic and vagus nerves. Extensive previous cardiac surgery has been associated with a poor outcome in most patients who have undergone heart-lung transplantation with this preoperative factor.

The patient with primary pulmonary hypertension may have a variable course, and it is sometimes difficult to determine when heart-lung transplantation should be recommended. A generally poor prognosis is present when severe right-sided heart failure develops with significant tricuspid insufficiency, syncope, or hemoptysis. These patients are often young and, because of a lack of previous thoracic surgery, are particularly good operative candidates.[6] The pretransplant chest roentgenogram of a 37-year-old patient who received a heart-lung transplant at The Johns Hopkins Hospital in March 1985 is shown in Figure 5–1. He had a large aortopulmonary window, Eisenmenger's syndrome, and a large aneurysm of the pulmonary artery.

At the present time, the centers performing heart-lung transplantation are limited and include Stanford University, The University of Pittsburgh, and The Johns Hopkins University.

Several other centers have performed transplants, and a number of those centers now performing heart transplantation anticipate beginning programs in combined heart-lung transplantation in the next few years. Thus, this potential therapy will be increasingly available to patients who might benefit from it.

DONORS

It is now clear that donors suitable for heart-lung transplantation will be found less frequently than those for heart transplantation. Brain death itself may be accompanied by neurogenic pulmonary edema, or pulmonary contusion may result from thoracic trauma. Cadaver donors all receive ventilatory support and are thus at risk of tracheobronchial infection or nosocomial pneumonia. Requirements for the heart-lung donor in-

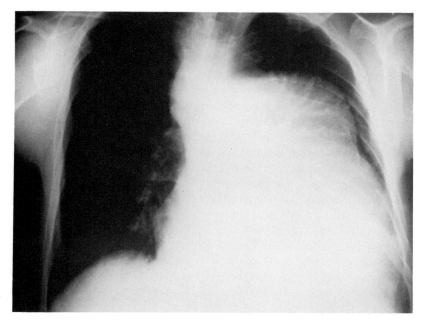

FIG. 5–1. Preoperative chest roentgenogram of a 37-year-old patient with a large aortopulmonary window, pulmonary artery aneurysm, and Eisenmenger's syndrome.

clude age less than 40 years, a close size match with the recipient to approximate lung volumes, and a completely clear chest roentgenogram. It may be necessary to treat the donor with antibiotics and vigorous pulmonary physiotherapy to accomplish this. The arterial PO_2 should be greater than 350 mm Hg on 100% oxygen, and pulmonary secretions should be free of gross infection. Approximately 20% of donors who are suitable for heart transplantation meet these stringent criteria, and this has limited the number of transplant procedures performed.

The preservation of the combined heart-lung graft is more difficult than that of the heart alone.[7] Methods of cardioplegia effective for the heart are not suitable for preservation of lung tissue. The only successful long-term preservation has resulted from maintaining a working heart-lung preparation, with the heart perfused and beating and with warm blood circulating to a reservoir and then returning to the right side of the heart, where the lung is perfused.[8,9] The lung is continuously ventilated, and the graft is transported in a sterile container with the heart beating. This type of preservation has been used by the group at the University of Pittsburgh and has been successful in several instances. Other attempts at extended static lung preservation by cold perfusion have not been successful to date, although preliminary laboratory work is encouraging.[10,11] Only when practical and effective long-term preservation has been obtained will there be any improvement in the number of potential donors, and thus the number of patients, who can be treated by transplantation.

Several important management principles differ from those used for cardiac transplant donors. Every effort should be made to maintain pulmonary sterility and optimum pulmonary function. Careful attention should be given to respiratory settings, maintaining the FIO_2 at the lowest tolerable level to give a satisfactory arterial PO_2. Fluid balance is important to ensure that the donor does not develop pulmonary edema. Appropriate cultures should be obtained by tracheal aspiration to treat early infection that may be developing in the recipient.

The method of heart-lung removal in the donor is similar to the dissection employed in the recipient. After median sternotomy, the entire pericardium is removed anteriorly, and the superior and inferior venae cavae as well as the ascending aorta are dissected free. The patient is then cannulated for cardiopulmonary bypass, and while on bypass, the patient's body temperature is cooled to between 10°C and 15°C. Ventilation is discontinued, and further dissection in the posterior mediastinum is carried out prior to removal of the graft. The heart alone undergoes selective cardioplegia followed by excision of the graft at the aorta, trachea, and both venae cavae. The heart-lung block is then ready for implantation.

THE OPERATION

The details of the operative procedure are briefly described below. The recipient is prepared in the same manner as for standard cardiac surgery and, through a median sternotomy incision, is placed on cardiopulmonary bypass. Both phrenic nerves are carefully dissected free on pedicles of pericardium as shown in Figure 5–2. The heart is excised, leaving a remnant of pulmonary artery adjacent to the aorta in the region of the recurrent laryngeal nerve. The left pulmonary artery and vein are divided in the hilus, and the bronchus of the left lung is stapled and cut, thereby allowing removal of the lung itself. The right lung is removed in the same way. At this time, all of the potential bleeding points in the posterior mediastinum are carefully controlled. The right and left bronchi are dissected back to the carina, and the trachea is divided one ring above the carina.

The graft is then inserted by performing a con-

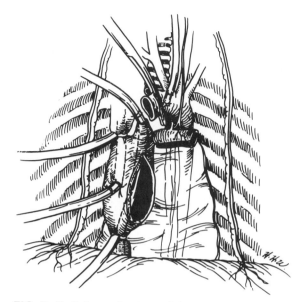

FIG. 5–2. *Schematic view of the empty thorax after heart and lung removal. Cardiopulmonary bypass is provided by cannulas positioned in the aorta and both venae cavae. The phrenic nerves are protected on pedicles of pericardium.*

tinuous anastomosis of the trachea with a monofilament suture. This is followed by an anastomosis of the right atrial cuff and a final anastomosis of the ascending aorta (Fig. 5–3). Air is aspirated from the heart and lung, and the aortic cross-clamp is removed, allowing resuscitation of the heart to occur. After satisfactory function has returned, bypass is discontinued and the chest is drained and closed routinely.

EARLY POSTOPERATIVE MANAGEMENT

In addition to standard postoperative cardiac-surgery care, special measures include pulmonary and immunosuppressive management. The recipient receives endotracheal suctioning when appropriate and is weaned from the ventilator according to standard protocols. When satisfac-

tory blood gases are obtained with good ventilatory mechanics, the patient is extubated. Close attention is given to fluid balance, and immunosuppressive drugs are started immediately. Typical drug regimens include cyclosporine, perioperative methylprednisolone, and azathioprine. The immunosuppressive regimen currently used at our institution is summarized in Table 5–1. Careful attention to cyclosporine serum levels and close monitoring of the white blood cell count are required. Perioperative antibiotics are continued for 48 hours and then are discontinued unless a specific pathogen has been identified in the donor tracheal cultures. Intense efforts in physical rehabilitation are begun, and the patient is mobilized as soon as possible.

Monitoring for allograft rejection includes frequent physical examination, chest roentgenogram, and endomyocardial biopsy. The transvenous endomyocardial biopsy is performed 1 week postoperatively and at weekly intervals for surveillance or for the follow-up of antirejection therapy. In general, the endomyocardial biopsy has been most useful for the detection of graft rejection. When a significant amount of infiltrate of mononuclear cells is identified together with myocyte necrosis, augmented immunosuppressive therapy is given. This usually consists of methylprednisolone (1 g intravenously) given daily for 3 days. Particularly severe rejection is also treated with rabbit anti–human thymocyte globulin. Rarely, allograft rejection may occur in the lung and may not be present simultaneously in the heart.[12] In this case, the endomyocardial biopsy is normal, but there is a significant amount of diffuse infiltrate in both lung fields. An open lung biopsy may be required to detect isolated pulmonary rejection, and it will show severe interstitial infiltrates of mononuclear cells and interstitial hemorrhage or edema. It is not associated with infected sputum, and it reverses readily with antirejection therapy.

In general, the heart-lung transplant recipient

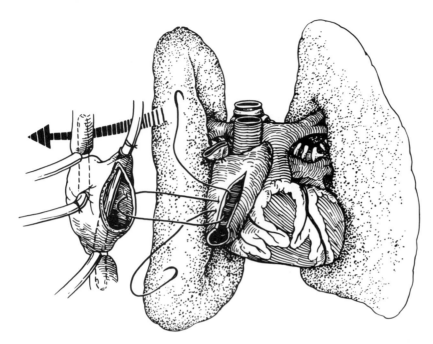

FIG. 5–3. The reanastomosis of the right atrium. The right lung lies in its normal anatomical position.

has the most severe rejection episodes within the first 3 months following transplantation, with gradual immune tolerance developing after that time. Rejection has not been particularly difficult to diagnose or treat, and maintenance immunosuppression can be gradually tapered to a fairly low and acceptable level (see Table 5–1).

In the first few weeks after lung transplantation, a picture consistent with an adult respiratory distress syndrome (ARDS) may develop. This is associated with poor pulmonary gas exchange and decreased lung compliance and has been termed the "reimplantation response."[13] Multiple factors may contribute to the development of ARDS, including ischemic injury at the time of transplantation, preexisting disease in the donor, operative trauma, denervation, and the interruption of pulmonary lymphatics. With improved preservation techniques, the incidence and severity of this complication have decreased markedly. When it occurs, the patient may require assisted ventilation, vigorous diuresis, and physiotherapy. Frequent pleural effusions may occur and are aspirated as necessary.

LATE MANAGEMENT

After hospital discharge, the patient is followed at weekly intervals. Transvenous endomyocardial biopsy is performed as an outpatient procedure at progressively increasing intervals: monthly for the first 6 months posttransplant and every 3 to 6 months thereafter. When the patient is stabilized on a chronic immunosuppressive drug regimen, he may return home if he lives outside the transplant center. Readmission is most frequently necessary for the treatment of rejection or infection.

A frequency posttransplant complication is nephrotoxicity associated with cyclosporine. Pa-

TABLE 5-1
IMMUNOSUPPRESSIVE DRUG THERAPY FOR HEART-LUNG TRANSPLANTATION

Drug	Dose	Frequency	Route	Comments
Early Postoperatively				
Cyclosporine	10 mg/kg	Daily	Oral	Serum levels between 100 ng–150 ng/ml
Solumedrol	125 mg/kg	q12h × 3	IV	Short perioperative course
Azathioprine	1 mg–2 mg/kg	Daily	Oral	White blood cell count >4000/mm³
Late Postoperatively (> 3 months)				
Cyclosporine	10 mg/kg	Daily	Oral	Serum levels between 50 ng–100 ng/ml
Azathioprine	1 mg–2 mg/kg	Daily	Oral	White blood cell count >4000/mm³
(+/−)Prednisone	0.2 mg/kg	Daily	Oral	Add only if a third agent is required to treat rejection

tients may develop hypertension or a rising creatinine level, which responds to decreasing the amount of cyclosporine administered. Serum levels are maintained at approximately 100 ng to 200 ng/ml in the early posttransplant period and between 50 ng and 100 ng/ml after several months of treatment. Other side-effects include a slight tremor and mild hirsutism. Abnormalities in hepatic enzymes occur infrequently and are also treated by decreasing the administered dose of cyclosporine.

RESULTS

Death in the early posttransplant period has usually been caused by multisystem failure. This may be initiated by a difficult operative procedure with excessive bleeding or by poor graft function. With preexistent severe liver enlargement and dysfunction, renal dysfunction, and severe weakness, the patient may have difficulty overcoming complications. However, the majority of patients do recover satisfactorily and are discharged after a hospital stay of 3 to 6 weeks.

Hospital mortality is approximately 20%, with 70% of patients alive at 1 year. The early functional results have been extremely gratifying. Patients who have been debilitated and chronically ill have returned to vigorous physical activity with rehabilitation similar to that of heart transplant patients.

For the most part, morbidity and mortality following combined heart-lung transplantation are similar to those after cardiac transplantation. The development of graft atherosclerosis, continued susceptibility to opportunistic infections, and other complications secondary to chronic corticosteroid administration have occurred in these patients. Because cyclosporine is continued indefinitely, late complications associated with this drug have also occurred. The most frequent of these are hypertension and declining renal function. Further tapering of immunosuppressive drugs is required long term, and attempts are made to keep the levels at the lowest tolerable amount.

Early pulmonary function tests are encouraging. There is commonly a decrease in most measured lung volumes, resulting in a moderately severe restrictive ventilatory defect. Arterial oxygen tensions are maintained in the normal range, and there is generally a progressive improvement in lung function for the first 1 or 2 years. Pulmonary function is consistent with an adequate functional state and with a sufficient capacity to sustain normal activities.[14]

Long-term problems with lung function have been reported. The most common are bronchitis and a mild to severe obstructive lung disease that is characterized histologically as bronchiolitis obliterans.[15] Although it is not proven, this bronchial disease may be a manifestation of chronic rejection occurring in the lung transplant, equivalent to the graft arteriosclerosis seen in heart transplants. In almost all cases, the development of bronchial disease has been simultaneous with the development of significant arterial disease in the heart. In a series of fourteen late survivors reported from Stanford, five developed some degree of bronchial disease after 2 years and one required retransplantation at 3 years. Measurement of the FEV_1 is a useful pulmonary function test for the early detection of this complication.

The late chest roentgenogram is usually normal (Fig. 5–4), unless significant bronchial disease has developed.[16] Serial right-sided heart catheterizations have shown normal pulmonary artery pressures and pulmonary vascular resistance.[17] Idiopathic pulmonary hypertension has not recurred in any patient to date.

SUMMARY

Despite limited experience, heart-lung transplantation has clearly been therapeutic for patients who were terminally ill with pulmonary vascular disease. Hemodynamics have returned to normal, and there is marked functional improvement. Allograft rejection has not been inordinately difficult to diagnose or treat, and the

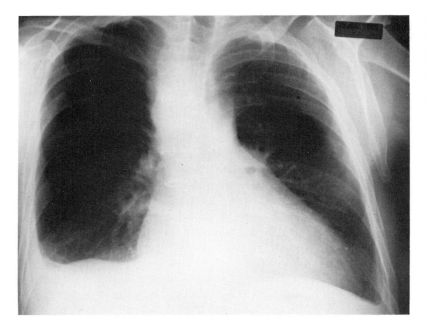

FIG. 5–4. Posttransplant chest roentgenogram of the patient shown in Figure 5–1, 2 months later. Note the right aortic arch, which presented no difficulties in the reimplantation of the trachea.

endomyocardial biopsy has been useful in this regard. Tracheal healing is satisfactory, and pulmonary infections have been manageable. With further experience, heart-lung transplantation may be extended to patients with other diffuse lung diseases. Such illnesses as emphysema, cystic fibrosis, and idiopathic pulmonary fibrosis might be treated.

The heart-lung transplant patient is unique because of cardiopulmonary denervation, and studies may provide useful physiologic information. Because there is little likelihood of a suitable mechanical replacement for the entire cardiopulmonary axis, this type of transplant will play a role in the treatment of patients with pulmonary vascular disease for many years to come. It is anticipated that results will continue to be equivalent to those presently being achieved for heart transplantation alone.

REFERENCES

1. Reitz BA, Wallwork JL, Hunt SA et al: Heart-lung transplantation: Successful therapy for patients with pulmonary vascular disease. N Engl J Med 306:557, 1982
2. Lower RR, Stofer RC, Hurley EJ, Shumway NE: Complete homograft replacement of the heart and both lungs. Surgery 50:842, 1961
3. Veith FJ: Lung transplantation. Surg Clin North Am 58:357, 1979
4. Reitz BA, Burton NA, Jamieson SW et al: Heart and lung transplantation, autotransplantation and allotransplantation in primates with extended survival. J Thorac Cardiovasc Surg 80:360, 1980
5. Pennock JL, Oyer PE, Reitz BA et al: Heart transplantation in perspective for the future: Survival, complications, rehabilitation and cost. J Thorac Cardiovasc Surg 83:168–177, 1982
6. Jamieson SW, Stinson EB, Oyer PE et al: Heart and lung transplantation for pulmonary hypertension. Am J Surg 147:740–742, June 1984
7. Haverich A, Scott WC, and Jamieson SW: Twenty years of lung preservation—A review. Heart Transplantation 4:234–240, 1985
8. Ladowski JS, Kapelanski DP, Teodori MF et al: Use of autoperfusion for distant procurement of heart-lung allograft preservation prior to heart-lung transplantation. Heart Transplantation 4:330–333, 1985
9. Robicsek F, Masters T, Duncan GD et al: An autoperfused heart-lung–preparation metabolism and function. Heart Transplantation 4:334–338, 1985
10. Stuart RS, Baumgartner WA, Borkon AM et al: Five-hour hypothermic lung preservation with oxygen free-radical scavengers. Transplant Proc 17:1454–1456, 1985
11. Breda MA, Hall TS, Stuart RS et al: Twenty-four hour lung preservation with hypothermia and leukocyte depletion. Heart Transplantation 4:325–329, 1985
12. Griffith B, Hardesty R, Trento A et al: Asynchronous heart and lung rejection following cardiopulmonary transplantation. Ann Thorac Surg (in press)
13. Siegelman SS, Sinha BB, Veith FJ: Pulmonary reimplantation response. Ann Surg 177:30–36, 1973
14. Theodore J, Jamieson SW, Burke CM et al: Physiologic aspects of human heart-lung transplantation: Pulmonary function status of the post-transplanted lung. Chest 86:349, 1984
15. Dawkins KD, Burke CM, Baldwin JC et al: Long-term complications of combined heart and lung transplantation. Circulation 70:II–690, 1984
16. Chiles C, Guthaner D, Jamieson SW et al: Heart-lung transplantation: The postoperative chest radiograph. Radiology 154:299–304
17. Dawkins KD, Hunt SA, Jamieson SW et al: Heart-lung transplantation for pulmonary vascular disease: Follow-up hemodynamic data (abstr). J Am Coll Cardiol 3:596, February 1984

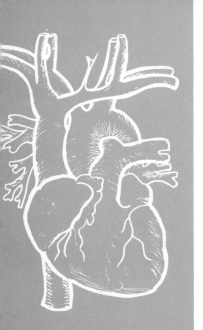

6

MITRAL VALVULOPLASTY

Robert W. M. Frater

Mitral commissurotomy was the first consistently successful operation for acquired valvular heart disease. As this operation was developed, it was soon clear that there were heavily diseased stenotic cases that were not suitable for commissurotomy and that there were cases of mitral insufficiency for which an entirely different approach was needed. Indeed, bold and imaginative surgeons were devising extraordinary procedures for attempting to correct mitral and aortic insufficiency. With the advent of cardiopulmonary bypass, progress to the development of effective artificial heart valves was rapid. However, it became apparent that, for the mitral valve at any rate, there remained a gap in the surgical armamentarium between the operation of commissurotomy for mitral stenosis, with the pathology confined to fusion of the cusps, and mitral valve replacement (with imperfect devices) for more extensive pathology and for cases of insufficiency.

The initial approach to filling the gap between simple commissurotomy and replacement was to add tissue.[1,2] Unfortunately, the tissue used, autogenous pericardium, proved unsuitable as a result of an excessive function-destroying healing process. The development of annuloplasty, which reduces the orifice to the dimensions of the existing cusp tissue rather than enlarges the cusps to cover a widened annulus, was a critical addition to the techniques for repair of mitral insufficiency.[3] Strenuous efforts were also made to increase the scope of mitral valve surgery for stenosis.[4] Despite all of this effort and even though artificial heart valves were admittedly imperfect, most cardiac surgeons continued to have at their disposal only two operations for mitral valve disease: commissurotomy for cases with pure cusp fusion and replacement for all the rest. Over the last 15 years, Alain Carpentier, an innovative French heart surgeon, has changed this by his persistent advocacy of new techniques for the extension of mitral valve repair.[5,6]

This chapter describes my efforts to widen the scope of valvular repair and to evaluate its worth as objectively as possible.

MITRAL VALVE ANATOMY AND FUNCTION

An absolute prerequisite for mitral valve repair is an understanding of the anatomy and function of the valve and the cardiac structures related to it.[7,8,9]

ANATOMY

The mitral valve is a continuous curtain of tissue attached to the subaortic curtain, and together with the left atrium and ventricle is connected to the atrioventricular membrane.

Cardiac Skeleton. The cardiac skeleton is a fibrous structure attached to the ostium of the left ventricle. A bar of fibrous tissue (the intervalvular trigone or the subaortic curtain) crosses the ostium and divides it unevenly into an inflow mitral portion and an outflow aortic portion. At the site of this division, the membrane is thickened into two distinct nodules, known as the left and right fibrous trigones. The three U-shaped cords of the aortic annulus are attached, at the base of the left coronary cusp, to the left fibrous trigone and, at the base of the right coronary cusp, to the right fibrous trigone. The depth of the intervalvular trigone is such that together with the trigones, it tilts the aortic orifice so that the plane of this orifice is always at an angle with the plane of the mitral orifice. From the right and left fibrous trigones, the atrioventricular membrane sweeps around the ventricular ostium posteriorly. Close to the trigones, it is ribbonlike. Posteriorly, it is more cordlike and may have very little depth. It serves to connect the left ventricular ostium to the left atrial wall and the mitral valve. The ventricle thus has a definable fibrous membrane separating it from the left ostium and mitral cusps. This is often seen as a cul-de-sac under the posterior cusp of the mitral valve in the right anterior oblique projection of a ventriculogram. Anteriorly, the mitral valve and left atrium are attached to each trigone and the subaortic curtain. Finally, the right fibrous trigone is the most substantial part of the skeleton connecting the mitral, aortic, and tricuspid parts of the skeleton. Behind it, the artery to the atrioventricular node is located quite close to the mitral part of the atrioventricular membrane. The node itself is located toward the tricuspid side of the artery, also behind the right fibrous trigone.

The location of the skeleton is commonly discernible as a fine indentation at the junction of the atrium and posterior cusp. The right fibrous trigone is deep to a dimple in the atrial wall adjacent to the anterior cusp about a centimeter in front and to the right of the medial commissure.

As a consequence of the attachment of the posterior cusp to the atrium and ventricle, two thirds of the mitral orifice is dynamic. The basis for this is the attachment of the ventricular and atrial

muscles and the posterior cusp of the mitral valve to the skeleton of the heart. The sphincteric action of the mitral orifice is crucial to both free diastolic flow and good apposition during systole. The average minimum systolic orifice area is 5.2 cm², and the average maximum diastolic area is 7.1 cm², thus giving a systolic area reduction of 26%.[10] The sphincter is sensitive to alterations in preload, afterload, and inotropy.[11-13]

The cusp tissue is scalloped so that its free-edge length is much greater than the circumference of the atrioventricular orifice. A large deep anterior cusp swings from the fibrous trigones to form a curved line of closure with the generally triscalloped posterior cusp. The free edge of the posterior cusp is longer than that of the semicircular anterior cusp, but in closure the scallops meet each other as well as the anterior cusp, producing the characteristic curved closure line and a closed orifice in which the anterior cusp is dominant. Thirty percent of the anterior cusp area is in contact with 50% of the posterior cusp during systole. The cusp tissue forms a continuous curtain around the orifice. Even at the commissure, it is at least 5 mm in depth and may be more than 10 mm.

There are three types of chordae tendineae:

Free-edge chordae originating from one side of a papillary muscle to the anterior cusp and from the other side to the posterior cusp

Appositional area chordae attached away from the free edge, a few of which may arise directly from the posterior ventricular wall. These chordae mark the division between the part of the cusp that is in contact with its opposite member during systole and that which is not. They have also been called strut chordae, rough-zone chordae, and second-order chordae.[14]

Commisural chordae, which differ from all

other chordae in that they fan out from a single origin on the papillary muscle to insert into *both* anterior and posterior cusps. These serve as the definitive marker of the commissures.

Casual observation of the chordae tendineae reveals great variability in length between the free-edge insertion and the papillary muscle origin. Despite this apparent variability, the chordae function to keep the free edges of opposing cusps at the same level relative to each other throughout systole and diastole. In doing so, they are always under some tension. In diastole, as the posterior ventricular wall lengthens and the papillary muscles move away from the atrioventricular ring, the chordae are kept taut and the cusps are pulled down. The papillary muscles also restrain the cusps so that the anterior cusp, in particular, is prevented from moving out to the septum. In systole, the free edges are always kept below the plane of the atrioventricular orifice.[7]

The papillary muscles are probably shock absorbers. They vary anatomically from flat and sessile to tall and protuberant and to having from one to several heads. The forces in the closed valve during systole can be calculated. In a two-dimensional model, the forces in the chordae are half those in the cusps. The greater the area of the cusps, the greater are the forces they experience.

Finally, the tissues of the mitral valve are thin and pliable. In the open heart, they assume a position entirely related to the effects of gravity.

MECHANISMS OF MITRAL INSUFFICIENCY

The mechanisms of mitral insufficiency are classified under the following headings: cusps, chordae, and mural annulus and ventricular wall (Fig. 6–1).

Cusps. Reduction in cusp area in the presence of a normal systolic annular area is a feature of rheumatic pathology. Characteristically, the posterior cusp loses its separation into identifiable separate scallops and becomes reduced in area. Shortening of the free edge of the anterior cusp may cause it to lose appositional area.

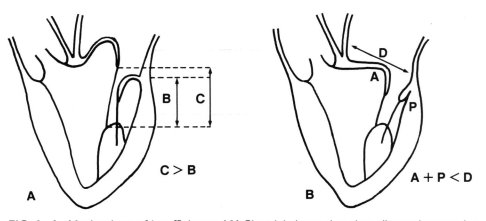

FIG. 6–1. Mechanisms of insufficiency. **(A)** Chordal elongation that allows the anterior cusp to rise above the atrioventricular plane. **(B)** Disproportion between systolic atrioventricular orifice area and the cusp area. This is due to either cusp shrinkage (as shown here) or failure of systolic ring contraction.

Cusp tears and perforations as a result of infection, jet lesions from infected aortic valves, and trauma are obvious additional causes of insufficiency. Irregularity and notching of the thickened free edges of rheumatic cusps can prevent good apposition and result in considerable insufficiency.

Chordae. Elongation of chordae, allowing the free edge of the cusps to fail to be consistently parallel to each other and, in particular, allowing one or more free edges to rise above the plane of the atrioventricular ring, must result in insufficiency.[7] Rupture of chordae obviously results in insufficiency and, in fact, if only one free-edge chorda is cut, there will be insufficiency at that point along the closure line.[15] It takes the rupture of one main chorda of the anterior cusp or the chordae to one half of one scallop of the posterior cusp to produce gross mitral incompetence. Shortening and thickening with loss of mobility of chordae may restrain a cusp of reasonable area so that it cannot rise to meet its opposite number. This can apply to both free-edge and appositional chordae. Today, degenerative pathology is the most common cause of elongated or ruptured chordae, but elongated anterior chordae are seen quite often with rheumatic disease. A particular deformation that is seen in some cases of both rheumatic and degenerative pathology is an alteration in the relationship between first- and second-order chordae of the anterior cusp. In this deformation, while the second-order chordae seem to be of reasonable length, the free-edge chordae appear to have elongated, allowing the edge to rise toward the plane of the atrioventricular orifice, thus changing the normal right-angle bend of the closed valve into one in which the free edge slips back toward the atrium, allowing insufficiency. Sometimes this is seen when both the free-edge chordae and the appositional chordae actually arise from the main chordae.

When considering the mitral valve prolapse syndrome, it is useful to distinguish between billowing of the valve, in which the body of the cusp rises above the plane of the ring but the edges are held below it, and prolapse, in which it is the edges that rise beyond this plane.

Mural Annulus and Ventricular Wall. If the mural annulus is dilated and, in particular, if it fails to shorten, the area of the orifice in systole may exceed that of cusps of normal area and insufficiency results. Dilatation of the mural annulus can occur during the acute stage of rheumatic fever and cause insufficiency. This may then persist after resolution of the rheumatic fever because the insufficiency itself causes the ventricular dilation to persist. If the free wall of the ventricle to which the papillary muscles are attached moves paradoxically in systole, tension on the chordae will pull the cusp edges apart. If the portion of the posterior ventricular wall between the atrioventricular junction and the papillary muscles is elongated enough, the movement of the chordal orifices away from the plane of the atrioventricular ring will pull the cusp edges apart. If the ring is dilated as this chordal pull takes place, the papillary muscle excursion needed to pull the cusp edges apart decreases. Permanent elongation of this portion of the posterior wall due to cardiomyopathy or previous infarction will result in this mechanism of insufficiency.

INTRAOPERATIVE EVALUATION: MITRAL INSUFFICIENCY

For the surgeon, inspection of the valve is through the atrium and, for proper evaluation of the mechanisms of insufficiency, must be done segment by segment. There are six valvular segments. The anterior cusp has two of them, anterolateral and posteromedial, defined by the origin of the chordae from one or other papillary muscle. On each side of the central bare area are main chordae leading to their respective papillary muscles. Between the commissure and the main chordae are the paramedial chordae. The posterior cusp has three scallops, but the central or middle scallop can also be divided, like the anterior cusp, into an anterolateral and a posteromedial half because of the fact that the chorda of each half lead to separate papillary muscles. For each of these segments, the evaluation proceeds as follows:

> *Cusps:* area; pliability (free edge, appositional, and nonappositional parts); restriction of mobility. The area of the cusps must be related to the dimension of the annulus.
> *Chordae:* length (short or long); integrity (intact or ruptured); consistency (thickened and immobile or normally thin and pliable). Gentle tension of the free edge of anterior and posterior cusps at points opposite each other will determine whether the crucial free-edge relationships have been altered and will determine whether the free edges rise above the plane of the atrioventricular ring.
> Gentleness is the key to this assessment, but in the paralyzed heart it also may be necessary to pass a suction catheter down to the apex of the heart and to hold it in place to prevent the ventricular muscle from being everted.
> *Annulus:* size relative to anterior cusp area is evaluated

MANEUVERS AVAILABLE FOR REPAIR OF MITRAL INSUFFICIENCY

The maneuvers used to repair mitral insufficiency are described below. Methods used to repair mitral insufficiency caused by cusp pathology include the following: (1) excision or exclusion, the former popularized by Carpentier for the treatment of ruptured chordae and the latter first introduced by McGoon for the same purpose; (2) cusp extension using additional material; and (3) cusp and chordal replacement, which was first used by us in the 1960s. Originally, we used autogenous pericardium for this and found it unsatisfactory, but more recently other materials have been used both experimentally and clinically.[1,2,6,7,16,17]

Methods used to repair mitral insufficiency caused by chordal pathology include the following: (1) chordal shortening, which was introduced by Carpentier; (2) chordal replacement, which was done experimentally very early in the history of open-heart surgery and which we used back in the 1960s and, subsequently, reintroduced more recently; (3) transposition of chordae; and (4) section of shrunken appositional chordae restricting posterior cusp mobility, popularized by Carpentier and his disciples (Fig. 6–2).[6,7,18,19]

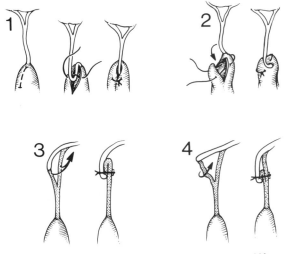

FIG. 6–2. Shortening of elongated chordae. **(1)** Carpentier technique for chordal shortening. **(2)** Duran method. **(3)** Cusp level shortening used in some rheumatic cases. **(4)** Disproportionate elongation of anterior cusp free-edge chordae and method of correction.

Finally, annuloplasty is the method used to reduce the size of the annulus to the size of the available cusps.[3,5,20] Whatever the method used, it is basically the mural muscular part of the mitral orifice that is being reduced either completely or partially.

Cusp Excision. The excision of cusps for chordal rupture works well for rupture of segments of the posterior cusps because usually there is an elongation of the mural annulus in these cases and its shortening is easy to do. By contrast, when the anterior cusp has ruptured chordae, it has been suggested that no more than one quarter or one sixth of this cusp should be excised and this in a triangular wedge. The point is that as soon as excision of the anterior cusp is practiced, the free edge is shortened. The crucial semicircular shape of the anterior cusp that is essential for proper apposition with the posterior cusp is thereby lost. Shortening of the mural annulus does not necessarily bring the posterior cusp to meet this shortened, straightened anterior cusp edge, and this is not compensated for by any attempts to shorten the distance between the trigones at the base of the anterior cusp, because not only will this *not* elongate the anterior free edge, it will also distort the aortic root and the aortic valve. For these reasons, I have abandoned anterior cusp excision. An alternative to cusp excision with anterior cusp chordal pathology is replacement of chordae.

Chordal Replacement. In our original experimental work years ago, we used autogenous pericardium for chordal replacement.[18] More recently, we have used tanned xenograft pericardium and have shown that it heals well to both papillary muscle and cusp, and, furthermore, during implantations of as long as 3 years in animals, it neither elongated nor shortened. Thus, whatever relationship of cusp edges we established at surgery would be preserved. Fibrous thickening and some calcification, particu-

larly at the healing ends, were seen, but this loss of chordal flexibility, especially in the setting of degenerative disease in which the rest of the chordae and cusps are normally pliant, did not affect competence.

The proper length of a new chorda is achieved as follows. After stitching the xenograft strip to the papillary muscle, the new chorda and the existing normal posterior cusp chordae opposite the point of anterior chordal rupture are put under slight tension. The level of the edge of the posterior cusp is then marked with a stitch on the new chorda, and this is used as the point of attachment to the free edge of the anterior cusp. The maintenance of the proper parallel relationship of anterior and posterior opposing points is thereby established, and competence is guaranteed. Instead of chordal replacement, posterior chordae can be transposed. When we used this years ago, we had a dilated annulus and a dilated orifice, and rather than reducing the annulus size, we added tissue.[7] Posterior-to-anterior chordal transposition has been effectively combined with annuloplasty by Carpentier and Lessana.

Chordal Shortening. Chordal shortening as practiced by Carpentier and Lessana and others involves the folding over and securing of an elongated chorda into a longitudinal trench cut in the papillary muscle (see Fig. 6–2).[6,19] A transverse incision with a folding over of the apex of the papillary muscle and its attached elongated chorda down into the bottom of this incision is used by Duran (see Fig. 6–2).[20] We have used both of these techniques and found both to work. We judge the degree of folding needed by first establishing the difference between the free edges with the chordae under gentle tension.

Another technique that we have used and have found particularly useful with somewhat thickened rheumatic chordae is to fold them up behind the free edge of the cusp to shorten them. This may be needed because a sessile papillary muscle does not allow shortening by other techniques. The differential elongation of free-edge chordae that we have already described may be overcome by suturing the cusp free edge down to the chorda (see Fig. 6–2).

Multiple chordal shortenings can be performed, but we have also used the insertion of multibranched new chordae to manage a long length of free-edge prolapse. Alternatively, we have used a strip of felt to turn over several paramedial anterior cusp chordae. Multiple mattress sutures through the papillary muscle base anchor the strip in place.

Annuloplasty. The goal of mitral annuloplasty is to fix the systolic dimension at a size that will be closed by the area of available cusp tissue. This can be done with relatively rigid (Carpentier) or more flexible (Duran) rings. However, the same effect is achieved by a mural shortening stitch crisscrossing through the atrioventricular junction, taking in 1 mm of cusps and 2 mm of atrium, starting at the left fibrous trigone and ending at the right, with the actual shortening being done with an obturator in the orifice. The size of the obturator is determined by the size of the anterior cusp. Although on occasion in rheumatic cases we have been forced to use less than a 25-mm diameter obturator, generally it should not be necessary to do this except in patients of small stature. A 25-mm obturator of my design, with one side partially cut off, has an area of 4 cm² while a No. 18 Hegar dilator has an area of 2.5 cm². By comparison, the geometric areas (which, of course, are always larger than the effective orifice areas) of 25-mm (mounting size) artificial mitral valves range from less than 2.5 to a little more than 3 cm². It is important to recognize, however, that when the systolic dimension is fixed by an annuloplasty, so also is the diastolic size. Note that an orifice of 4 cm² is only 56% of the normal average diastolic dimension. Some mitral obstruction is inevitably produced by fixing the annulus at a systolic dimension.

MECHANISMS OF MITRAL STENOSIS

Rheumatic pathology produces obstruction of flow in a number of ways (Fig. 6–3).

1. *Reduction of orifice at free-edge level.* In essentially all cases of rheumatic disease, the separate definition of the posterior cusp scallops is lost. This occurs even without fusion between the anterior and posterior cusps and is always evident after successful commissurotomy. In addition there appears to be, in some cases, a

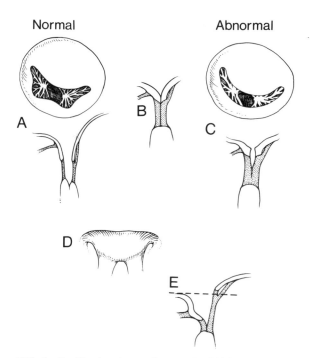

FIG. 6–3. Mechanisms of stenosis. **(A)** Normal valve. Posterior scallops are defined. Chordae and cusps are thin and pliable. **(B)** Cusps and chordae are thickened and stiffened and fused. **(C)** Separation of fused cusps and chordae does not restore the orifice to normal because of fusion of posterior scallops. **(D)** Anterior chordal fusion. **(E)** Posterior cusp restrained by third-order chorda. Elongation of anterior cusp chordae.

further shortening of the length of the free edge, as though a purse string suture running through it had been tightened (Fig. 6–3C).

2. *Cusp fusion.* This occurs between the chordally supported parts of the opposing cusps, leaving only the central bare areas open (Fig. 6–3B).

3. *Chordal fusion.* Chordal fusion occurs between anterior and posterior cusp chordae (Fig. 6–2B).

4. *Chordal shortening and thickening.* In patients with this pathology, cusp motion is inevitably restricted by both the reduced arc through which the chordae can move and by their inability to flex at their papillary muscle attachment.

5. *Cusp fibrosis and calcification producing loss of pliability.* Cusp fibrosis largely produces thickening of the appositional parts of the cusps. An anterior cusp afflicted in this way will hold its bowed systolic form against the influence of gravity (Fig. 6–4). Calcification occurs most prominently at the commissures. It may be on the cusps with a definable plane of dissection or within their substance.

6. *Fusion of adjacent anterior cusp chordae.* This type of fusion confines flow to the central space between the papillary muscles (Fig. 6–3D).

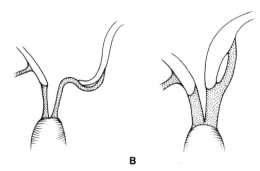

A   **B**

FIG. 6–4. *Cusp stiffness. **(A)** Gravity determines the position of the cusp. **(B)** Tissue stiffness causes the cusp to resist gravity.*

EXPERIMENTAL MODELS OF RHEUMATIC MITRAL OBSTRUCTION

Although reduction of the orifice is the obvious and easily understood mechanism of rheumatic mitral obstruction, other factors seem to play a role. In an animal model we have tried to isolate cusp stiffness, chordal stiffness, and anterior cusp chordal fusion as factors in mitral obstruction. In all of the animals a piece of curved felt was sutured to the posterior cusp to imitate the thickened, fibrosed (no longer scalloped) rheumatic posterior cusp. Curved, bow-shaped, rigid plastic inserts were attached behind the anterior cusp to make it rigid either from commissure to commissure or, more extensively, from ring to ring. Fused anterior cusp chordae were imitated by sheets of pericardium sutured, on each side, between the papillary muscles and the anterior cusp edge. Stiff chordae were reproduced by four plastic rods pushed into the papillary muscles in a closed position and sutured to the edges of the anterior cusps. Some mild obstruction was produced by all of these measures; most seemed to result when the anterior cusp was made stiff from ring to ring. One implication is that if the chordae were flexible and good hinge action remained at the periphery, central stiffening or bowing would not produce significant obstruction. This, of course, is a rare combination, but the corollary is that a mobile chordal–papillary complex and free hinging between the commissure and ring will compensate for central cusp thickening.

METHODS FOR RELIEF OF STENOSIS

Separation of Fusion. In the classic case of pure mitral stenosis with pliable cusps and unfused pliable chordae, separation of fused cusps is all that is needed (Fig. 6–5). But in cases with more extensive pathology, which might ordinarily be considered for replacement, the essential point is that pliable tissue must be reached so that despite

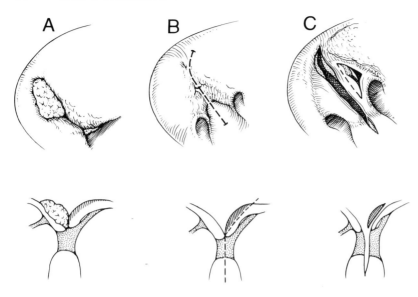

FIG. 6–5. Mitral valve plasty. **(A)** Interior commissure calcific nodule, cusp fusion, chordal fusion, cusp thickening, and chordal thickening and shortening. **(B)** Calcium removed. Incision is made between cusps, through fused chordae into papillary muscle. **(C)** Extension into thin cusp tissue and pliable muscle, fenestration of fused anterior chordae, and thinning of the cusp.

the degree of stiffness that remains in the anterior cusp, it will hang from good hinges and will be able to swing open and closed with minimal restriction. To achieve this, it is necessary to go beyond the fan chordae at each commissure and down into the papillary muscles. Thickened fan chordae can be split. If this is not possible, the cut extends out beyond the central branch. Thin pliable tissue is almost always reached by this maneuver. Similarly, the papillary muscles almost always remain muscular and, therefore, pliable, so that cutting them compensates for the stiffness and limited arc of short, thick chordae (Fig. 6–5B).

Decalcification and Thinning of Cusps and Chordae. Surface calcific nodules can frequently be removed by incising endothelium at the base of the nodule and finding a plane of dissection. The cusps are commonly remarkably pliable under such nodules. Calcification within the cusp, of course, is not treatable without cusp destruction. Fibrous thickening and, in particular, the buildup of scar within the appositional area can be shaved off until the cusps and chordae no longer maintain their form in resistance to gravity. A plane may be found between fibrous thickening and quite thin and pliable cusps (Fig. 6–5B).

Fenestration of Fused Anterior Chordae. Quadrangles of tissue approximately 2-mm wide are excised between the papillary muscle and the cusp edge, leaving chordae that are themselves 2-mm wide. If two such openings with an average length of 4 mm are made on each side, the potential gain in flow area would be 0.32 cm². This is, obviously, a modest return for a significant amount of quite delicate work, and unless the chordae and cusps were rendered pliable at the same time a benefit might not be realized (Fig. 6–5C).

MITRAL STENOSIS AND INSUFFICIENCY

I have discussed rheumatic mitral stenosis in isolation, but, of course, in many of the cases at issue in this presentation, namely those that might ordinarily be treated by replacement, there is a combination of stenosis and insufficiency. Treatment of the insufficiency involves shortening of chordae and/or adjusting the relative areas of the cusps and the systolic orifice. In the early days, we added tissue in the form of autogenous pericardium, but pliability was lost in the healing process. We have, of course, used tanned xenograft pericardium for chordal replacement. The fact that, particularly at the healing ends, it becomes thickened and stiff does not matter because the chordae are not required to bend to fulfill their function. However, because of this tendency to thicken at the healing margins, we have been more cautious about using it as a substitute for cusps. We have recently begun to use it cautiously as a material for cusp advancement or extension, particularly when it is possible to do so without intruding on a flexion area. For the most part, we continue to rely on mural annulus reduction or annuloplasty to achieve a proper systolic orifice to cusp area ratio. In the common absence of a dilated atrioventricular annulus in cases of combined stenosis and insufficiency, the latitude available to the surgeon for reducing the area of the systolic orifice is small. For this maneuver to be useful, there must be an anterior cusp with enough depth to form a semicircular line of closure in systole.

Modest improvements in systolic apposition may be achieved by maneuvers that improve cusp flexibility. Cutting posterior cusp appositional chordae has been disappointing in our experience.

Intraoperative Testing. The testing of insuficiency is a critical step in all cases. There are many ways of doing this. It is convenient to do the testing in the arrested heart, and if, after forceable injection of fluid into the ventricular cavity (either through the orifice, the ventricular apex, or the aorta and aortic valve), the valve is competent with no more than small, very circumscribed jets of insufficiency, then that valve will be competent when the heart is beating. Any testing system must avoid the risk of pumping air into the coronary arteries, and there must be a way of clearing air from the ascending aorta and the ventricular cavity before applying pressure to the ventricular cavity. After removing the patient from bypass, it is essential to measure transvalvular pressures and cardiac outputs not only for the demonstration of the relief of insufficiency, but also for the avoidance of excessive obstruction. If cardiac output is very low, it may, in fact, be difficult to judge the degree of obstruction, and this emphasizes even more the importance of good myocardial protection to be able to evaluate the valvuloplasties effectively. If the result is not satisfactory, then it is appropriate to go back on bypass and either correct the problem or replace the valve. Two-dimensional echocardiography is of great value both in the operating room and postoperatively, again to define the state of anatomy after correction, to measure the orifice and the degree of residual insufficiency. In our early experience, we used M-mode echocardiography with saline injection into the left ventricular cavity as a test of residual insufficiency. Although this is of some value, two-dimensional studies certainly show more and can help to define inadequacies such as residual prolapse. The major contribution of postbypass intraoperative imaging techniques is to clarify the status of the valve when pressure injection of fluid into the ventricle has yielded an equivocal result. Sometimes distortion of the skeletal framework is necessary to achieve enough visibility to see the entire valve. The injection test may then show significant regurgitation. Contrast echocardiography with the beating, undistorted heart may then be most valuable either to confirm success or to determine the need for immediate resumption of bypass and further valve surgery.

These initial evaluations, whether intra- or postoperative, are of great importance to the later assessment of the course of the patient. Baseline observations make subsequent observations all the more valuable.

Without these measurements, no quality control of the surgeon's performance is possible. Such quality control is an essential part of this branch of cardiac surgery. Nothing less than this is acceptable for evaluation of the immediate mechanical results of the operations. Comparison with the preoperative observations, and the intraoperative descriptions of pathology and the maneuvers used to correct them, will then allow the establishment of the limits and potential benefits of reparative surgery in that surgeon's hands.

Clinical Material and Results. For this discussion, patients with pure mitral stenosis requiring no more than cusp separation for the relief of obstruction are excluded. During the last 12 years, I have operated on 483 diseased mitral valves. A small number of patients with aortic valve disease and secondary dilatation of the atrioventricular orifice in whom a mitral annuloplasty was performed together with aortic valve replacement have been excluded. Also excluded are patients with congenital atrioventricular defects who underwent primary mitral and tricuspid repairs. Included are patients who received coronary artery bypass grafts, patients operated on as emergencies, all patients with class-IV disability, patients who had tricuspid valve surgery, patients with aortic valve disease who had primary pathology of the mitral valve, patients with previous mitral valve surgery, and finally, patients with gross mitral insufficiency *following* atrioventricular defect repairs.

Over the last 12 years, since restarting an active program of mitral valve repair, I have performed 242 conservative mitral valve operations for primary mitral valve disease. Eight-eight of these patients had simple commissurotomies and are by the definition already given excluded from analysis. Thus there were 155 patients who had

repair who might quite reasonably have had their valve replaced.

Of these 155 patients, 65 had dominant insufficiency. A majority of this group had degenerative disease, but a substantial minority had rheumatic pathology as defined by a history of rheumatic fever, thickened cusp tissue, loss of posterior scallop definition, and thickened, elongated chordae. In this group there were seven miscellaneous patients: two with prolapse of medial commissural tissue accompanying ostium secundum defects, three with gross mitral insufficiency after repair of atrioventricular defects, and two with healed endocarditis with cusp defects. The patients' ages ranged from 5 months to 81 years with a mean of 57 years.

Ninety patients had rheumatic disease with stenosis or stenosis and insufficiency. The patients' ages ranged from 15 years to 78 years with a mean of 58 years.

Of the 155 patients, 52 were symptomatically in class IV, 96 in class III, and 7 in class II of the New York Medical Association (NYMA) classification. Coronary artery surgery was performed in 25 patients, tricuspid valve surgery in 24, and aortic valve surgery in 18. Twenty-five patients had had previous cardiac surgery.

Mortality. Thirty-day hospital mortality for the 88 commissurotomy patients was zero. There were six such deaths among the 155 patients undergoing repair, an incidence of 3.9%. Three of these deaths were neurologic. They occurred in the first half of the study period and probably would be less likely to occur today with the development of improved techniques of detecting and eliminating retained intracardiac air. Two patients with significant coronary artery disease and mitral insufficiency with flail anterior cusps died with evidence of perioperative myocardial infarction. One patient died after reattachment of a papillary muscle and placement of four coronary bypass grafts. He developed a severe bleeding disorder in the early period and was reoperated on three times for this. At some point in the course, a severe myocardial infarction developed. The other patient with the flail mitral cusp was treated by triangular cusp excision and two coronary bypass grafts. She sustained a perioperative myocardial infarction and died several days later from progressive myocardial failure. It is not certain whether these patients would have fared better with valve replacement. Finally, one patient died of progressive right-sided heart failure due to complete failure of resolution of systemic levels of pulmonary hypertension, despite a satisfactory valve repair. Thus the hospital mortality for the 155 patients with valve repair was 3.9%.

Hemodynamic Performance. Intraoperative hemodynamic measurements were made in 76 patients, and two-dimensional Doppler echocardiographic examinations were made in 64, with some patients getting one or the other of the examinations, rather than both. Obstruction to forward flow has been expressed as an effective orifice area obtained from intraoperative hemodynamic measurements, as a planimetric orifice measurement in the echocardiographic short-axis view of the open mitral valve, and as a measurement obtained by halftime continuous-wave Doppler methods. Correction of mitral insufficiency is judged by the presence and size of a V wave in the simultaneously obtained left atrial and ventricular pressures, by intraoperative contrast echocardiography, by echocardiographic observation of changes in cusp motion and Doppler-detectable insufficiency, by echocardiographic observation of the changes in left atrial and ventricular systolic and diastolic dimensions that occur with correction of mitral insufficiency and, of course, by auscultation. Clinically "good" results are judged in the conventional manner by improvement in exercise capacity and by auscultatory evidence of the presence or absence of stenosis and insufficiency.

Thirty-three stenosis and stenosis and insufficiency patients with transvalvular flows of more than 100 ml/second had an average effective orifice area of 1.8 cm² (1.3 cm² to 2.1 cm²), while thirty-four pure insufficiency patients had an average effective orifice area of 2.8 cm².

Among patients with flows of more than 100 ml/second, there were five in which different sets of cardiac outputs were obtained with markedly different rates of transvalvular flow. In every case, at the higher flows, the orifice areas were proportionally higher than they were at lower flows. The early two-dimensional echocardiographic data also show a marked difference between 35 patients with stenosis and insufficiency and 25 with pure insufficiency with average values of 1.8 cm² and 3 cm², respectively.

In seeking an explanation for the difference between stenosis and insufficiency patients and the failure to achieve normal hemodynamic function, there are several possibilities to discuss. These include the orifice size at the free-edge level, the orifice size at the atrioventricular level, and the degree of stiffness of the valve tissues.

There is no doubt that the pathology of rheumatic disease produces a shortening of the free edge. At the completion of a simple commissurotomy in which the chordae are normal and the cusps only somewhat thickened, it is always evident that the size of the orifice at the free-edge level is less than that at the ring. The implication of this is that the benefit to forward flow provided by diastolic dilatation of the ring is lost and that there will be some measurable reduction of the orifice. For the rheumatic stenotic cases under discussion, invariably there are changes in the consistency of cusps and chordae in addition to fusion, so that whatever the size of the orifice obtained by separation of fused structures, there is the potential for a significant extra interference with flow as a result of stiffness of the tissues.

In Table 6–1, the effective orifice areas obtained by hemodynamic measurements in 12 patients are compared with the size of the orifice

TABLE 6-1
SIZE OF HOLE AT FREE-EDGE LEVEL

Obturator Size		Hemodynamic Area (cm²)	No. of Patients
Diameter (mm)	Area (cm²)		
18	2.54	1.76	5
22	3.8	1.35	1
23	4.1	1.62	2
25	4.9	1.6	2
2 (fingers)	4.0	1.54	2

measured by an obturator at the free-edge level at surgery. The hemodynamic area is invariably less than the area measured by the obturator, and the areas in general do not correlate well with the varying areas of the different-sized obturators. The explanation for this must be related to cusp and chordal stiffness.

Fixing the diastolic dimension at an end systolic size by annuloplasty also produces some orifice obstruction. A 25-mm obturator (area 4 cm²) was used to control the size of annulus reduction in 4 patients with stenosis and in 13 with insufficiency. All had effective orifice areas less than 4 cm², presumably related to fixing the diastolic atrioventricular size at less than normal systolic level, but whereas the average area for the stenosis cases was 1.6 cm², the average for the insufficiency cases was 3 cm². Tissue stiffness presumably accounts for this difference.

Alternatively, when only stenosis cases were examined, eight patients who had annuloplasty in addition to other procedures had a mean effective orifice area of 1.46 cm², while 27 without had a mean area of 1.9 cm², suggesting that the addition of annuloplasty in cases of stenosis produced an additional measure of obstruction.

THROMBOEMBOLISM AND DURABILITY

Comparison of Valve Repair with Valve Replacement. Since all of the cases considered would, in some surgeons' hands, have been re-placed, it is appropriate to compare the results of valve repair with those of valve replacement.

For comparisons between valve repair and replacement to be valid, we contend that the cases must be contemporaneous and from the same institution; that all patients must be followed at least annually by direct contact; and that during this contact, all patients must receive the same detailed questionnaire designed to assess their symptomatic status and to determine, as precisely as possible the occurrence of transient ischemic attacks and other embolic episodes. This questionnaire has been published before.[21] Major embolic episodes are defined as strokes, especially those that leave residua, or produce symptoms for at least 5 days. Minor episodes are characteristically episodic; they should be clearly defined and, of course, transient. There are obvious difficulties in these definitions: patients with migraine equivalents, Meniere's syndrome, and previous strokes are commonly quite difficult to analyze. We have chosen to regard scintillation scotomata as evidence of emboli, but there are many patients in whom events occur that we classify as "possible." In this discussion we shall exclude the "possible" episodes from analysis and look only at those with major and minor episodes. Because we are taking cohorts of patients followed 8 to 10 years, we have only 39 of the valvuloplasty patients to be compared with 29 patients with Starr ball valve replacements and 59 with bioprosthetic replacements. The percentage of patients with atrial fibrillation is the same for all three groups: 90% of the mechanical valve recipients, 47% of the bioprosthetic recipients, but only 21% of those who had valvuloplasties were anticoagulated. At 8 years, 52% of the mechanical valve recipients, 75% of those with bioprostheses, and 89% of those with plasties were free of emboli. These differences were significant. Further examination of the data shows that Coumadin has no effect on the incidence of emboli in the valvuloplasty cases. Whereas the bioprosthetic patients have a significant incidence of reoperation accelerating from the sixth year, the valvuloplasty and mechanical valve cases have a very low incidence of reoperation. Patient survival, however, is lowest for the mechanical prostheses and is best for the valvuloplasties.

Current Practice. The comparative data presented above refer to cohorts of patients from 1975, 1976, and 1977. There is no doubt that there has been an evolution in practice, particularly in the aggressiveness with which repair is pursued. The last 100 cases of primary mitral valve surgery other than commissurotomy give a better idea of practice in the 1980s.

Of the first 50 patients, 29 had repair and 21 had valve replacement. During this time, another 8 patients had prosthetic valve re-replacements. No repair patients died, but three came to reoperation, all within 2 years of surgery. In two of these, organic tricuspid disease was the major problem, but their valve repairs were imperfect because of tissue stiffness. In the remaining patient with coronary disease and cardiomyopathic ventricle, triple anterior chordal shortening held but the annuloplasty stitch tore out. This was the only incidence of suture dehiscence in 50 cases.

Of the next 50 patients, there were 39 who had repairs and 11 who had replacements. Two of the latter had an initial attempt at repair that was judged unsuccessful in the operating room. An-

other 17 had prosthetic valve re-replacements. One repair patient died, and two subsequently came to valve replacement within 1 year of the previous surgery. One of these had multiple shortenings of thickened rheumatic chordae with some apparent distortion of the anterior cusp. The other patient had multiple coronary bypass grafts in the past and had a myopathic ventricle. At the second operation, rheumatic mitral insufficiency of the classic sort was found and treated by annuloplasty. Intermittent cardiac failure accompanied by mitral insufficiency recurred postoperatively. At reoperation the mechanism for insufficiency was not clear. Replacement by a mechanical valve has been accompanied by continued episodes of pulmonary congestion. There have been no late deaths in any of the repair patients.

DISCUSSION AND CONCLUSIONS

The subject of repair can be discussed under several headings: techniques, causes of failure, comparison with replacement, and learning.

TECHNIQUES

Annuloplasty fixes the diastolic dimension at a less than normal systolic size; it must thereby produce some stenosis. It would seem inappropriate to use it in every case. By itself, it is seldom the answer for insufficiency. Suture annuloplasty is effective, easy, and apparently durable. The increased use of cusp enlargement by appropriate material would lessen the need for annuloplasty and would result in valves with larger orifice areas.

Chordal replacement is an excellent answer for anterior chordal rupture. *Chordal shortening* at cusp level is an appropriate alternative to papillary infolding techniques. *Calcium and fibrous tissue removal* can be done with remarkable early benefit but inevitably leaves a question of recurrence.

CAUSES OF FAILURE

Art continues to dominate science in mitral valve repair and therefore the causes of failure remain anecdotal. Underestimated tissue stiffness and unrecognized chordal elongation are problems in rheumatic cases. Right ventricular dysfunction, with or without organic tricuspid disease, produces residual disability in the presence of a less than perfect mitral result.

The ischemic cardiomyopathic ventricle may cause repair of organic mitral pathology to fail, perhaps as a result of incoordinate ventricular contraction.

COMPARISON WITH REPLACEMENT

The data presented here are borne out by Perier's comparison of valve repair patients with those having various forms of valve replacement. The patients with repaired valves live longer, have fewer complications, and have no more reoperations than those with valve replacements.[22]

LEARNING

Learning to perform mitral valve repair presents many difficulties. The first of these is that it is much easier and demands less from the surgeon to take a competent and mildly stenotic valve from a shelf than to create one from diseased tissue at the operating table. Failure of an artificial device can be laid at the manufacturer's door. Failure of a repair will be seen as a failure of either surgical technique or surgical judgment. Secondly, the surgeon practicing in a modern industrial state, embarking on the task of learning mitral valve repair, is faced with the obvious problems that learning is directly linked to experience, that the volume of mitral valve surgery is generally too low to provide optimal experience, and that failures along the way are likely to cause voluntary or involuntary termination of the venture.

Modern cardioplegic protection is helpful; it allows the surgeon to safely spend time on a repair, to decide that it has failed, and to proceed to valve replacement. Combining methodical evaluation of pathology, meticulous intraoperative testing and rigorous recording and follow-up can make it possible for surgeons with quite modest volumes to learn valve repair and, in so doing, provide their patients with significant benefit.

REFERENCES

1. Frater RWM, Berghuis J, Brown AL, Ellis FH, Jr: Autogenous pericardium for posterior mitral leaflet replacement. Surgery 84:260, 1963
2. Bailey CP, Zimmerman J, Merose T, Folk FS: Reconstruction of the mitral valve with autologous tissue. Ann Thorac Surg 9:103, 1970
3. Wooler GH, Nixon GPF, Grimshaw VA, Watson DA: Experience with repair of the mitral valve in mitral incompetence. Thorax 17:49, 1962
4. Bailey CP, Zimmerman J, Likott W: The complete relief of mitral stenosis: Ten years in progress toward this goal. Dis Chest 37:1, 1960
5. Carpentier A: La valvuloplastie reconstitutive. Une nouvelle technique de valvuloplastie mitrale. Presse Med 77:251, 1969
6. Carpentier A: Cardiac valve surgery—the "French Correction." J Thorac Cardiovasc Surg 86:323, 1983
7. Frater RWM: Anatomical rules for the plastic repair of the mitral valve. Thorax 19:458, 1964
8. Frater RWM: Functional anatomy of the mitral valve. In Ionescu M, Cohn L (eds): Mitral Valve Disease. Diagnosis and Treatment, p 127. London, Butterworths, 1985
9. McAlpine WA: Heart and Coronary Arteries. Berlin, Springer-Verlag, 1975
10. Ormiston JA, Shah PM, Tei C, Wong M: Size and motion of the mitral annulus in man. Circulation 64:113, 1981
11. Yellin EL, Yoran C, Sonnenblick EH et al: Dynamic changes in the canine mitral regurgitant orifice during ventricular ejection. Circ Res 45:667, 1979
12. Yoran C, Yellin EL, Becker RM et al: Mechanism for reduction of mitral regurgitation with vasodilator therapy. Am J Cardiol 43:773, 1979

13. Yoran C, Yellin EL, Becker RM et al: Dynamic aspects of mitral regurgitation: Effects of ventricular volume, pressure and contractility on the effective regurgitant area. Circulation 60:170, 1979

14. Lam JHC, Ranganathan W, Wigle ED, Silver MD: Morphology of the human mitral valve: J Chordae Tendineae: A new classification. Circulation 41:449, 1970

15. Frater RWM, Ellis FH: The anatomy of the canine mitral valve: With notes on function and comparisons with other mammalian mitral valves. J Surg Res 1:171, 1961

16. McGoon DC: Repair of mitral insufficiency due to ruptured chordae tendineae. J Thorac Cardiovasc Surg 39:357, 1960

17. Van der Spuy JC, Meintjies FA, Human G: The surgical approach to the mitral valve and the technique of correcting insufficiency of the anterior and of the posterior cusp with pericardium. S Afr Med J 38:554, 1964

18. Frater RWM, Gabbay S, Shore D et al: Reproducible replacement of elongated or ruptured mitral valve chordae. Ann Thorac Surg 35:14, 1983

19. Lessana A, Herreman F, Boffety C et al: Hemodynamic and cineangiographic study before and after mitral valvuloplasty. Circulation II(64):195, 1981

20. Duran CMG, Ubago JL: Clinical and hemodynamic performance of a totally flexible prosthetic ring for atrioventricular reconstruction. Ann Thorac Surg 22:458, 1976

21. Becker RM, Sandor L, Tindel M, Frater RWM: Medium-term follow-up of Ionescu–Shiley heterograft valve. Ann Thorac Surg 32(2):120–126, 1981

22. Perier P, Deloche A, Chauvaud S et al: Comparative evaluation of mitral valve repair and replacement with Starr, Björk, and porcine valve prostheses. Circulation 70(I):187, 1984

7

EVALUATION OF NEWER HEART VALVE PROSTHESES

Alexander S. Geha

Anatomic intracardiac replacement of diseased cardiac valves with valvular prostheses became a successful reality shortly after the development of open intracardiac surgery in the 1950s. The earlier replacements of diseased heart valves were characterized by attempts to duplicate the design of the human cardiac valves, using a variety of prosthetic textile material to construct leaflets and cusps for this purpose. It did not take long, however, to realize that these prosthetic materials fashioned in the form of valvular leaflets and cusps did not have the structural characteristics of the human valvular tissue and therefore were doomed to structural failure within a relatively short period. Since then, numerous prosthetic valvular designs have been developed and applied, spanning a wide spectrum from totally mechanical prostheses, with no resemblance to the normal human anatomy, to biologic valvular prostheses using valvular allografts. These heterografts or bioprostheses are constructed from other biologic tissue. By establishing the practicality of the surgical approach to intracardiac valves under direct vision, the advent of reliable methods of cardiopulmonary bypass and the improvement in the methods of myocardial protection during intracardiac surgery have resulted in an overwhelmingly high early operative survival following cardiac valvular replacement.

Although the availability of several excellent valvular prostheses offers a variety of options almost beyond our hopes just over a decade ago, and despite the tremendous early success following operation, all available cardiac valve substitutes, either mechanical or tissue valves, have limitations. Therefore, it remains true that when one replaces a dysfunctional cardiac valve, he is trading one disease for another, because the ideal replacement does not yet exist.[1]

The search for the ideal cardiac valve substitute, therefore, continues. The cardiovascular professional community, and in particular the cardiac surgical community, is continuously bombarded by the prosthetic valve industry with models of newer heart valve prostheses claiming newer designs, modifications of previous designs, improvements in well-tested previous valves, and numerous other advances in search of the ideal prosthetic valve. With more stringent regulations being imposed before approval is granted for the unrestricted use of new valvular designs, the cardiac surgeon is frequently asked to participate in the evaluation of newer heart valve prostheses.

This chaper reviews the requirements and characteristics of the ideal prosthetic valve and examines the methods of evaluation of how such newer heart valve prostheses meet the requirements of the ideal prosthetic valve.

CHARACTERISTICS OF THE IDEAL PROSTHETIC VALVE

There are six characteristics of a good substitute prosthetic cardiac valve[2]:

> It should have good hemodynamic characteristics, thus being nonobstructive and completely competent.

It should be nonthrombogenic.

It should have infinite durability and structural performance.

It should not significantly alter blood components.

It should be amenable to easy implantation without undue technical difficulties.

It should not be an annoyance to the patient.

The evaluation of each of these characteristics may be relatively easy and attainable within a short period, or it may be extremely complex, requiring many years of testing and trial before reaching the exact answer.

HEMODYNAMIC CHARACTERISTICS

Two approaches are used in this evaluation, and usually both are required in the evaluation of a newer prosthesis. These approaches are *in vitro* testing of the valve and *in vivo* testing of the hemodynamic characteristics.

In Vitro **Testing of the Valve.** These studies include a bioengineering evaluation of the design of the valve; its theoretical blood compatibility; its strength, fatigue failure, and wear resistance; its mechanics; and its hydrodynamics. These studies usually are carried out by mechanical engineers and bioengineers, often with input from surgeons, who function as consultants to the project. This evaluation requires the use of a number of approaches, including stress and strain testing, testing of the opening and closure mechanism of the valve, and accelerated life-cycle testing and high-pressure failure-mode testing. Accelerated life-cycle testing usually is conducted using a tuned oscillating test apparatus at rates up to 1500 bpm and a transvalvular pressure of approximately 200 mm Hg. This allows some extrapolation regarding the durability of the valve design. High-pressure failure-mode testing usually is conducted in a test apparatus that cycles valves at a physiologic rate and at an increasing closure pressure to determine the

pressure required to disrupt the valve or to damage it structurally.

The hydrodynamics of the valve are tested *in vitro* in mock circulatory systems using steady-state flow and pulsatile flow with flow visualization studies. Transvalvular pressure drop, regurgitation on closure, and leakage during closure should be determined over a broad range of physiologic conditions of pulse rate and cardiac output. The percentage of ventricular energy loss can be computed, combining the factors of pressure drop, regurgitant fraction, and leakage fraction, to provide a single measurement that represents the overall hemodynamic efficiency of a cardiac valve; lower values of ventricular energy loss correspond to a more efficient cardiac valve.

In Vivo **Hemodynamic Evaluation.** Having been satisfied with the *in vitro* hemodynamic characteristic of the valve, as well as its structural and mechanical performance and its projected durability, one is ready to begin *in vivo* testing. Again, this could be carried out in animals, but ultimately, the answer will have to come from human clinical trials. A rigorous protocol by an internal review group in the surgeon's institution, including a detailed patient consent form, is mandatory to ensure the patient's protection, cooperation, and understanding. The hemodynamic information is similar to that described above for *in vitro* testing and, as of this writing, still requires postoperative catheterization at intervals and pressure and flow determinations over a broad range of physiologic conditions of pulse rate and cardiac output. Controlled intraoperative hemodynamic readings and perioperative echo-Doppler flow studies are other means to obtain important *in vivo* information.

The hemodynamic data obtained from the clinical human trial, along with the data about other characteristics of the valve that are concomitantly and simultaneously accumulated during this phase, form the backdrop for acceptance of the valve and its release for clinical use.

THROMBOGENICITY

Any valvular prosthesis is a foreign body implanted within the circulatory system and is continuously exposed to a blood–prosthetic interface. Thrombogenicity, therefore, can be very variable, depending on the characteristics of the prosthetic component of this interface. When biologic tissue is used for the valvular prosthesis, this thrombogenicity tends to be quite low. Nevertheless, it can still exist and precipitate thrombus formation on the prosthesis. Thrombogenicity is much more prominent when totally prosthetic material is used, and it can change substantially with various types of mechanical prosthetic material. Metal and metal alloys are usually more thrombus prone than is pyrolytic carbon. However, although pyrolytic carbon was introduced and touted as a nonthrombogenic surface, this has not been true, and thrombogenicity remains a characteristic of all nonbiologic prostheses.

Animal models are notoriously poor in evaluating thrombogenicity because the thrombotic characteristics of the blood component of the blood–prosthesis interface is quite different from those of humans. In evaluating the thrombogenicity of a valve, the picture is further complicated by the patient's own cardiac disease and cardiac arrhythmias, which may lead to thromboembolic complications arising from thrombus formation within the cardiac chambers themselves rather than on the valvular prosthesis. Thus, thrombogenicity and thromboembolic manifestations accompanying a prosthetic valve are extremely difficult to evaluate. Nevertheless, a higher rate of thromboembolic complications associated with any valve being tried certainly indicates this valve's propensity for thrombogenicity. When other characteristics of the valve are overwhelmingly attractive, one can resort to altering the blood component of the blood–prosthesis interface by the administration of anticoagulant medications. Such alterations can take the form of interference with the platelet function or with the mechanism of clotting itself by the use of Dicumarol and its derivatives. One should keep in mind, however, that anticoagulant-related hemorrhage is a significant complication of the administration of anticoagulant agents and should be incorporated into the evaluation of a newer prosthetic heart valve from the point of view of thrombogenicity.

STRUCTURAL FAILURE

Although *in vitro* testing can give us a good idea about the durability of the valve and its propensity for structural failure, such testing can never replace human clinical trials and tests. The composition of the *in vitro* bath varies from that of blood. Furthermore, the composition of blood varies among patients, as was well illustrated in the cases of bioprosthetic valves in children and in patients undergoing hemodialysis for chronic renal falure.[3–6] Durability may take many years to evaluate accurately, and several aspects of it should be examined and kept in mind. A propensity to develop periprosthetic valvular leaks should always be kept in mind, and such events should be analyzed to determine whether they relate to the patient's tissue or to the prosthesis itself. Blatant mechanical or structural failure of the valve itself is easily appreciated, but subtle changes and wear may be much more difficult to detect. Nevertheless, they can eventually lead to diastrous and fatal developments, and methods to detect them are required to attract attention to the need for elective replacement in such instances and to obviate unnecessary catastrophes. It behooves the prosthetic valve industry to analyze every instance of structural or tissue failure of one of their prostheses and to be forthright and open about such complications.

Durability probably remains the most difficult characteristic to evaluate and answer accurately.

It takes many years of clinical trial and testing before one realizes some of the subtle changes in durability and performance. A recent analysis of all surviving patients between 18 and 88 years of age receiving biologic or mechanical valves at our institution from January 1974 through January 1985 has been carried out with a complete follow-up.[7] Factors analyzed included thromboembolism, anticoagulation-related hemorrhage, endocarditis, perivalvular leak, valve failure, need for reoperation, and late cardiac death. The occurrence rates of these events were analyzed in linear ([%/patient-year]) and actuarial terms over the 11-year period. Six hundred six biologic valves (328 aortic, 252 mitral, 24 tricuspid, 2 pulmonary, consisting of 482 Carpentier–Edwards valves, 108 Hancock valves, 15 Ionescu–Shiley valves, and 1 fascia lata valve) and 510 mechanical valves (330 aortic, 175 mitral, 5 tricuspid, consisting of 178 Starr–Edwards valves, 164 Bjork–Shiley valves, and 166 St. Jude Medical valves, 1 Kay–Shiley valve, and 1 Smelloff–Cutter valve) were inserted. The data are summarized in Table 7–1.

This analysis provides some interesting insights into the performance of these valves, which have been in use for a range of many years. Such a review illustrates the need for long-term evaluation of valvular prostheses, with careful documentation and complete follow-up being absolutely mandatory. Such documentation is time-consuming and expensive but absolutely essential to reach meaningful conclusions about durability and long-term functioning of prosthetic cardiac valves. Computerization of patient records simplifies this task somewhat. It is extremely important for various centers to analyze their experience and to report it in a standardized fashion so that these important issues related to the performance of cardiac valvular prostheses can be addressed.

ALTERATION OF BLOOD COMPONENTS

Hemolysis due to red cell fragmentation is a recognized complication of prosthetic heart valve implantation. Improvement in valve material and perfection of valve design facilitate smooth hemodynamics and have lessened the trauma to red cells. Nevertheless, hemolysis continues to characterize prosthetic valves, particularly the mechanical prostheses. In addition, platelets

TABLE 7–1
OCCURRENCE RATES OF BIOLOGIC AND MECHANICAL VALVE COMPLICATIONS

Event	Biologic Valves (N = 606)		Mechanical Valves (N = 510)	
	λ/Patient-year (%)	% Free*	λ/Patient-year (%)	% Free
Thromboembolism	0.7	95 ± 1.5% (10 yr)	2.0	74 ± 3.9% (10 yr)
Anticoagulation hemorrhage	0.2	96 ± 2.8% (10 yr)	0.5	94 ± 3.9% (10 yr)
Endocarditis	0.9	94 ± 1.5% (10 yr)	1.1	89 ± 1.9% (10yr)
Replacement for perivalvular leak	0.3	98 ± 1.1% (10 yr)	1.0	95 ± 1.3% (10 yr)
Replacement for valve failure	2.4	75 ± 4.0% (9 yr)	0.7	94 ± 2.0% (10 yr)
Cardiac death	4.2	44 ± 3.7% (10 yr)	4.8	54 ± 4.2% (10 yr)
Valve-related death	0.9	92 ± 2.0% (8 yr)	1.2	92 ± 1.7% (10 yr)
All morbidity and mortality	4.0	58 ± 4.2% (8 yr)	5.4	57 ± 4.2% (10 yr)

may sometimes be affected by the prosthetic valves. Thus, it is extremely important that the *in vivo* evaluation of a valve undergoing clinical investigation include longitudinal studies to determine hemoglobin content, reticulocyte count, platelet count, haptoglobin, lactate dehydrogenase, hemosiderinuria, and red cell survival time (using radioactive-labeled autologous red cells).

EASE OF INSERTION

Any prosthetic valve that would be associated with undue difficulty in insertion would be easily recognized and quickly excluded from use. However, in addition to the ease of suturing the valve in its anatomical position, ease of insertion should take into consideration the orientation of the valve, any propensity of the valve mechanism to become caught up with or jam on tissue, or to be amenable to jamming on or catching dangling sutures. Ideally, a valve that could be quickly inserted in which a mechanism would be implanted instantaneously into the cardiac valvular annulus would be a very attractive one. However, past experience with such designs (Magovern–Cromie) has been disappointing, and suturing the valve in place remains the favored approach because it allows secure attachment to the tissue. Nevertheless, it is conceivable that newer designs that address this issue may develop with improvements in technology and bioengineering.

PATIENT ACCEPTANCE

The newer prosthetic valve should cause no annoyance to the patient. Obviously, a noisy valve that keeps the patient awake is a major annoyance and will be quickly rejected. Patients adjust to the noise of a mechanial valvular prosthesis remarkably well, but some complain about such noise.

More subtle annoyances include the need to monitor anticoagulant levels in the blood and to take medications continuously to prevent thromboembolic or other complications of the valve. In the long run, patient compliance can be taxed despite the best intentions, and thus the search of a valve that is free of major as well as minor annoyances should continue.

SUMMARY

None of the cardiac valve substitutes currently available conforms with all of the requirements of an ideal substitute for destroyed or damaged human heart valves. Despite the advantages and improvement in prosthetic heart valve design, complications after valve replacement remain a substantial source of late morbidity and mortality. Systemic arterial embolization and obstruction of valve prostheses due to thrombus formation, prosthetic valve endocarditis, mechanical failure, and perivalvular leakage are potentially life-threatening problems.

The need for continuing research and development of a more ideal cardiac valve substitute is obvious. The bioengineering profession and the valve industry continue to develop and evaluate newer prostheses, and the role of the surgeon and the cardiovascular profession in contributing to and participating in these evaluations is an extremely important one. Careful documentation and patient follow-up are absolutely mandatory and eventually will be the basis on which the identification and acceptance of a better newer prosthesis hinges and rests.

REFERENCES

1. Geha AS: Selection of heart valve. In Roberts AJ (ed): Difficult Problems in Adult Cardiac Surgery. Chicago, Year Book Medical Publishers, 1985

2. Roberts WC: Choosing a substitute cardiac valve: Type, size, surgeon. Am J Cardiol 38:633, 1976

3. Geha AS, Laks H, Stansel HC et al: Late failure of porcine valve heterografts in children. J Thorac Cardiovasc Surg 78:351, 1979

4. Kopf GS, Geha AS, Hellenbrand WE et al: Fate of leftsided cardiac bioprosthesis valves in children. Arch Surg 121:488, 1986

5. Williams WG, Pollock JC, Geiss DM et al: Experience with aortic and mitral valve replacement in children. J Thorac Cardiovasc Surg 81:326–333, 1981

6. Oyer PE, Miller DC, Stinson EB et al: Clinical durability of the Hancock porcine bioprosthetic valve. J Thorac Cardiovasc Surg 80:824, 1980

7. Hammond GL, Geha AS, Kopf GS et al: Biological vs. mechanical valves: Analysis of 1116 valves inserted in 1012 adult patients with a 4192 patient year and 4646 valve year follow-up. J Thorac Cardiovasc Surg (in press)

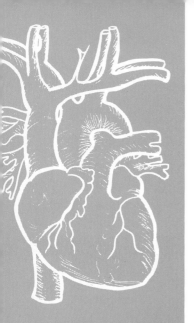

8

ASSIST DEVICES FOR LEFT- AND RIGHT-SIDED HEART SUPPORT

William F. Bernhard

Frederick J. Schoen

Warren Clay

James G. Carr

Nancy A. Howell

Thomas Hougen

A PNEUMATIC VENTRICULAR ASSIST SYSTEM FOR TEMPORARY CIRCULATORY SUPPORT

Ventricular assist devices (VADs) for temporary and permanent circulatory support are under development for patients with severe cardiac failure (acute or chronic) that is unresponsive to standard methods of management. The acute category includes 1% to 2% of postcardiotomy patients exhibiting left or right ventricular dysfunction, following an otherwise technically successful procedure. These individuals cannot be separated from cardiopulmonary bypass (CPB) using various catecholamines and a 60-minute trial of intra-aortic balloon counterpulsation (IABP). Also included are patients who develop cardiogenic shock within 72 hours postoperatively, occasional transplant candidates who decompensate while awaiting a donor organ, and others with acute myocardial infarction after surgical or medical reperfusion. For these individuals, circulatory support may be provided by pneumatic, paracorporeal VADs, with inflow and outflow conduits interposed between the left ventricular (LV) apex and ascending aorta, or between the left or right atria and aorta or pulmonary artery.

The chronic failure category comprises a larger number of refractory patients with end-stage coronary artery disease or irreversible cardiomyopathy. They require a permanent form of circulatory support, consisting of an implantable, multicomponent ventricular assist system (VAS) that is powered electrically.§ The device receives energy by way of a transcutaneous energy transmission system (TETS), eliminating percutaneous wires and tubes and employing either a portable battery pack or a conventional electrical outlet. Other VAS components include a blood pump and contiguous electromechanical energy converter (motor), a controller/internal battery pack, and a variable volume compliance chamber. The latter provides a reservoir for air displaced during each pump cycle.

Three VAD models designed for temporary use have been evaluated in an NHLBI clinical trial* that employed a carefully structured patient-selection protocol. Data from 41 device implantation cases recently reviewed by four pa-

* Investigation sponsored by the National Heart, Lung, and Blood Institute (NHLBI), National Institutes of Health (NIH), Bethesda, MD.

† The principal investigators of the NHLBI Temporary VAD Clinical Trial were Drs. William F. Bernhard, Robert L. Berger, Leonard R. Golding, and D. Glenn Pennington.

‡ The authors are indebted to Robert Valeri, M.D. (Hematology Consultant) and Victor L. Poirier, David Burke, David Gernes, Andy H. Levine, Alan L. Oslan, and Stanley Buczak for engineering contributions to these studies; and to Drs. Shukri F. Khuri, Ronald M. Weintraub, J. Kenneth Koster, Ernest Barsamian, and Steven J. VanDevanter for referring patients to the Children's Hospital VAD Program. We also are indebted to Francis and Gerard Tucker for technical assistance.

§ Cleveland Clinic Foundation and Hospital, Boston University Hospital, St. Louis University Hospital, Boston Children's Hospital Program

thologists from participating hospitals will be summarized in this chapter.[1] Finally, the current status of an electrical VAS under development in the laboratory will be reviewed.

MATERIALS AND METHODS

Three different temporary VADs employing either Dacron-valved (inflow and outflow) conduits or a pair of catheters with an attached vascular graft (for anastomosis to the ascending aorta or pulmonary artery) were evaluated. The first device, a Model XI axisymmetric pulsatile pump (designed by Thermedics, Inc.)* was implanted in 24 patients, 22 in the Children's Hospital Program and two others at Boston University Hospital. Although the VAD engineering specifications and pneumatic control system have been described previously, certain information is worthy of brief review.[2-6] The device consists of a titanium housing containing a cylindric, polyurethane bladder (Biomer)† with a stroke volume of 75 ml. Metal elbows join the housing to a pair of Dacron conduits, each containing a glutaraldehyde-preserved bioprosthetic valve. The pump bladder surface of this VAD differs from the two other devices in that it is integrally textured (fibrillar) rather than smooth. It consists of a tangled matrix of polyurethane fibrils, approximately 18 microns in diameter and 300 microns in length, and it immediately attracts a fibrin-cellular coagulum after exposure to blood (Fig. 8–1). The autologous lining is firmly attached to the surface, and it functions as a blood-contacting layer without the need for anticoagulant agents (until flow weaning is initiated).

A second VAD, designed by Thoratec,‡ was a sac-type prosthesis used to support 14 patients at

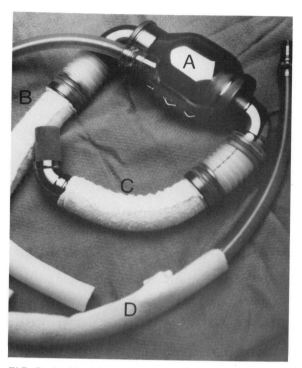

FIG. 8–1. Model #11 Axisymmetric, temporary VAD, designed by Thermedics, Inc. Pump parts include **(A)** the titanium housing that encloses a cylindric polyurethane bladder; **(B)** outflow-valved conduit and attached Dacron graft; **(C)** inflow-valved conduit and curved titanium apical cannula (18 mm ID); and **(D)** percutaneous tube for connection to the pneumatic control system.

St. Louis University Hospital. The device consisted of a polycarbonate housing and a smooth-surfaced polyurethane sac (stroke volume 65 ml), and incorporated two Bjork–Shiley valves.§ Blood inflow was conducted through a large-bore, right-angled (51F), wire-wound, polyurethane tube, and outflow was ejected through a graft anastomosed to the aorta or pulmonary artery. A pneumatic control system set in

* Thermedics Inc., Woburn, MA
† Ethicon, Inc., Somerville, NJ
‡ Thoratec Inc., Berkeley, CA

§ Shiley Corporation, Irvine, CA

the asynchronous mode delivered pulsatile flow to these patients.* The final device, employed in three Cleveland Clinic cases, was also a sac-type VAD with a smooth, biolized, gelatin lining.[7-9] Catheters were used for inflow drainage (LV apex or left atrium), and outflow was directed to the ascending aorta.

In most cases, VADs were implanted through a previously created median sternotomy incision during continuous CPB. After connection of conduits or catheters to the heart, VAD flow was established (uniformly) in the asynchronous mode while CPB flow was gradually reduced. Continuous monitoring of left atrial (LA) pressure and total VAD output was used to achieve a flow rate of 2 liters/minute/M^2, and an LA pressure reduction below 20 mm Hg. Because an element of right ventricular (RV) failure was present in most patients, vasoactive agents were infused to increase ventricular contractility. In addition, rhythmic manual compression of the RV was undertaken (intermittently) to maintain an adequate pulmonary blood flow.

Postoperative monitoring in the intensive care unit (ICU) was not significantly different from that employed in other patients receiving IABP support. It consisted of cardiac output (CO) determinations, and measurements of right and left atrial pressures (RAP and LAP), aortic pressure, pulmonary artery (PA) pressure, and continuous VAD flow.

Only asynchronous pumping was possible during the initial 24 hours of circulatory support because of the presence of atrial and ventricular tachyarrhythmias. However, ECG synchronization was undertaken as soon as possible (24 to 36 hours) in one of the hospital programs (Children's Hospital). Patients in the other two VAD programs were assisted asynchronously throughout the interval of circulatory support.

When patients had improved sufficiently (72

* Vitamek, Inc., Houston, TX

to 96 hours) to maintain a cardiac index of 2 liters/minute/M^2 (in the presence of 50% VAD flow reduction), complete weaning from the device was pursued (over a 4- to 8-hour interval). Heparin was administered (300 units/kg) when the pump flow dropped below 2 liters/minute and was reversed immediately after removal of the conduits or catheters. Continuous monitoring of LAP, arterial pressure, and CO provided sufficient information for patient management. Experience indicated that an increase in LAP, with accompanying VAD flow reduction, was the most reliable indicator of cardiac failure and of the need to return to a maximum perfusion rate for an additional period (4 to 8 hours).

The ability to maintain stable hemodynamics at reduced flows (for several hours) was sufficient evidence to proceed with device retrieval.

RESULTS

Temporary VAD support was employed in a total of 41 patients: in 39 immediately after a cardiac surgical procedure, and in 2 cardiomyopathy patients who had no previous cardiac operations (Table 8-1).

Of the postcardiotomy cases, three developed acute LV failure in the ICU, while 36 patients were in the operating room (on CPB) receiving counterpulsation with IABP. Improvement in cardiac function was noted within 48 to 72 hours in 16 of 41 patients (group I), while 25 others (group II) failed to demonstrate hemodynamic improvement and died within 120 hours (Table 8-2). Unfortunately, all patients were subjected to prolonged CPB during the initial phase of cardiac resuscitation (prior to VAD implantation). The duration of perfusion in group I ranged from 69 to 540 minutes (mean 245 minutes), and from 175 to 600 minutes (mean 355 minutes) in group II. Ventricular assistance was maintained for a mean of 127 hours in group I and 19 hours in group II.

TABLE 8–1

SEPARATION OF 41 TEMPORARY VAD RECIPIENTS INTO TWO GROUPS
DEPENDING UPON EVIDENCE OF HEMODYNAMIC IMPROVEMENT*

	Group I Hemodynamic Improvement	Group II No Improvement
No. of Patients	16	25
Age (yr)		
Mean	49	56
Range	27–69	15–72
Surgical Procedures		
MVR	2	0
AVR	0	2
CABG	8	14
CABG + other procedures†	3	7
Cardiomyopathy (No previous surgery)	2	0
Other‡	1	1
Duration of CPB (min)		
Mean	245	355
Range	69–540	175–600
Development of shock		
Preexisting§	2	0
Operating room	11	24
Intensive care unit	3	0

Abbreviations: CABG, coronary artery bypass graft; MVR, mitral valve replacement; AVR, aortic valve replacement; LVA, left ventricular aneurysm; CPB, cardiopulmonary bypass.

* NHLBI-sponsored clinical VAD trials in four cooperating institutions.

†CABG + MVR (3), CABG + AVR (5), CABG + LVA (1), CABG + MVR + LVA (1).

‡ Atrial septal defect with anomalous pulmonary venous return (1); repair of aortic aneurysm (1).

§ Patients with cardiomyopathy only.

Weaning and device retrieval were possible in 11 of 16 group-I patients. Seven of these had predominantly LV failure (managed with a left VAD); two who demonstrated RV failure were treated with a right VAD (RA to PA); and two with biventricular decompensation received right and left VADs. Six of eleven were long-term survivors (2 to 6 years), while five died 5 to 30 days later. Deaths were secondary to low output cardiac failure associated with myocardial necrosis (MN) (two); to multiple organ failure and associated sepsis (two); and to sudden exsanguination 30 days postoperatively in one ambulatory patient (with *Aspergillus aortitis* and aortic rupture). The remaining five died before VAD weaning, because of pulmonary emboli (two), intracerebral hemorrhage (two), and MN (one). Some individuals undergoing left VAD support had associated RV failure as a significant complicating factor. Finally, persistent postoperative mediastinal hemorrhage (of a diffuse nature) was responsible for the deaths of 9 of 25 patients (group II), despite massive blood replacement therapy (Table 8–3).

Cardiac Pathology. Myocardium was available for histologic study in 33 patients (23 biopsies taken at the time of VAD implantation and 24 autopsies). Myocardial necrosis (MN) was noted by biopsy or autopsy in 28 of 33 cases (85%)—

TABLE 8–2
TEMPORARY VAD EXPERIENCE IN 41 PATIENTS*

	Group I Improvement on VAD	Group II No Improvement on VAD
No. of patients	16	25
Expired without weaning	5	25
Successful weaning from VAD	11	0
Expired 5 to 30 days later	5	0
Long-term survivors	6	0

* NHLBI-sponsored clinical VAD trials in four cooperating institutions. (CHMC Program)

10 patients in group I and 18 in group II. In addition, pre-VAD biopsy revealed MN in 2 of 6 long-term survivors. Eleven patients demonstrated MN with prominent contraction bands (three in group I and eight in group II), an injury associated with severe myocardial ischemia occurring during CPB (followed by reperfusion).

Patient/Device Interactions. Three smooth-surfaced VAD sacs contained small, focal, fibrin thrombi, and one device was associated with a large, loosely adherent apical thrombus. Pump bladders with textured (fibrillar) surfaces contained a thin pseudointimal (PI) membrane (10 to 300 microns thick), varying among patients and sites on the bladder surface. It consisted of fibrin with numerous, randomly oriented polymorphonuclear and mononuclear leukocytes, as well as many trapped erythrocytes (Fig. 8–2). The layer was firmly adherent to the underlying fibrillar matrix. No evidence of calcification or infection was noted on any bladder.

VAD-related complications included one fatal *Aspergillus aortitis* at the CPB aortic cannulation site in one patient and extensive pulmonary emboli in a second patient. The latter was supported with a smooth-surfaced right VAD, interposed between the RA and PA. In this case, mural thrombus was evident in the RA and PA, adjacent to cannulation sites. No foreign-material emboli were encountered in any of the organs examined during 24 autopsies.

Hematology. Severe hemolysis and thrombocytopenia were noted in all of these cases prior to VAD implantation and for 12 to 24 hours postoperatively. The presence of markedly elevated plasma hemoglobins (greater than 100 mg/dl) was routine, and these values declined rapidly if renal function was unimpaired. However, reduced platelet counts (less than 50,000 mm³) required daily platelet transfusions, and this condition generally persisted until the VAD was removed.

Clotting studies performed postoperatively revealed prolonged, activated partial thromboplastin times, prothrombin times, and thrombin times, which contributed to active bleeding. In addition, severe hypofibrinogenemia was detected in two patients in group II and one patient in group I. The problem may have been caused by either primary or secondary fibrinolysis.

DISCUSSION

Early death after cardiac surgery occurs in at least 1% to 2% of patients today despite major advances in myocardial preservation methods. Studies indicate a high frequency of acute MN in nonsurvivors; in many cases, this is an injury

TABLE 8–3
CAUSES OF DEATH IN 35 TEMPORARY VAD PATIENTS*

Cause	Hemodynamic Improvement	No Hemodynamic Improvement
Myocardial necrosis	3	11
Hemorrhage (persistent, postoperative)	0	9
Cerebrovascular accident	2	1
Pulmonary emboli	2	0
Infection	3	0
Technical error	0	1
No anatomic lesion noted†	0	3
Total	10	25

*NHBLI-sponsored clinical VAD trials in four cooperating institutions.
† Pump failure in operating room.

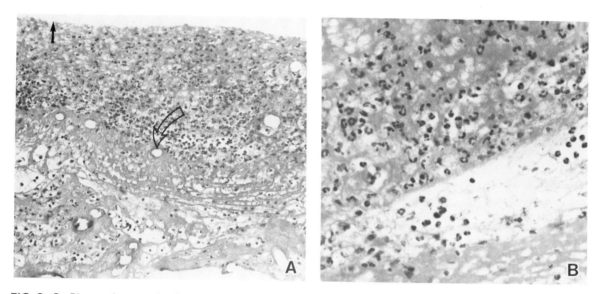

FIG. 8–2. Photomicrograph of a cross section of pseudointima formed on the pumping bladder of a device used in a patient for 109 hours. **(A)** Overview of fibrin/platelet/inflammatory cell accumulation. The luminal surface is at the top **(closed arrow),** and the overall thickness is approximately 500 μm (0.5 mm). Holes produced by the fibrils of the textured bladder surface are seen within the deposit **(open arrow).** (Hematoxylin-eosin × 150). **(B)** High-magnification photomicrograph of bladder thrombotic deposit, illustrating polymorphonuclear leukocytes, mononuclear phagocytes, and the underlying fibrin/platelet matrix. (Hematoxylin-eosin × 375)

related to severe ischemia (during CPB) followed by restoration of circulation.[10,11,13] However, an investigation of some patients with postcardiotomy ventricular dysfunction revealed no apparent myocardial abnormalities by gross inspection or light microscopy.[12,13] These lesions either had insufficient time to develop a recognizable morphologic appearance, or the injuries were confined to the ultrastructural level. A final possibility is that there is no known morphological correlate to the myocardial dysfunction in such patients.

Although the presence of myocardial necrosis at the time of VAD implantation did not preclude long-term survival in the NIH clinical trial, most patients with extensive damage did poorly. Existing necrosis is unaffected by VAD-augmented perfusion or a reduction of myocardial work; therefore, a reversible type of cardiac functional abnormality must involve other factors. Likely processes include resolution of myocardial edema (intracellular or interstitial), or subendocardial hemorrhage in areas of otherwise viable myocardium. On the basis of severe ischemic injury, return of contractility to muscle with depressed function would be another possibility.[12]

Defective cell-volume regulation with consequent modest cell swelling is one of the earliest abnormalities noted in lethal acute myocardial ischemia.[14] In addition, reperfusion of ischemic areas accentuates increases in tissue water and electrolytes.[15,16] Significant intracellular (mitochondrial) edema has been noted in patients following global ischemia, produced by temporarily cross-clamping the ascending aorta.[17] Finally, swelling of cells and interstitium may magnify ischemic tissue injury through vascular compression and subsequent reduction in tissue perfusion. In the presence of adequate circulatory support, resolution of edema and improved ventricular compliance could be accomplished within several days following injury.

Investigations of LV bypass have demonstrated the feasibility of myocardial salvage

through reduction of oxygen utilization (in the nonischemic heart), as well as a beneficial effect on myocardial ischemia and evolving infarction.[18,19] Nevertheless, studies of myocardium subjected to severe ischemia, followed by reperfusion, have indicated that return of normal metabolic activity and function may be delayed after sublethal cellular damage (no necrosis).[16,20] In effect, the myocardium is viable but "stunned."[21] Morphologic correlates of this damage or its recovery are unknown; however, the time course for return of myocardial contractility after restoration of adequate perfusion is compatible with the temporary VAD experience.

A number of patients in the clinical trial demonstrated severe RV failure, a process in which the pathogenesis is unclear and the potential for recovery uncertain.[22-24] Reversible RV dysfunction could relate to myocardial ischemia or necrosis, particularly if hypothermic protection of the anterior (right) ventricle was incomplete during the period of temporary aortic cross-clamping. Another possibility might be a complement-mediated polymorphonuclear leukocyte activation, with stasis of these cells in the pulmonary capillaries and arterioles (producing acute pulmonary hypertension).[25,26] In addition, several investigators have observed C5a activation during CPB, but the role of such mediator-release-stimulated effects on cardiopulmonary function (after cardiac surgery) has not been elucidated.[26,27] Whatever the cause of the injury, patients with acute RV dysfunction may also be successfully resuscitated using temporary VAD support.

An improved understanding of the pathogenesis of this form of cardiac decompensation should improve patient selection for VAD resuscitation and uncover additional pathophysiological effects of CPB. It is also apparent that VAD implantation earlier in the cardiac resuscitation process should significantly enhance patient salvage.

Information derived from the recently completed NHLBI clinical trial indicated that resuscitation could be achieved with several VAD models. In addition, modest flow rates (2 liters/minute/M²) proved to be adequate for the task in patients at bed rest, rather than the much higher perfusion rates anticipated in pretrial discussions. Surprisingly, synchronization of the VAD (with the heart) was not essential for patient survival. However, the competitive systolic ejection associated with random VAD function *cannot* possibly contribute to myocardial recovery from injury.

Postoperative management of patients with functioning paracorporeal VADs required continued vigilance to avoid contamination or obstruction of conduits connected to the heart. Otherwise, nursing activities in the ICU were similar to those provided for patients receiving IABP support, including VAD weaning and the hemodynamic monitoring practiced during device removal.

AN ELECTRICAL VENTRICULAR ASSIST SYSTEM FOR PROLONGED CIRCULATORY SUPPORT

A multicomponent ventricular assist system (VAS)* designed for use in older patients with end-stage cardiac disease is in the final stages of development. The electrically actuated device consists of a pusher-plate blood pump and Dacron-valved conduits coupled to a low-speed torque motor. An internal variable volume chamber attached to the motor serves as a reservoir for air displaced during each pump cycle; and synchronization of the system with the heart is provided by a controller/internal energy storage unit. A transcutaneous energy transmission

* Thermedics, Inc., Woburn, MA, and Cardiovascular Surgical Research Laboratory, Children's Hospital, Boston, MA

system (TETS) conducts electrical power to the motor (across intact skin), avoiding use of percutaneous tubes or wires with their attendant hazard of infection (Fig. 8–3).

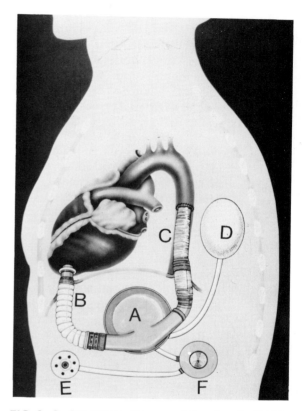

FIG. 8–3. *Schematic diagram of the electrical VAS with the pump, energy converter, and controller attached to the ninth and tenth ribs. System components include* **(A)** *pusher-plate pump and contiguous motor;* **(B,C)** *dacron-valved inflow and outflow conduits;* **(D)** *variable-volume chamber in the left pleural space;* **(E)** *secondary coil of the TETS; and* **(F)** *the controller. The VAS may be implanted through either a left lateral thoracotomy incision or a median sternotomy incision, with extension to the upper abdomen.*

MATERIALS AND METHODS

Blood Pump and Contiguous Energy Converter. The pusher-plate blood pump (stroke volume 85 ml) and an attached electromechanical energy converter (motor), weighing a total of 0.87 kg, were capable of ejecting a pulsatile flow of 10 liters/minute.[28,29] The rigid pump housing and energy converter were fabricated from a titanium alloy and contained a flexible polyurethane diaphragm (Biomer)* that isolated one component from the other. Upward displacement of the diaphragm by the motor produced systolic ejection, whereas diastolic filling occurred passively. The diaphragm had a textured blood-contacting surface identical to that found in the temporary VAD.[6] The internal surface of the adjacent pump housing was covered by a powdered metallurgy (PM) layer that consisted of masses of interconnected titanium microspheres approximately 140 microns in diameter. The sintered surface was porous and attracted a fibrin-cellular coagulum after contact with blood.

The low-speed torque motor operated on a beat-to-beat basis and had only four moving parts. Upon receipt of an ejection signal, the rotor of the unit turned one revolution and stopped (systolic ejection), employing solid-state electronic commutation. A magnet mounted on the pusher-plate and a Hall-effect sensor located in the center shaft of the rotor permitted monitoring (electronically) of the pusher-plate position to provide a measurement of stroke volume (Fig. 8–4).

Variable Volume Chamber. In the absence of an external vent between the motor and external environment, a chamber was used to maintain a constant gas volume within the motor during systolic ejection and diastolic filling. The

* Ethicon Inc., Somerville, NJ

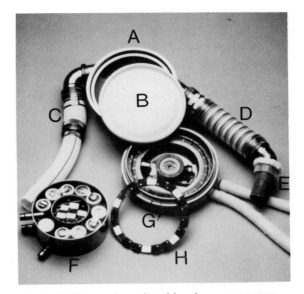

FIG. 8–4. The pusher-plate blood pump, energy converter, and controller prior to final assembly. **(A,B)** Pump housing and polymer diaphragm. **(C,D)** Valved outflow and inflow conduits with **(E)** the titanium apical inflow cannula. **(F)** Controller with ten internal batteries and interconnected circuit boards. **(G,H)** Parts of the low-speed, torque motor.

chamber consisted of a rigid backplate and a flexible discoid sac covered with Dacron velour fabric. The presence of the velour layer promoted formation of a thin capsule at the sac surface in contact with visceral pleura. During VAS function, the chamber inflated with air as blood flowed into the pump and deflated into the motor section during synchronized ejection of blood. The fibrous capsule inhibited formation of thick pleural adhesions, which could restrict the motion of the chamber, limiting pump output.

Control System/Internal Energy Storage Unit. The control unit was encased in a titanium housing and consisted of three interconnected, printed circuit boards (3.8 cm in diameter) wrapped in a plastic liner. Ten nickel-cadmium batteries were included in the housing, forming a battery with a capacity of 4.5 watt-hours (supplying 8 watts of power). They constituted an emergency backup capability for the VAS in case of power failure and had a discharge time in excess of 30 minutes.

Three operating modes were possible within the controller: synchronous counterpulsation, fixed-volume asynchronous pumping, and fixed-rate operation. Synchronization of the device was accomplished by detecting changes in pump fill-rate, corresponding to the rate of descent of the pusher-plate following ventricular systole. ECG signals were not utilized because of the inherent potential for fatigue-fracture of myocardial leads.

Transcutaneous Energy Transmission System (TETS). The TETS consisted of a power oscillator; a tuned transcutaneous transformer; and output power-conditioning circuitry. The oscillator converted DC power from external batteries to an AC voltage of 160 kHz. During pump function, AC current was conducted to a superficial primary coil on the external chest wall and was inductively coupled with an implanted, subcutaneous secondary coil. High-frequency magnetic fields were capable of transmitting power through an unbroken layer of skin (approximately 1.5-cm thick) and was approximately 75% efficient. The technique was important because it eliminated percutaneous tubes or wires and the risk of bacterial infection. AC power was converted to the DC voltage necessary for actuation of the pump and support electronics (approximately 7 watts) by a power-conditioning module in the energy storage unit.

During these investigations, some studies were performed with only the compliance chamber and blood pump-motor unit (energy converter) requiring the use of a cable attached to an external electrical power system; however, several animal implants were carried out with the total VAS.

External Battery Capacity and Power Requirements. The external battery power source (carried in a shoulder holster) provided 10 hours of pump function at a nominal flow rate of 7 liters/minute, 120 mm Hg mean pressure. Blood flow of this magnitude constituted a 5-watt power drain and must be added to the 1.74 watts necessary for implanted electronics as well as for internal battery charging. Additional small power losses were incurred in transferring energy across the intact skin, resulting in a total power requirement of 7.8 watts (10 hours of operation). Batteries must be replaced with an alternate unit every 8 to 10 hours and recharged every 24 hours using a recharger unit powered from a conventional wall outlet.

VAS Implantation. Implantation of VAS components was undertaken in calves (90 kg to 110 kg), and all animals received humane care in compliance with *Principles of Laboratory Care.** Attachment of the inflow and outflow conduits (containing bioprosthetic valves) was accomplished through a left lateral thoracotomy, and an additional subcostal incision permitted abdominal location and fixation of the pump housing and controller (ninth and tenth ribs). In two experiments, the secondary TETS coil was implanted in a dorsally located (tenth rib) subcutaneous pocket, and the primary coil was taped to the skin for AC current induction. The valved conduits (inflow and outflow) were directed superiorly to the LV apex and descending thoracic aorta (level of the eighth rib posteriorly) through incisions in the left hemidiaphragm. The curved

* Formulated by the National Society for Medical Research and the Guide for Care and Use of Laboratory Animals prepared by The National Academy of Sciences and published by The National Institutes of Health (NIH, publication 80-23) (revised), 1978.

titanium cannula at the end of the inflow conduit had an internal diameter of 18 mm and contained a powdered metallurgy surface that encouraged tissue ingrowth. There was never any evidence of blood flow obstruction through a conduit caused by cannula impingement on the interventricular septum.

Inoculation of Textured Surfaces with Bovine Fetal Fibroblasts. The textured blood-contacting surfaces of the pump were seeded with cultured fetal fibroblasts to accelerate development of a thin, collagenous, nonthrombogenic lining.[30-34] Cells were distributed over the surface during rotation of a sterile sealed pump for 2 hours (ambient temperature).[35,36] Firm cell attachment to the fibrillar diaphragm and PM surfaces occurred during this interval, employing 30×10^6 cells suspended in complete media (Fig. 8–5). The fibroblasts were stored in liquid nitrogen ($-195°C$), until needed, and were thawed, plated, and incubated for 48 hours at $37°C$ prior to use.

In anticipation of preparing (seeding) pump

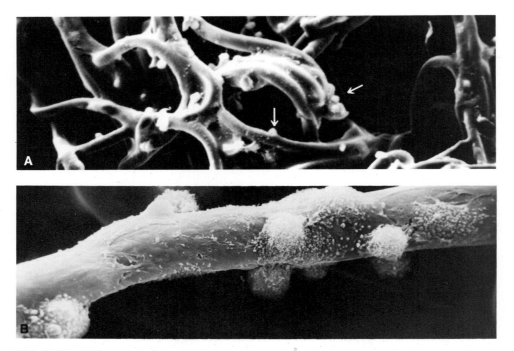

FIG. 8–5. (A) Scanning electron micrograph demonstrating a textured polyurethane fibrillar surface. Numerous fetal (allogeneic) fibroblasts can be seen attached to the polymer fibrils. (**Arrows** indicate representative cells.) ($\times$ 200) **(B)** Scanning electron micrograph showing fetal fibroblasts attached to a fibril following brief preimplant rotation (approximately 6 to 8 revolutions per hour). ($\times$ 2000)

surfaces with fibroblasts prior to clinical use, a series of *in vitro* experiments was conducted with human cells (WI-38).* These cells, free of contaminating viruses and microorganisms, were a diploid fibroblast strain derived from embryonic lung tissue. Of importance, they had the capacity to form a multilayered membrane and to produce collagen (*in vitro*) throughout their life cycle.[37–39] For practical purposes, fibroblast-seeded surfaces must be prepared prior to use in the operating room, with cell viability maintained (devoid of media) until pump connection to the circulation.

To investigate the viability requirement, cell studies were conducted using 12 sealed sterile blood pumps, each containing 30×10^6 fibroblasts. The devices remained at ambient temperature for periods up to 24 hours, prior to chemical removal of cells (trypsinization) and reculture (37°C). The end point for each experiment was identification of 75% or more of the original fibroblasts capable of monolayer formation.

RESULTS

Partial LV bypass (4 to 5 liters/minute) was established in 11 calves (50 to 150 days) employing electrical VAS components. In nine experiments, an external electrical power system was employed, but in two others, a TETS delivered AC power to an implanted secondary coil. In simultaneous *in vitro* engineering investigations, evaluation of motors (in continuous operation) was carried out for periods exceeding 2 years.[28] Although no motor-related abnormalities developed during the *in vivo* experiments, other problems were encountered that prompted premature termination of some experiments. In general, the failures were minor, consisting of broken wires, malfunction of a Hall-effect sensor and pusher-plate, partial-valved–conduit ob-

* American Type Culture Collection, Rockville, MD 20852

structions due to kinking, and one severe soft tissue infection.

Few hematologic abnormalities were noted; the most significant one was a mild thrombocytopenia, which disappeared within 7 to 10 days. Plasma hemoglobin values were unchanged from preoperative levels, and occult erythrocyte membrane damage did not occur, as evidenced by unchanged mechanical fragility values. Previous red cell and platelet survival studies did not reveal evidence of chronic hemolysis or platelet destruction.[29]

Examination of blood-pump surfaces demonstrated the presence of a thin, collagen membrane attached both to the fibrillar surface of the polymer diaphragm and the PM surface of the housing. No embolic organ damage was noted during autopsy examination, and all Dacron-valved graft conduits were free of obstructing thrombus. One partially calcified bioprosthetic valve (inflow) was discovered after 67 days, but other porcine-valve specimens were unchanged by the period of implantation. Granular calcific deposits were noted at the diaphragm/pseudointima junction in some specimens, but these did not penetrate the surface integrity of the lining (Fig. 8–6).

In vitro studies performed with human fibroblasts seeded on 12 blood-pump surfaces revealed an abundance of viable cells upon reculture and incubation. Three experiments were continued for 24 hours before trypsinization was undertaken, indicating that in the future, surface preparation can be undertaken within very reasonable time limits.

DISCUSSION

A clinical trial of prolonged ventricular bypass for patients with end-stage coronary disease or decompensated cardiomyopathy appears feasible within 3 years. Efforts to achieve this objective have resulted in the development of a multi-

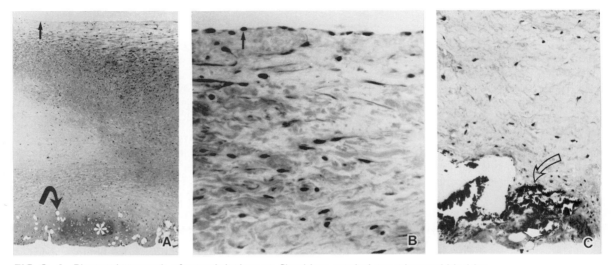

FIG. 8–6. Photomicrograph of pseudointima on fibroblast-seeded experimental bladder surface in a calf that was pumped for 159 days. **(A)** Overview of fibrous pseudointima. The thickness of this tissue layer is approximately 1 mm. The luminal surface is at the top **(straight arrow).** Spaces left by fibrils of the integrally textured bladder surface are noted in the nonluminal portion of the fibrous deposit **(closed arrow).** An area of cartilaginous metaplasia **(asterisk)** is noted near the deepest portion of the tissue layer. (Hematoxylin-eosin × 60) **(B)** High-power photomicrograph of luminal surface demonstrating collagenous connective tissue structure with predominant spindle cells (most likely fibroblasts), occasional inflammatory cells, and an endothelial-like cellular layer at the luminal surface **(arrow).** **(C)** High-power photomicrograph of the antiluminal portion of pseudointima demonstrating focal calcification **(open arrow)** associated with fibrils from the textured bladder surface **(light arrow).** (B and C, hematoxylin-eosin × 375)

component, electrical VAS that provides patient mobility without tethering by transcutaneous tubes and wires. The prosthetic system consists of a pusher-plate blood-pump, electric motor, electronic controller, variable volume compliance chmber, and TETS, all designed for at least 2 years of continuous function. Location of most components within the abdomen makes repair or replacement of parts, when necessary, a less hazardous procedure.

Engineering progress during the investigation has been accompanied by efforts in the surgical laboratory to develop a textured, nonthrombogenic, blood-contacting surface.[29] Acceleration of PI development by inoculating textured surfaces with allogenic, cultured fetal fibroblasts resulted in the formation of a thin collagenous membrane within several weeks following implantation. Fibroblasts attach firmly to the fibrillar matrix and are *not* displaced by forces created by systolic flexion of the polymer diaphragm. Within 3 to 5 months, a spontaneous reduction in the metabolic activity of donor fibroblasts appears to occur, avoiding excessive collagen buildup and reduced compliance of the diaphragm. Sheets of dense, mature collagen develop on the pump surface with increased cellularity at the luminal and basal areas of the matrix. The thickness of the lining seldom exceeds 1 mm in either inflow, middle, or outflow areas of the device. Granular calcification does occur at the junction between the surface material and the PI, but has never interrupted surface integrity.

Previous immunologic studies undertaken in our laboratory failed to demonstrate evidence of cytotoxicity against cultured allogenic fibroblasts.[36] This lack of immune response was believed to be related either to the dense collagenous layer inhibiting fibroblast recognition by the host immune system or to the fact that fetal fibroblasts may be relatively nonimmunogenic.

Clinical investigations done previously have confirmed the long-term viability of allogenic fibroblasts in patients undergoing aortic valve replacement with fresh homograft valves.[40–46] Efforts to determine donor fibroblast viability (after implantation) consisted of excising tissue from a homograft valve and growing the cells in tissue culture. In addition, histologic sections of homograft valves demonstrated the persistence of viable fibroblasts, but the absolute number of cells decreased with time. Specimens removed after 2 to 4 years revealed a small fibroblast population, which would grow actively in tissue culture, and a larger acellular valve area. Host (autologous) fibroblasts appeared in a sheath at the base of a donor aortic cusp, and these cells were distinct morphologically from the original donor cells. The chromatin-Barr body could be identified, establishing the presence of "female" donor cells, and was obtained when a homograft valve (excised from a female donor) was inserted in a "male"-valve recipient.

Currently, several pump development programs are proceeding toward clinical trials. For those who are successful, many class-IV cardiac patients await palliation and a chance to return to productive living.

REFERENCES

1. Schoen FJ, Palmer DC, Haudenschild CC et al: Pathologic findings and their implications in patients managed with temporary ventricular assist. Trans Am Soc Artif Intern Organs 31:66, 1985
2. Filler RN, Bernhard WF, Robinson T et al: An implantable left ventricular-aortic assist device. J Thorac Cardiovasc Surg 54:795–806, 1967
3. Bernhard WF, Poirier V, LaFarge CG, Carr JG: A new method for temporary left ventricular bypass: Preclinical appraisal. J Thorac Cardiovasc Surg 70:880, 1975
4. Bernhard WF, Stetz J, Carr JG et al: Temporary left-ventricular bypass: Factors affecting patient survival. Circulation (Suppl I) 60:I–131, 1979
5. Bernhard WF, Poirier VL, Carr JG: A paracorporeal left ventricular assist device. In Encyclopedia of Thoracic Surgery-Modern Techniques in Surgery. Cardio-Thoracic Surgery 28:1, 1980
6. Bernhard WF, Clay W, Gernes D et al: Temporary and permanent left ventricular bypass: Laboratory and clinical observations. World J Surg 9:54, 1985
7. Pennington DG, Bernhard WF, Golding LR et al: Long-term followup of postcardiotomy patients with profound cardiogenic shock salvaged by ventricular assist devices. Circulation (Suppl II) 70:216, September 1985
8. Pennock JL, Pierce WS, Wisman CB et al: Survival and complications following ventricular assist pumping for cardiogenic shock. Ann Surg 198:469, 1983
9. Yozu R, Golding LAR, Jacobs G et al: Preclinical evaluation of a biolized temporary ventricular assist device. Cleve Clin Q 51:119, 1984
10. Schoen FJ, Bernhard WF, Khuri SF et al: Pathologic findings in postcardiotomy patients managed with a temporary left ventricular assist pump. Am J Surg 143:508, 1982
11. Gotlieb A, Masse S, Allard J et al: Concentric hemorrhagic necrosis of the myocardium. A morphological and clinical study. Human Pathol 8:27, 1977
12. Bulkley BH, Hutchins GM: Myocardial consequences of coronary artery bypass graft surgery: The paradox of necrosis in areas of revascularization. Circulation 56:906, 1977
13. Schoen FJ, Titus JL, Lawrie GM: Autopsy-determined causes of death after cardiac valve replacement. JAMA 249:899, 1983
14. Leaf A: Cell swelling. A factor in ischemic tissue injury. Circulation 48:455, 1973
15. Willerson JT, Scales F, Mukherjee A et al: Abnormal myocardial fluid retention as an early manifestation of ischemic injury. Am J Pathol 87:159, 1977
16. Jennings RB, Reimer KA: Factors involved in salvaging

ischemic myocardium: Effect of reperfusion of arterial blood. Circulation (Suppl I) 68:1–25, 1983

17. Schaper J, Schwarz F, Kittstein H et al: The effects of global ischemia and reperfusion on human myocardium: Quantitative evaluation by electron microscopic morphometry. Ann Thorac Surg 33:116, 1982

18. Dennis C, Hall DP, Moreno JR, Senning A: Reduction of the oxygen utilization of the heart by left heart bypass. Circ Res 10:298, 1962

19. Pennock JL, Pae WE, Pierce WS, Waldausen JA: Reduction of myocardial infarct size: Comparison between left atrial and left ventricular bypass. Circulation 59:275, 1979

20. Kloner RA, Ellis SG, Lange R, Braunwald E: Studies of experimental coronary artery reperfusion. Effects on infarct size, myocardial function, biochemistry, ultrastructure and microvascular damage. Circulation (Suppl I) 68:I–15, 1983

21. Braunwald E, Kloner RA: The stunned myocardium: Prolonged, post-ischemic ventricular dysfunction. Circulation 66:1146, 1982

22. Laks H, Berger RL, Parr CVS, Pennington DG: Acute cardiac failure: The importance of the right ventricle. Trans Am Soc Artif Intern Organs 28:678, 1982

23. Pennington DG, Merjavy JP, Swartz MT et al: The importance of biventricular failure in patients with postoperative cardiogenic shock. Ann Thorac Surg 39:16, 1985

24. O'Neill MJ, Pierce WS, Wisman CB et al: Successful management of right ventricular failure with the ventricular assist pump following aortic valve replacement and coronary bypass grafting. J Thorac Cardiovasc Surg 87:106, 1984

25. Jacob HS, Craddock PR, Hammerschmidt DE, Modlow CF: Complement-induced granulocyte aggregation. An unsuspected mechanism of disease. N Engl J Med 302:789, 190

26. Hammerschmidt DE, Stroncek DF, Bowers TK et al: Complement activation and neutropenia occurring during cardiopulmonary bypass. J Thorac Cardiovasc Surg 81:370, 1981

27. Kirklin JK, Westaby S, Blackstone EH et al: Complement and the damaging effects of cardiopulmonary bypass. J Thorac Cardiovasc Surg 86:845, 1983

28. Bernhard WF, Clay W, Schoen FJ et al: Clinical and laboratory investigations related to temporary and permanent ventricular bypass. Heart Transplantation 3:16, 1983

29. Bernhard WF, Gernes DG, Clay WC et al: Investigations with an implantable electrically-actuated ventricular assist device. J Thorac Cardiovasc Surg 88:11, 1984

30. Liotta D, Hall CW, DeBakey ME: A permanent autologous lining for implantable blood pumps. Cardiovasc Res Cent Bull 4:69, 1966

31. Gidoni J, Liotta D, Hall CW, DeBakey ME: Healing of pseudointima in velour-lined arterial prostheses. Am J Pathol 53:375, 1968

32. Bernhard WF, LaFarge CG, Robinson T, Carr JG: An improved blood pump interface for left ventricular bypass. Ann Surg 168:750, 1968

33. Bernhard WF, Husain M, Curtis GW, Carr JG: Fetal fibroblasts as a substratum for pseudoendothelial development on prosthetic surfaces. Surgery 66:284, 1969

34. Bernhard WF, LaFarge CG, Liss RH et al: An appraisal of blood trauma and the prosthetic interface during left ventricular bypass in the calf and in humans. Ann Thorac Surg 26:427, 1978

35. Bernhard WF, Colo NA, Wesolowski JS et al: Development of collagenous linings on impermeable prosthetic surfaces. J Thorac Cardiovasc Surg 79:552, 1980

36. Bernhard WF, Colo NA, Szycher M et al: Development of a nonthrombogenic collagenous blood-prosthetic interface. Ann Surg 192:369, 1980

37. Hayflick L, Moorhead PS: The serial cultivation of human diploid cell strains. Exp Cell Res 25:585, 1961

38. Paz MA, Gallop PM: Collagen synthesized and modified by aging fibroblasts in culture. In Vitro 11(5):302, 1975

39. Green H, Goldberg B: Kinetics of collagen synthesis by established mammalian cell lines, Nature 200:1097, 1963

40. Angell WW, Shumway NE, Kosek JC: A five-year study of viable aortic valve homografts. J Thorac Cardiovasc Surg 64:329, September 1972

41. Barratt–Boyes BG: Long-term follow-up of aortic valvar grafts. Br Heart J (Suppl)33:60, 1971

42. Kosek JC, Iben AB, Shumway NE, Angell WW: Morphology of fresh heart valve homografts. Surgery 66:269, July 1969

43. Davies D, Missen GAK, Blandford G et al: Homograft replacement of the aortic valves: A clinical and pathologic study. Am J Cardiol 22:195, August 1968

44. Ross DN, Yacoub MH: Homograft replacement of the aortic valve: A critical review. Prog Cardiovasc Dis XI:275, January 1969

45. Bodnar E, Wain WH, Martelli V, Ross DN: Long-term performance of 580 homograft and autograft valves used for aortic valve replacement. J Thorac Cardiovasc Surg 27:31, 1979

46. Ionescu MI, Ross DN, Wooler GH (eds): Tissue Heart Valves, Sevenoaks, England, Buttersworths & Co, Ltd, 1972

9

SURGICAL TREATMENT OF SUPRAVENTRICULAR ARRHYTHMIAS

Will C. Sealy

Jay G. Selle

Direct operations for supraventricular arrhythmias are now well established for patients with disabling or life-threatening symptoms that will not respond to conservative measures. The indications for surgery and a brief description of the surgical procedures will be reviewed in this chapter. The operations are considered to be direct because they divide a normal and an abnormal conduction pathway, alter normal conduction, ablate an arrhythmogenic area, or isolate the area from the remainder of the heart. Indirect operations, on the other hand, include pacemaker implantation, aneurysmectomy, coronary artery bypass, and sympathectomy.

Reentrant and automatic tachycardias occur in the supraventricular area, and both may be amenable to surgical treatment. A reentrant or circus movement tachycardia occurs only when there are two pathways of conduction with different electrophysiologic properties connected both proximally and distally. The classic example is found in patients with Wolff–Parkinson–White (WPW) syndrome, in which there are two pathways of atrioventricular (AV) conduction: the His bundle and the Kent bundle. The reentry or circus movement tachycardia is initiated by an atrial premature depolarization (Fig. 9–1). The impulse is blocked in the Kent bundle because of its long effective refractory period but excites the AV node His bundle because of its short effective refractory period. Because the impulse is normally delayed in its passage through the AV node and His bundle, the impulse arrives at the ventricular end of the Kent bundle after it has recovered its excitability. This allows the impulse

to reenter the atrium, starting the circus movement. This results in a narrow QRS tachycardia. The sinoatrial (SA) node, rarely, and the AV node, more commonly, may be the site of reentry. The normal AV node may be composed of two distinct physiologic pathways that can support a reentry tachycardia. The third circumstance is reentry that occurs in scarred areas of atrial myocardium, which usually results in atrial flutter and then fibrillation.

An automatic or focal tachycardia may be considered the manifestation, under certain circumstances, of the innate ability of all myocardial cells to depolarize spontaneously. When the depolarization rate of an atrial myocardial cell is faster than that of the sinus node, an automatic atrial tachycardia occurs. The tachycardia has characteristics similar to those of a normal sinus node taking over after a pause in that there is a warm-up at the onset of the tachycardia. The P waves are different from those in sinus rhythm. It is believed that automatic tachycardias occur only in the presence of diffuse myocarditis or myocardial scarring.

Clinical electrophysiologic studies are required before direct arrhythmia surgery can be carried out.[1] These studies, performed in the cardiac catheterization laboratory, are long and complex and require the insertion of multiple cardiac catheters carrying stimulating and sensing electrodes. The examinations will determine the exact type of tachycardia, its characteristics, the area of origin, and whether or not the arrhythmia can be controlled with medication. An important step in this evaluation is programmed stimula-

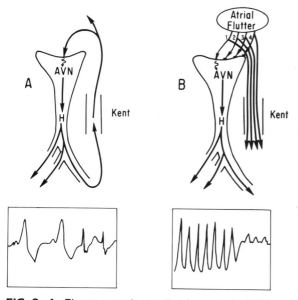

FIG. 9–1. *The two tachycardias found in WPW patients are shown.* **(A)** *Reentry type.* **(Box)** *The wide QRS of preexcitation changes to a narrow QRS during the reentry tachycardia.* **(B)** *Fast ventricular response during atrial flutter.* **(Box)** *The rhythm strip shows the rapid ventricular response progressing to ventricular fibrillation.*

tion. This is done by pacing the atria at a fixed cycle length. Then, one or more stimuli are added within the cycle at selected times after the pacing stimulus. The clinical definition of a reentry tachycardia is based on the ability to induce and revert the tachycardia with this method. Automatic tachycardias usually are not induced this way.

ARRHYTHMIAS TREATED BY OPERATION

The most frequent supraventricular arrhythmia treated by operation was described by Doctors Wolff, Parkinson, and White[2] and occurs as a part of WPW syndrome. Dr. Francis Wood[3]

sometime later found the cause to be a Kent bundle, also called as accessory pathway of AV conduction, which is the reason for a short PR interval and a wide QRS complex on the ECG. This is also called *preexcitation.* The Kent bundles are congenital anomalies and probably represent the remnants of the continuity between the atria and ventricles that is present in the embryo.[4] Thus, it is not unexpected that the fibers can be found in the septum and around the right and left free walls. There may be more than one pathway. We have divided three separate pathways in three patients.[5] The number of anatomical specimens of Kent bundles studied is not great; however, it is now well established that there may be multiple fibers of working myocardium in the bundle. Their size is 0.5 mm to 1 mm in diameter, making them invisible and not palpable.

After a review of all the reports of the anatomical studies as well as an extensive clinical experience, the following classifications have been devised for accessory pathways of the Kent type (Fig. 9–2): left free wall, right free wall, anterior septal, and posterior septal. These are illustrated in Figure 9–2. This classification has supplanted the old one, which was based on the surface ECG of type A for left-sided pathways and type B for right-sided ones. Left free wall pathways are present in about 50% of surgical patients, posterior septal in about 25%, anterior septal in 5% to 10%, and right free wall in 15%.

From an electrophysiologic point of view, the pathways nearly always exhibit the characteristics of working myocardium. Some pathways, found in 25% of patients in our surgical series, conduct a fast atrial rhythm such as occurs in flutter fibrillation one-to-one to the ventricle (see Fig. 9–1).[6] The pathways have a short effective refractory period. In contrast, about 75% of the surgical patients with pathways having a long effective refractory period have only reentry tachycardia. Among the other physiologic variations have been those that will conduct only in one direction.[7] Approximately 15% of the pa-

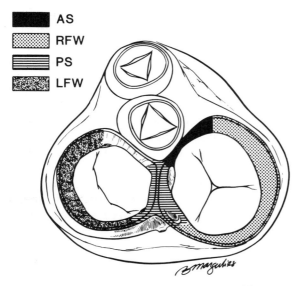

■ AS
▨ RFW
▤ PS
▨ LFW

FIG. 9–2. Classification of Kent bundles. (**AS,** anterior septal; **RFW,** right free wall; **PS,** posterior septal; **LFW,** left free wall)

tients in our series had pathways that would conduct only in a retrograde manner. Occasionally, a pathway will be found that will conduct only in an antegrade direction; obviously, a patient with this condition would still be subject to a lethal arrhythmia, provided that the pathway had a short effective refractory period. The retrograde pathways do not cause preexcitation, and for this reason they are called *concealed pathways.* Approximately 30% to 40% of reentry supraventricular tachycardias that are not associated with preexcitation are due to Kent bundles with only retrograde conduction capacity.[1]

The reason for operation in about 75% of patients with WPW syndrome is recurrent tachycardia. In others, the problem will be an episode of ventricular tachycardia or fibrillation often requiring cardiac resuscitation. In our experience there have been many harrowing incidents of this problem in young patients. Such an episode

may be the first indication that the patient has a Kent bundle. The mechanism for the atrial fibrillation and flutter, the usual cause of the problem, can be in a spontaneous episode of this arrhythmia, or it can occur in a young person after a very fast reentry tachycardia that degenerates into atrial fibrillation and flutter.

Other patients are referred for operation only because of reentry tachycardia that is resistant to treatment, or because the drugs that are needed to control it are poorly tolerated. All young patients who need daily drugs to control the tachycardia should be offered surgical treatment. The burden of a lifetime program of medication as well as the possible risk of years of drug treatment is too great to impose on a young patient. Additional congenital lesions or acquired heart disease may add to the effect of the arrhythmia, making the fast heart rate poorly tolerated. Ebstein's anomaly is found to be present in nearly 10% of patients. Hypertrophic cardiomyopathy is not an uncommon associated problem.

SURGICAL TREATMENT OF TACHYCARDIAS CAUSED BY KENT BUNDLES

The two tachycardias, the reentry and the potentially lethal one, associated with a Kent bundle can be corrected by interruption of the Kent bundle. The reentry circuit can also be interrupted by His bundle ablation. This would not correct the potentially lethal type of tachycardia. Early in our experience, some poor-risk patients were electively treated by His bundle interruption, while in others, the His bundle was interrupted when the Kent bundle could not be found.[8]

The first step in the operation for interruption of a Kent bundle is to locate the pathway. This is done by modification of the clinical electrophysiologic study called *mapping* (Fig. 9–3).[9] In brief, a stimulating and a recording electrode are placed on the atrium and on the ventricle on the side of the suspected pathway. Using a hand-

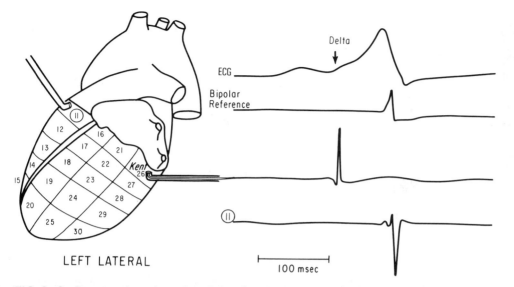

FIG. 9–3. For mapping, the epicardial surface is divided into an arbitrary grid. With a single hand-held electrode, the epicardial activation times are recorded during atrial pacing. The electrogram resulting when the pathway crosses grid square 26 on the left free wall occurs simultaneously with the delta wave on the ECG, before the bipolar reference (electrode not shown) and the electrogram at grid square 11, which is recorded at another beat.

held electrode, the activation sequence of the ventricles is plotted on an arbitrary grid. The heart rate is controlled by atrial pacing. The point of earliest activation found along the ventricular side of the coronary sulcus points to the pathway's crossing. A complete surface map is done to exclude the presence of a Mahaim fiber or other Kent bundles. Then with either ventricular pacing or during reentry tachycardia, the atrial end of the pathway is identified. Retrograde mapping may require cardiopulmonary bypass. The method requires about 15 to 20 minutes with only 4 or 5 minutes of bypass time and with relatively simple instrumentation.

The steps in interruption of left free wall pathways demonstrate the basic principles used at operation on these invisible and nonpalpable structures (Figs. 9–4 and 9–5).[10] The surgical approach is through a mediastinotomy. Mapping

is done after the patient is connected to the pump oxygenator, which is achieved using the aorta and right atrium. The aorta is cross-clamped and cardioplegia is induced. The heart is cooled and perfusion hypothermia maintained. The left atrium is opened by an atriotomy similar to that used for mitral valve replacement. The pathway's crossing point is identified within the left atrium by passing a suture through the area where the atrial end of the pathway was found. Following this, a generous incision is made 2 mm to 3 mm above the annulus fibrosus of the mitral valve, exposing the coronary sulcus fat. This includes almost all of the mitral annulus. In carrying out the dissection of the pathway after the endocardial incision, the assumption is made that the Kent bundles may originate in the atrium and pass through the ventricle, hugging the mitral annulus, or pass to the ventricle in the coro-

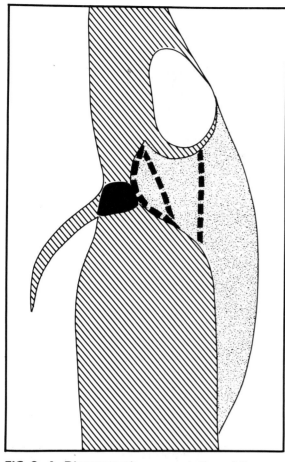

FIG. 9–4. Diagrammatic representation of the three possible courses of a left free wall from the atrium to the ventricle as follows: from the coronary sinus **(dotted line at right)**; from the atrium through the sulcus fat to the ventricle; and adjacent to the mitral annulus. The mitral valve is to the left, the atrium above, and the ventricle below.

nary sulcus fat, or it may originate from the coronary vein, which is surrounded by atrial muscle. Blunt dissection is then used to separate the fat from the atrium, the annulus fibrosus, and finally the top of the ventricle almost to the epicar-

dium. A blunt nerve hook has been found to be ideal for this purpose. Sharp dissection tends to lead the surgeon out into the sulcus fat. The myocardial surface must be kept in view at all times. The endocardial incision and then the atriotomy are carefully closed. The aortic cross-clamp time for most operations varies from 35 to 40 minutes. Exposure can be difficult because the atrial cavity is normal and thus small.

Right free wall pathways are approached in slightly different ways.[11] The right atrium is the site for both the superior and inferior catheter placement so that both cavae can be occluded. It is convenient, and perhaps just as safe, to use the aortic cross-clamping and cardioplegia for the few minutes that it takes to interrupt the pathway. The surgeon can perform a right atriotomy first and then make a wide endocardial incision centered at the pathways' crossing point, 2 mm above the tricuspid annulus. The atrial epicardium is then divided just above the coronary sulcus fat, and the fat pad is carefully separated from the atrial wall, the external aspect of the triscupid annulus, and finally down below the ventricular summit. This exposes the endocardial incision. Another method is to make the epicardial incision first, separating the atrial fat and exposing the annulus of the tricuspid valve and the ventricle. On two occasions at this stage, I have not done an atriotomy but have used cryothermia for ablation using three to five freezes. There is no great advantage in this. The two or three incisions that are made are closed with running sutures.

In anterior septal pathways, the mapping shows the site of early ventricular activation on the outflow track of the right ventricle, which may be distant from its crossing point.[12] However, on retrograde mapping, the exact crossing point of the pathway from atrium to ventricle can be easily demonstrated. The approach is by a right atriotomy. An endocardial incision is then made from above the tricuspid annulus to the

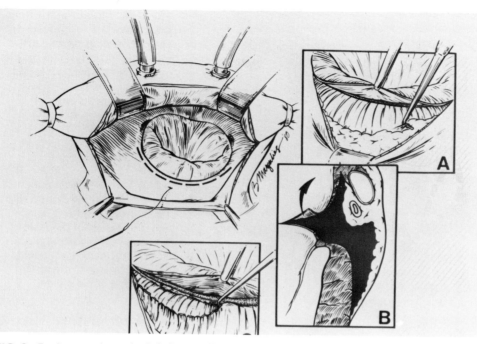

FIG. 9–5. Approach to the left free wall pathway as described in the text. **(A)** Separation of the coronary sulcus fat away from the ventricular myocardium with a blunt nerve hook. **(B)** The extent of the separation of the coronary sulcus fat from the atrium, annulus of mitral valve, and ventricle is indicated by the black area. **(*Box, bottom center*)** The interruption of the superficial fibers of the ventricular myocardium at the annulus is achieved with a sharp nerve hook.

membranous ventricular septum to divide pathways coursing adjacent to the septum (Fig. 9–6). A few fibers of the septum may be teased away. Although the maps may show that the Kent bundle is just 2 mm to 3 mm from the His bundle, the latter is protected by the right fibrous trigone. The AV node is protected by the atrial septum as shown in Figure 9–6.

Posterior septal Kent bundles are more complicated and more difficult surgical problems.[13] The cannulas for venous return are placed in the superior vena cava through the right atrium and in the inferior cava through the femoral vein. This is worth the trouble because a great advantage is gained in exposure, even though a groin incision has to be made. Identification of the crossing point of the pathway is not accurate. The early area of ventricular activation is at the crux, or just to the right or left ot it. Following a right atriotomy, an endocardial incision is made that begins beneath the orifice of the coronary sinus and extends posteriorly to the right free wall. Figure 9–6 shows the interior of the right atrial cavity and the landmarks used for the operation. The incision is then carried forward until the posterior aspect of the atrial septum is encountered at the point where it is inserted into the right fibrous trigone. This must be clearly identified

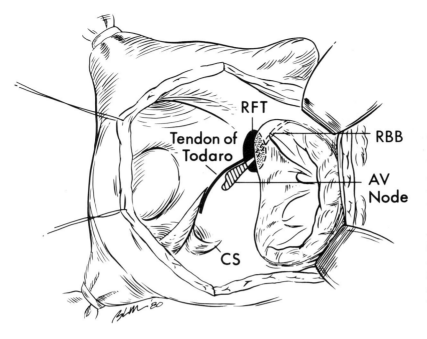

RFT

Tendon of Todaro

RBB

AV Node

CS

FIG. 9–6. *Interior of the right atrium. The anterior aspect of the right fibrous trigone* **(RFT)** *marks the posterior limit of the incision for an anterior septal pathway, whereas its posterior aspect marks anterior limits of incision for posterior septal pathways. The AV node is in the atrial septum above the RFT. The RFT and atrial septum thus protect the node and His bundle from injury. Cryothermia for AV node–His interruption is applied at the superior aspect of the membranous septal portion of the RFT. To divide the His bundle by sharp incision, the atrial septum has to be divided at the RFT.*

because the AV node is within the atrial septum. The dissection is based on the following possible crossing patterns of pathways (Fig. 9–7): adjacent to the membranous ventricular septum coursing with the His bundle, from right atrium to ventricular septum; from the atrial septum arising anywhere along its posterior course to the crux to the muscular ventricular septum; from the left atrium to the ventricular septum or from the right atrium to the ventricular septum; and lastly, from the coronary sinus and possibly from the first part posterior descending coronary vein to the ventricular septum. Following the endocardial incision, the fat in the pyramidal space on top of the muscular ventricular septum is separated from the right atrium and carried back well away from this structure. Then the dissection is carried anteriorly, where the surgeon can usually identify the artery to the AV node. This is usually not divided, but it may be, as has occurred several times without any damage to the AV node.

Then the dissection is extended toward the left, and the fat is dissected away from the undersurface of the atrial septum as it ascends posteriorly. This exposes the left atrial wall. The dissection is then carried down until the annulus of the mitral valve is clearly seen, and the fat is then dissected well away from the annulus and the left atrium. The undersurface of the coronary sinus, beginning at its orifice, is then cleared of fat. At this point, an incision is made externally through the epicardium at its junction with the atrium, crossing the crux to the left free wall. The fat is dissected from the coronary sinus, exposing the posterior descending coronary vein, which is then divided. This gives access to the right endocardial incision and exposes the pyramidal space on the summit of the muscular ventricular septum completely. The fat is carefully cleared from the undersurface of the coronary sinus, which is then reflected upward. The fat is further dissected away from the left atrial wall by exposing the

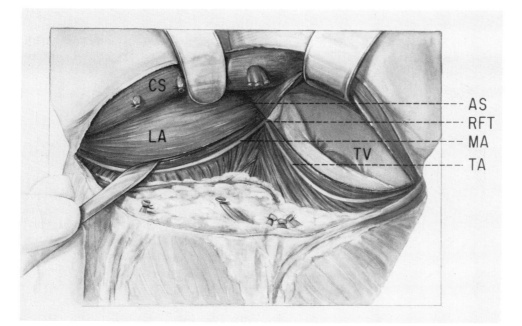

FIG. 9–7. The extent of the dissection used for interruption of posterior septal Kent bundles is shown. The incision made from the right atrial approach in the first step is shown on the right. The tricuspid valve **(TV)** can be seen. The apex of pyramidal space is shown and is the right fibrous trigone **(RFT)**. The coronary sinus **(CS)** is deflected upward and the posterior descending coronary vein is divided. An incision is shown in the left atrium **(LA)**. Now this area would be frozen. The posterior descending coronary vein is shown divided; there is no need to divide the other branches of the coronary sinus. (**MA,** mitral annulus; **TA,** tricuspid annulus; **AS,** atrial septum)

posterior portion of the muscular ventricular septum, beyond the first part of the left free wall. Formerly, in patients in whom we suspected that the pathway crossed at the junction between the free wall and the posterior septal area, we would incise the left atrium at this point. We subsequently found that cryothermia was satisfactory, with freezes being placed along the left free wall and the posterior aspect of the septal portion of the left atrium. One has to carefully identify the point at which the arial septum inserts into the right fibrous trigone. This contains the compact AV node. Although extensive, the incisions are easily closed and injury to the coronary sinus corrected by including the tears in the epicardial incisions.

OTHER METHODS

Another approach to right and left free wall pathways is that of Klein and Guiraudon and colleagues,[14] which is done without an atriotomy but with standby cardiopulmonary bypass. For left free wall pathways, the coronary sinus, the sulcus fat, and coronary artery are deflected downward, exposing the left atrium, the mitral annulus, and the top of the ventricle. Using cryothermia, the crossing point is frozen. This is similar to a method that we have reported for use in the correction of right free wall pathways.

There have been numerous case reports in which ablation of a pathway has been attempted using controlled electrical burns inflicted with an ordinary clinical defribrillator.[15-21] Unfortunately, the extent of the electrical burn is not easily controllable. When this method is used for right free wall pathways, there is a real danger of injuring the right coronary artery. The coronary sinus, the place for cautery insertion, is too high above the mitral annulus to interrupt left free wall pathways, perhaps with the exception of those that originate in the coronary sinus wall. Burns with necrosis of the epicardial surface of the coronary sinus are a hazard that precludes use of this defibrillator method beyond the orifice of the sinus.

RESULTS OF SURGERY FOR WOLFF – PARKINSON – WHITE SYNDROME

The risk of operation to correct the tachycardias associated with Kent bundles is similar to that associated with any open-heart operation plus the increased risk in the few patients who have associated heart diseases. The latter may make the operation mandatory. Beginning with the first reported successful case, the mortality in the patients that we have been associated with, which now number nearly 300, has been less than 3%. In the last 100 patients, mortality has been 1%. The deaths, with two exceptions, usually have been of patients with associated cardiac problems such as hypertrophic cardiomyopathy or coronary artery disease. In the last 100 patients, there was one AV node His bundle injury following reoperation in a patient with an anterior septal pathway. In a second patient, the

His and Kent bundles coursed so close together that both had to be divided. Additional operations have been necessary for two patients with posterior septal pathways. All right and left free wall operations have been successful.

OTHER SUPRAVENTRICULAR ARRHYTHMIAS

The most common site of origin of a supraventricular reentry tachycardia, exclusive of those due to Kent bundles, is in the AV node. In Josephson's series, 58% of 150 patients had reentry in the AV node; some of these 150 patients had Kent bundles with only retrograde function.[1] The explanation for the AV nodal reentry tachycardia is that there are two separate electrophysiologic pathways, a slow one and a fast one, within the node. Under certain circumstances, this difference widens, and the pathways become able to support a reentry circuit. The tachycardia can be induced by a premature depolarization. Although drugs will nearly always control AV nodal reentry tachycardia, occasionally there are patients in whom these drugs are not effective or cannot be tolerated. The arrhythmia can be treated by His bundle interruption, which is an operation of last resort.[22] Perhaps there will be other less drastic methods devised to correct this problem. In one case, the partial division of the approaches to the compact AV node resulted in correction of an AV nodal reentry tachycardia.[23] For the future, it is expected that a precise incision with a knife will be required instead of the imprecise approach that results when either cryothermia or electrical burns are used.

Mahaim fibers, which are accessory conduction pathways connecting either the AV node or penetrating His bundle to the ventricle, may support a reentry tachycardia. Recently, German and associates have successfully interrupted conduction over the His bundle with an electrical burn and preserved the AV conduction over what was believed to be a Mahaim fiber.[24]

ENHANCED AV NODE CONDUCTION

Enhanced conduction through the AV node becomes surgically important when atrial tachycardia is conducted through the AV node at a rapid rate. The definition for enhanced AV node conduction includes the following: an atrial-to-His-bundle conduction time of 60 msec or less, one-to-one atrial-to-His-bundle conduction at pacing rates of 200 beats or more per minute, and failure of atrial-to-His-bundle interval to lengthen more than 100 msec over the value recorded during sinus rhythm at the shortest cycle length associated with one-to-one conduction. Castellanos and associates have offered several explanations for this problem and have stressed the point that occasionally a patient will develop ventricular fibrillation with atrial fibrillation.[25] In our clinical experience, most patients with supraventricular tachycardia needing AV-conduction interruption have had associated heart disease, such as cardiomyopathy or mitral valve disease. The arrhythmia must be both intolerable and uncontrollable.

Interruption of the His bundle is considered to be a direct operation because the His bundle interruption effectively isolates an arrhythmogenic area; in this instance, the atria is separated from electrical continuity with the ventricle. It substitutes a controllable ventricular rate and rhythm at the expense of sacrificing the physiologic effect of the "atrial kick." The methods used for atrial ventricular conduction interruption have undergone an interesting evolutionary process. Cardiologists now do most of the His bundle interruptions, although they may describe the operation as interventional cardiology or label the procedure as the nonpharmacologic therapy for arrhythmia.[26] Before transvenous His bundle

interruption was introduced, surgical attempts through an atriotomy included incision, suture ligation, and cautery. None of these was uniformly successful. Interruption of AV conduction by division of the penetrating His bundle at its junction with the AV node was employed next. This requires the division of the atrial septum as it is inserted into the central fibrous body. This is the only certain way, by surgical incision, of dividing the AV node His bundle. It is now rarely used, but there is a 10% failure rate with transvenous cauterization and cryothermia by way of atriotomy.

The next step was the use of cryothermia through right atriotomy.[27] The identification of the His bundle is done with the mapping probe. Three freezes are then applied to the area where the atrial deflection is the greatest, with care being taken not to extend it to the lower membranous septum to avoid the branching His bundle. This results in a junctional rhythm with a relatively short escape time and a rate of somewhere between 40 and 50 beats per minute. The results were successful in over 90% of the cases.

Recently, Scheinman and colleagues and Gallagher and his group have demonstrated the successful use of transvenous cauterization of the area containing the His bundle using equipment commonly employed for external cardiac defibrillation.[28-30] Guided by the usual method of His bundle identification, the electrode-bearing catheter is positioned over this area, usually where the greatest atrial deflection is associated with the His deflection. Then 200 joules of current is usually passed through the catheter. The second electrode is placed in the middle of the posterior thorax. Sometimes more than one shock is used, and an electrical burn results. Experimental studies showing the extent of injury caused by the electrical current have appeared in the literature.[31,32,34,35] In dogs an injury has been fairly well localized when the His bundle has been the object of electrical burn. When the left ventricle has been burned, the damage is extensive. At present, reports describing the use of this method in patients show that it has not been associated with any severe complications. The success rate for His bundle ablation is approximately 80% to 90%.

AUTOMATIC ATRIAL TACHYCARDIAS

Surprisingly enough, case reports describing successful operations for automatic atrial tachycardias are constantly appearing.[36-43] These have included excision of the right atrial appendage, catheter cauterization, ablation with cryothermia of an arrhythmogenic area, and exclusion of most of the left atrium from the right. Ott and colleagues have reported operations on eleven patients with nine successes.[40] Electrophysiologic study before operation has localized the area in most patients, although intraoperative mapping during persistent tachycardias has been possible.

Junctional tachycardia in infancy may be uncontrollable and lethal. This has been treated by Gillette and colleagues using transcatheter His bundle ablation of the AV node His bundle junction.[44]

SUMMARY

The place of surgery is now firmly established for treating a variety of drug-refractory supraventricular tachycardias and for the two tachycardias caused by Kent bundles. The operations are frequently done by cardiologists. Their participation is very likely to increase as more controlled methods of electrical burns and a practical method of intracardiac catheter control of laser energy are devised. A need exists for surgical studies of the atrial septum in the region of the AV node, because it is in the approaches to the compact AV node, an ill-defined anatomical area, that the exciting events occur in the AV node. Perhaps an alteration of this area with a cataract knife rather than the area destruction that occurs with an electrical burn or freezing would preserve AV conduction yet correct nodal reentry or enhanced conduction.

REFERENCES

1. Josephson ME, Seides SF: Clinical Cardiac Electrophysiology. Philadelphia, Lea & Febiger, 1984
2. Wolff L, Parkinson J, White PD: Bundle branch block with short P-R interval in healthy young people prone to paroxysmal tachycardia. Am Heart J 5:685, 1930
3. Wood FC, Wolferth CC, Geckeler GD: Histologic demonstration of accessory muscular connections between auricle and ventricle in a case of short P-R interval and prolonged QRS complex. Am Heart J 25:454, 1943
4. Truex RC, Bishof JK, Hoffman EL: Accessory atrioventricular bundles of the developing human heart. Anat Rec 131:45, 1958
5. Sealy WC, Gallagher JJ: Surgical problems with multiple accessory pathways of antrioventricular conduction. J Thorac Cardiovasc Surg 81:707, 1981
6. Dreifus LS, Haiat R, Watanabe Y et al: Ventricular fibrillation: A possible mechanism of sudden death in patients with Wolff–Parkinson–White Syndrome. Circulation 43:520, 1971
7. Sealy WC: Surgical treatment of the two types of tachycardia caused by Kent bundles with only retrograde function. J Thorac Cardiovasc Surg 85:746, 1983
8. Sealy WC: His bundle interruption for re-entry tachycardia in Wolff–Parkinson–White Syndrome. Ann Thorac Surg 36:345, 1983
9. Gallagher JJ, Sealy WC, Kasell J: Intraoperative mapping studies in the Wolff–Parkinson–White Syndrome. PACE 2:523, 1979
10. Sealy WC, Gallagher JJ: Surgical treatment of left free wall accessory pathways of atrioventricular conduction of the Kent type. J Thorac Cardiovasc Surg 81:698, 1981
11. Sealy WC: The evolution of the surgical methods for interruption of right free wall Kent bundles. Ann Thorac Surg 36:29, 1983
12. Sealy WC: Kent bundles in the anterior septal space. Ann Thorac Surg 36:180, 1983

13. Sealy WC, Mikat EM: Anatomical problems with identification and interruption of posterior septal Kent bundles. Ann Thorac Surg 36:584, 1983

14. Klein GJ, Guiraudon GM, Perkins DG et al: Surgical correction of the Wolff–Parkinson–White Syndrome in the closed heart using cryosurgery: A simplified approach. J Am Coll Cardiol 3:405, 1984

15. Fisher JD, Brodman R, Kim SG, Matos JA: Wolff–Parkinson–White Syndrome: Nonsurgical Kent bundle ablation via the coronary sinus (abstr). PACE 6:148, 1983

16. Brodman R, Fisher JD: Evaluation of a catheter technique for ablation of accessory pathways near the coronary sinus using a canine model. Circulation 67:923, 1983

17. Weber H, Schmitz L: Catheter technique for closed-chest ablation of an accessory atrioventricular pathway. N Engl J Med 308:653, 1983

18. Critelli G, Perticone F, Coltorti F et al: Antegrade slow bypass conduction after closed-chest ablation of the His bundle in permanent junctional reciprocating tachycardia. Circulation 67:687, 1983

19. Bardy GH, Poole JE, Coltorti F et al: Catheter ablation of a concealed accessory pathway. Am J Cardiol 54:1366, 1984

20. Morady F, Scheinman MM: Transvenous catheter ablation of a posteroseptal accessory pathway in a patient with the Wolff–Parkinson–White Syndrome. N Engl J Med 310:705, 1984

21. Critelli G, Gallagher JJ, Perticone F et al: Transvenous catheter ablation of the accessory atrioventricular pathway in the permanent form of junctional reciprocating tachycardia. Am J Cardiol 55:1639, 1985

22. Sealy WC, Gallagher JJ, Kasell J: His bundle interruption for control of inappropriate ventricular responses to atrial arrhythmias. Ann Thorac Surg 32:429, 1981

23. Pritchett ELC, Anderson RW, Benditt DG et al: Re-entry within the atrioventricular node: Surgical cure with preservation of atrioventricular conduction. Case report. Circulation 60:440, 1979

24. Ellenbogen KA, O'Callaghan WG, Colavita PG et al: Catheter atrioventricular junction ablation for recurrent supraventricular tachycardia with nodoventricular fibers. Am J Cardiol 55:1227, 1985

25. Castellanos A, Zaman L, Luceri RM, Myerburg RJ: Arrhythmias in patients with short P-R and narrow QRS complexes. In Josephson ME, Wellens HJJ: Tachycardia: Mechanisms, Diagnosis, Treatment, chap 7. Philadelphia, Lea & Febiger, 1984

26. Gallagher JJ, Cox JL, German LD, Kasell JH: Non-pharmacologic treatment of supraventricular tachycardia. In Josephson ME, Wellens HJJ: Tachycardia: Mechanisms, Diagnosis, Treatment, chap 12. Philadelphia, Lea & Febiger, 1984

27. Harrison L, Gallagher JJ, Kassel J: Cryosurgical ablation of the AV node-His bundle: A new method for producing AV block. Circulation 55:463, 1977

28. Scheinman MM, Morady F, Hess DS, Gonzalez R: Catheter induced ablation of the atrioventricular junction to control refractory supraventricular arrhythmia. JAMA 248:851, 1982

29. Scheinman MM, Evans–Bell T, and The Executive Committee of the Percutaneous Cardiac Mapping and Ablation Registry: Catheter ablation of the atrioventricular junction: A report of the percutaneous mapping and ablation registry. Circulation 70:1024, 1984

30. Gallagher JJ et al: Catheter technique for closed-chest ablation of the atrioventricular conduction system: A therapeutic alternative for the treatment of refractory supraventricular tachycardia. N Engl J Med 306:194, 1982

31. Coltorti F, Bardy GH, Reichenbach D et al: Catheter-mediated electrical ablation of the posterior septum via the coronary sinus: Electrophysiologic and histologic observations in dogs. Circulation 72:612, 1985

32. Westveer DC, Nelson T, Stewart JR et al: Sequelae of left ventricular electrical endocardial ablation. J Am Col Cardiol 5:956, 1985

33. Critelli G, Gallagher JJ, Thiene G et al: Hisologic observations after closed chest ablation of the atrioventricular conduction system. JAMA 252:2604, 1984

34. Lee BI, Gottdiener JS, Fletcher RD et al: Transcatheter ablation: Comparison between laser photoablation and electrode shock ablation in the dog. Circulation 71:579, 1985

35. Bardy GH, Ideker RE, Kasell J et al: Transvenous ablation of the atrioventricular conduction system in dogs: Electrophysiologic and histologic observations. Am J Cardiol 51:1775, 1983

36. Anderson KP, Stinson EB, Mason JW: Surgical excision of focal paroxysmal atrial tachycardia. Am J Cardiol 49:869, 1983

37. Marquez–Montes J. Rufilanchas JJ, Esteve JJ: Paroxysmal nodal reentrant tachycardia: Surgical cure with preservation of atrioventricular conduction. Chest 83:690, 1983

38. Olsson SB, Blomstrom P, Sabel KG, William–Olsson G: Incessant ectopic atrial tachycardia: Successful surgical treatment with regression of dilated cardiomyopathy picture. Am J Cardiol 53:1465, 1984

39. Yee R, Guiraudon GM, Gardner MJ et al: Refractory paroxysmal sinus tachycardia: Management by subtotal right atrial exclusion. J Am Coll Cardiol 3:400, 1984

40. Ott DA, Gillette PC, Garson A, Jr et al: Surgical manage-

ment of refractory supraventricular tachycardia in infants and children. J Am Coll Cardiol 5:124, 1985

41. Silka MJ, Gillette PC, Garson A, Jr, Zinner A: Transvenous catheter ablation of a right atrial automatic ectopic tachycardia. J Am Coll Cardiol 5:999, 1985

42. Smith DK, Holman WL, Cox JL: Surgical treatment of supraventricular tachycadia. Surg Clin N Am 65:553, 1985

43. Iwa T, Ichihashi T, Hashizume Y et al: Successful surgical treatment of left atrial tachycardia. Am Heart J 109:160, 1985

44. Gillette PC, Garson A, Jr, Coburn JP: Junctional automatic ectopic tachycardia: New proposed treatment by transcatheter His bundle ablation. Am Heart J 106:619, 1983

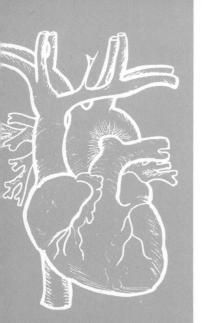

10

PERIOPERATIVE CORONARY ARTERY SPASM

Alfred E. Buxton

Coronary vasospasm has been implicated in the pathogenesis of multiple manifestations of acute myocardial ischemia, including angina at rest (both stable and unstable), exertional angina, sudden cardiac death, and myocardial infarction. The degree of ischemia resulting from acute spasm may be so mild that symptoms do not appear, or it may be severe enough to result in hemodynamic collapse. Recently, coronary artery spasm has been suggested as one cause of perioperative myocardial infarction and death following myocardial revascularization.[1-3] We have observed perioperative coronary artery spasm in nine patients following saphenous vein bypass grafting for fixed atherosclerotic ischemic heart disease.

We based the diagnosis of coronary artery spasm on the following criteria: reversible, transient ST-segment elevation of at least 2 mm in one or more ECG leads; and absence of significant (>60% reduction in diameter) atherosclerotic obstruction of the coronary artery supplying the ischemic area.

We observed nine cases of perioperative coronary spasm over 24 months.* This represented a 1% incidence of perioperative spasm at our institution in patients undergoing myocardial revascularization. These episodes occurred between 1978 and 1980 *before* calcium channel blockers

* The author acknowledges the collaboration of the members of the cardiothoracic surgery and cardiovascular sections of the Hospital of the University of Pennsylvania in the care of these patients.

and parenteral preparations of nitroglycerin had been released for general medical use. Over the 4½ years since the last reported case occurred, we have not observed any further symptomatic episodes. Although others have reported isolated cases of perioperative coronary vasospasm, we are aware of no other data regarding the prevalence of this condition.[1,2,4-7]

The purpose of this chapter is to describe the clinical manifestations, acute and chronic management, and long-term consequences of perioperative coronary artery spasm.

CLINICAL CHARACTERISTICS OF PATIENTS

Detailed case histories for six of the nine patients have been published previously.[2,8] Pertinent preoperative clinical characteristics and perioperative findings appear in Tables 10–1, 10–2, and 10–3. The nine patients ranged in age from 38 to 76 years, and there was an equal distribution among males and females. Six of the patients presented with exertional angina, and six had angina at rest. All but one of the patients (case 1) had an unstable pattern of angina; even those presenting with exertional angina only had rapidly progressing symptoms. Two patients had variant angina (episodes of rest angina associated with ST-segment elevation) and were strongly suspected of having coronary artery spasm prior to surgery. However, the five patients who un-

TABLE 10–1
PREOPERATIVE CHARACTERISTICS OF PATIENTS WITH PERIOPERATIVE CORONARY SPASM

Patient No.	Age (years)	Sex	Symptoms	Exercise Test	Preoperative Angiography	Ventriculogram	Preoperative Medication	
							Propranolol	Nitroglycerin
1	67	Male	Exertional angina X 3 yr	+ angina; 5 mm inferior and anterior ST depression	90% obstruction LMCA; 60% obstruction RCA; collaterals RCA to LAD	ND	80 mg/day	
2	53	Female	Rest angina with inferior ST elevation X 4 yr, exertional angina X 4 yr	Normal	80% obstruction LAD; RCA spasm in response to cold pressor test	Normal; EF = 57%		+
3	55	Female	Rest angina X 5 wk associated with anterior ST elevation	ND	95% obstruction LAD; cold pressor test negative	Normal; EF = 65%	120 mg/day	+
4	39	Female	Rest angina X 4 wk	ND	90% obstruction LMCA; 99% obstruction LAD; 90% LCFX	Normal, EF = 69%	80 mg/day	+
5	54	Male	Exertional angina X 1 yr	+ angina; 2-mm ST depression lateral leads; anteroseptal reversible thallium defect	Normal	240 mg/day	+
6	52	Male	Rest and exertional angina	+ angina; anterior reversible thallium defect	90% obstruction LAD; 70% obstruction diagonal artery	Normal; EF = 76%	80 mg/day	+
7	55	Male	Exertional angina X 2 wk	+ angina; 3-mm anterior ST depression	90% obstruction LMCA; 70% obstruction diagonal artery; 50% obstruction RCA	ND	80 mg/day	+
8	38	Female	Exertional and rest angina	ND	50% obstruction LMCA; 100% obstruction LAD; 50% obstruction RCA	Normal; EF = 75%		+
9	76	Female	Postinfarction rest angina (non-Q wave anterior MI)	ND	99% obstruction LAD	Apical akinesis; EF = 78%	80 mg/day	+

Abbreviations: ND, not done; LMCA, left main coronary artery; LAD, left anterior descending artery; LCFX, left circumflex artery; RCA, right coronary artery; EF, left ventricular ejection fraction.

119

most have
1 or 2 grafts!

TABLE 10–2
OPERATIVE PROCEDURES IN PATIENTS WITH PERIOPERATIVE
CORONARY SPASM

Patient No.	Anesthesia	No. of Grafts	Vessels Grafted
1	N$_2$O, halothane	2	LAD RCA
2	Unknown	2	LAD PDA
3	N$_2$O, halothane	1	LAD
4	N$_2$O, halothane	2	LAD LCFX
5	N$_2$O, halothane	2	LAD LCFX
6	Fentanyl	2	LAD Diagonal
7	Fentanyl	3	LAD Diagonal LCFX
8	N$_2$O, halothane	2	LAD LCFX
9	N$_2$O, halothane	1	LAD

Abbreviations: PDA, posterior descending artery. See other abbreviations listed in footnote to Table 10–1.

derwent preoperative exercise stress tests all had markedly positive results, consistent with myocardial ischemia resulting from fixed atherosclerotic coronary obstruction. Fixed obstructive disease in the left coronary system was confirmed in each case by the preoperative coronary angiograms. The two patients (cases 2 and 3) with documented or suspected variant angina underwent provocative testing for coronary artery spasm at the time of their preoperative catheterizations. The cold pressor test provoked coronary spasm in one of these two patients. Other than cases 2 and 3, there was no clinical suspicion prior to surgery that coronary artery spasm played a role in these patients' symptoms, nor was there any clue that they should have a pre-

disposition to developing perioperative coronary artery spasm.

The operative procedures were performed by a total of four different cardiac surgeons, but methods of anesthesia and cardioplegia were similar in all cases. General anesthesia was given, using either a combination of nitrous oxide and halothane, or fentanyl. All revascularization procedures were performed under systemic hypothermia (26°C to 30°C) and cold cardioplegic arrest (4°C, 20 mEq potassium/liter). Patients received between one and three saphenous vein bypass grafts. Only one patient (case 1) received a graft to the right coronary artery. In all other cases, grafts were restricted to the left coronary system (see Table 10–2).

TABLE 10–3
IMMEDIATE POSTOPERATIVE COURSE OF PATIENTS WITH PERIOPERATIVE CORONARY SPASM

Patient No.	Postbypass Hypertension Prior to Onset of Spasm	Time from End of Bypass to Onset of Spasm	Observations During Spasm			Treatment of Spasm	Peak Postoperative Serum CK (Day of Peak)	ECG Done 1 Week Postoperatively	Outcome
			Hypotension	AV Block	Ventricular Arrhythmias				
1	—	1 hr	+	—	—	Resumption of CPB; insertion of IABP, IV—NIG, nifedipine, epinephrine, isoproterenol	—	—	Death
2	—	.5 hr	+	—	—	SVG to RCA; IABP, IV—NIG	—	—	Death
3	—	Transient 2. hr; Sustained 2.5 hr	+	—	—	Open chest cardiac massage, IV—NIG, nitroprusside, phenotlamine isoproterenol, nifedipine	—	—	Death
4	+	2 hr	+	+	VT	IC and IV NIG, nifedipine	4014 (2)	Diffuse T wave inversions	Recovery
5	—	5 hr	+	+	—	TC—nitroprusside, IABP nifedipine; IV—NIG	15,100 (4)	New inferior Q waves	Recovery
6	+	1.5 hr	+	+	VT	IV—NIG, nifedipine phentolamine	526 (1)	Nonspecific ST–T abnormality	Recovery
7	+	2 hr	+	—	—	IV—NIG, nifedipine, phentolamine	491 (day of surgery)	Nonspecific ST–T abnormality	Recovery
8	—	1.5 hr	+	—	—	IV—NIG, nifedipine, dopamine	709 (2)	New inferior Q waves	Recovery
9	+	2 hr	—	—	—	IV—NIG, nifedipine	153 (1)	New inverior Q waves	Recovery

Abbreviations: CPB, cardiopulmonary bypass; IABP, intra-aortic balloon pump; IV, intravenous; IC, intracoronary; NIG, nitroglycerin; SVG, saphenous vein graft; CK, creatine kinase; VT, ventricular tachycardia.

121

MANIFESTATIONS OF PERIOPERATIVE SPASM

Cardiopulmonary bypass was terminated successfully in all patients. In four cases, postoperative systemic arterial hypertension requiring therapy with trimethaphan or nitroprusside developed (see Table 10-3). Thirty to 200 minutes after initial termination of bypass, all patients developed inferior ST-segment elevation. The duration of episodes of ST-segment elevation ranged from 10 minutes (cases 3 and 9) to as long as 5 hours. In all but one case (case 9), ST-segment elevation was associated with sudden marked systemic hypotension (systolic blood pressure <90 mm Hg). In addition, transient atrioventricular conduction block occurred in three patients, and paroxysms of ventricular tachycardia and fibrillation developed in two patients (Fig. 10-1).

TREATMENT OF PERIOPERATIVE SPASM

Hypotension was resistant to standard therapy with fluids and catecholamines in all cases (see Table 10-3). Three patients developed spasm while still in the operating room, and in each case, cardiopulmonary bypass was reinstituted. However, evidence of spasm recurred soon after multiple attempts to discontinue cardiopulmonary bypass in all three patients. Ancillary supportive measures included institution of intra-aortic balloon counterpulsation in three patients, phentolamine in three patients, and nifedipine in all. No definite beneficial effect was apparent from any of these measures, although in two patients spasm did not recur after administration of phentolamine.

All patients received intravenous nitroglycerin, without clear-cut beneficial effect. Two patients (cases 4 and 5) with persistent and recur-

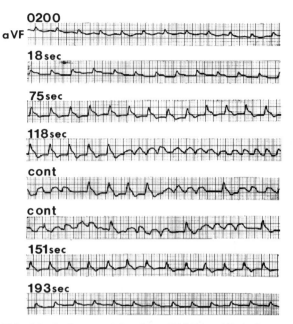

FIG. 10-1. Sequential strips of ECG lead II during postoperative spasm. As ST-segment elevation reaches a maximum, as shown in the strip obtained at 118 seconds after the onset of the episode of spasm, multiple episodes of polymorphic ventricular tachycardia occur, which abate as the ST segments return to baseline.

rent spasm associated with total hemodynamic collapse were given massive doses of intracoronary nitroglycerin (37 mg and 8 mg, respectively) before episodes of coronary spasm abated. Intracoronary nitroglycerin was administered in the catheterization laboratory in one of these patients, who first developed spasm in the surgical intensive care unit postoperatively. Coronary angiography prior to administration of intracoronary nitroglycerin confirmed the diagnosis of coronary vasospasm in this patient. The second patient developed spasm while in the operating room, and intracoronary nitroglycerin was administered through a 26-gauge needle inserted directly into the proximal right coronary artery.

Following resolution of clinical and electrocardiographic evidence of spasm, the survivors were placed on intravenous nitroglycerin, which was tapered slowly after 24 hours. In addition, all survivors were given nifedipine orally.

OUTCOME

The first three patients with coronary spasm in this series died of hemodynamic collapse caused by refractory coronary vasospasm. The hypotension in each of these cases occurred in the presence of sinus rhythm. An autopsy performed in case I showed no evidence of acute myocardial infarction and confirmed the presence of severe atherosclerotic lesions in the left coronary system. However, the right coronary artery lesion only decreased the lumenal diameter by 40%, rather than the 60% predicted angiographically prior to surgery.

None of the six survivors of the acute episode had recurrent angina, either in the early postoperative period or during long-term follow-up. Peak postoperative serum creatine kinase levels ranged from 153 to 15,100 (peaks occurred on the day of surgery to 4 days after surgery) in the survivors (see Table 10–3). Electrocardiographic changes following surgery included new inferior Q waves in three patients, diffuse T-wave inversions in one patient, and new nonspecific ST–T wave abnormalities in two patients.

LATE POSTOPERATIVE COURSE

Nifedipine was continued chronically in the six survivors for 3 to 12 months after surgery. Five patients were admitted to the hospital for reevaluation at that time (one patient refused restudy and continued to receive nifedipine). Under continuous electrocardiographic monitoring, nifedipine was discontinued. After 48 hours of moni-

toring, no patient had evidence of spontaneous recurrent coronary artery spasm, and all underwent cardiac catheterization with provocative testing. Hemodynamic measurements during catheterization were within normal limits and were unchanged from preoperative values in three patients. Two patients showed mild increases in the left ventricular end diastolic pressure to 18 mm Hg. One patient demonstrated an increase in right ventricular filling pressure (11 mm Hg) in addition to the increase in left ventricular filling pressure. Left ventricular ejection fractions calculated from the single-plane angiogram ranged from 47% to 77%, and all but one patient had new areas of inferior-wall hypokinesis. One patient had new anterior hypokinesis in addition to inferior hypokinesis (he had an episode of anterior ECG ST-segment elevation following the initial ST-segment elevation). All patients had patent saphenous vein grafts, and the right coronary artery remained unchanged from the appearance on the preoperative angiogram in all. Ergonovine maleate provocative testing (total of 0.2 mg) failed to provoke spasm in four patients. In one patient focal narrowing occurred at a 50% fixed lesion in the right coronary artery. However, no chest pain or electrocardiographic evidence of spasm was observed. The five patients who underwent catheterization remained off nifedipine and have had no clinical evidence of recurrent coronary spasm to date.

COMMENT

Coronary vasospasm is most often recognized when it causes the syndrome of variant (Prinzmetal's) angina, which is angina occurring at rest with ST-segment elevation. However, myocardial ischemia caused by coronary artery spasm may be expressed in a number of ways, ranging from Stokes–Adams attacks due to bradyarrhythmias to myocardial infarction resulting from prolonged ischemia, or sudden cardiac death as a result of ventricular fibrillation.[9-13] Our experience and that of others demonstrate one other setting in which coronary artery spasm may occur, that is, following myocardial revascularization procedures.[1-8] In this setting, it is important to note that coronary artery spasm may occur in patients with and without preoperative histories of variant angina. The manifestations of coronary artery spasm occurring after revascularization ranged from asymptomatic electrocardiographic changes to total hemodynamic collapse.

MECHANISMS UNDERLYING PERIOPERATIVE SPASM

The mechanisms underlying coronary artery spasm are not well understood at present. Although alterations in autonomic nervous system tone have been implicated frequently, evidence supporting their role is conflicting. For example, while increases in α-adrenergic tone may provoke coronary spasm, attempts to use prophylaxis against spontaneous episodes of spasm with α-adrenergic blockers have failed.[17-25] In addition, there is no evidence that a generalized increase in sympathetic nervous system function is present in patients with spontaneous episodes of spasm.[26] However, selective increases in discharge of some sympathetic nerve endings have been implicated, as have alterations in the balance between sympathetic and parasympathetic tone.[19,27] However, cardiac denervation may not prevent coronary vasospasm.[28]

Among the factors known to be capable of increasing coronary vascular resistance and provoking coronary spasm, many may be present in the perioperative period. Among these factors are increases in blood pH, cutaneous cold, α-adrenergic stimulation, and physical manipulation of coronary arteries.[29-32] In some cases, the balance between release of vasoconstrictor sub-

stances by platelets and release of vasodilators by the vascular endothelium may play a role.[33-35] It is intriguing that other manifestations of increased α-adrenergic activity such as systemic arterial hypertension frequently occur after myocardial revascularization.[36] Four patients in this series manifested arterial hypertension prior to the onset of spasm after cardiopulmonary bypass. Whether these two potential manifestations of increased sympathetic nervous system activity were related in these patients is unknown. Three patients were given phentolamine as part of their therapy, and in two, evidence of spasm abated after this drug was given. Because these patients received multiple therapies, it is difficult to know what role phentolamine played in terminating spasm.

A review of operative records failed to reveal any unique features of surgical procedures used in these patients that could permit us to identify why spasm developed. There was no difference in the methods of myocardial preservation or choice of anesthetic agents between these patients and others having surgery at the same time who did not develop spasm. The blood pH in these patients was not markedly alkalotic prior to developing spasm. Although physical manipulation of a coronary artery may provoke spasm, only one of nine patients had any direct manipulation by a saphenous vein graft to this vessel. Animal experiments have shown that reperfusion of the left coronary artery may result in a spinal sympathetic reflex.[37,38] Perhaps reperfusion using bypass grafts can trigger such a reflex in humans. If so, the increase in sympathetic tone might be enough to provoke coronary spasm in patients who are predisposed. However, this still does not explain why these nine patients in particular developed coronary spasm.

It is noteworthy that two of these nine patients had variant angina, which could have been provoked by coronary spasm prior to surgery. It appears that patients who have coronary spasm prior to surgery have a higher incidence of perioperative infarction and death and a lower operative success rate than do patients undergoing myocardial revascularization for fixed atherosclerotic lesions without histories suggestive of coronary spasm.[39-42] Perioperative myocardial infarction rates as high as 50% have been noted by other researchers when patients with variant angina undergo saphenous vein bypass grafting. Thus, there appears to be something "spasmogenic" about coronary artery bypass grafting that is especially likely to be expressed in patients with histories of variant angina. However, it is clear that this problem may develop in patients without any preoperative suggestion of a predisposition toward developing coronary artery spasm.

INCIDENCE OF PERIOPERATIVE SPASM

As noted above, the nine cases of perioperative coronary artery spasm that we observed were clustered over a 2-year period. Over the 4½ years since the last case occurred, we have not seen any clinically significant episodes. This dramatic decline appears to be the result of several factors. Shortly after the last of these cases was observed, calcium channel blockers became available for general clinical use. Today, most patients undergoing coronary bypass grafting for severe and unstable angina, as was the case with these patients, are receiving calcium channel blocking agents up until the time of surgery. Some effect of these agents may persist through the perioperative period, counteracting a tendency to develop spasm. A second and possibly more important factor is the availability of parenteral nitroglycerin preparations. Nitroglycerin for intravenous use did not become readily available until after the onset of this cluster of cases. After we observed these cases, our anesthesiologists became attuned to the possibility of coronary spasm occurring in the operating room and in the surgical intensive care unit immediately following surgery. The anesthesiologists developed a reflex to administer intravenous nitroglycerin promptly when any significant alteration in the appearance of the ST segments in the operating room occurred. It seems likely that systemic (intravenous) administration of nitroglycerin before systemic hypotension develops may prove to be more effective than when therapy is delayed. This approach may abort episodes of coronary artery spasm in the early stages that would otherwise develop into significant clinical problems.

RECOGNITION AND MANAGEMENT: IMPLICATIONS FOR THE PRACTITIONER

Our experience with this series of patients has shown that coronary vasospasm must be considered in the differential diagnosis of sudden hemodynamic collapse in patients following coronary artery bypass grafting. Even if ECG monitoring of a postoperative patient shows normal sinus rhythm in the presence of cardiovascular collapse, multiple standard ECG leads should be recorded because ST-segment elevation may occur in only a limited number of leads. If ST-segment elevation is recognized in this setting and if the vessel that serves the ischemic segment does not have significant obstructive lesions prior to surgery, the diagnosis of coronary spasm should be entertained and therapy with intravenous nitroglycerin instituted promptly. Recognition of the cause of hypotension is important because standard measures such as catecholamine and volume administration, or intra-aortic balloon counterpulsation will not reverse hypotension during severe episodes of spasm. Therapy must be directed toward the primary abnormality. If systemic administration of nitroglycerin does not reverse the evidence of spasm, intracoronary nitroglycerin should be administered, either directly if the patient's chest is still open in the operating room or by way of coronary catheters in the catheterization laboratory. Such therapy may reverse otherwise refractory and life-threatening spasm. Finally, the use of calcium channel blockers, especially as they become available in parenteral form, may prove to be a valuable form of adjunctive therapy to nitrates for acute reversal of coronary vasospasm.

REFERENCES

1. Pichard AD, Ambrose J, Mindich B et al: Coronary artery spasm and perioperative cardiac arrest. J Thorac Cardiovasc Surg 80:249–254, 1980
2. Tanimoto Y, Matsuda Y, Kobayashi Y et al: Coronary spasm as a cause of perioperative myocardial infarction. Jpn Heart J 25:275–281, 1984
3. Buxton AE, Goldberg S, Harken A et al: Coronary-artery spasm immediately after myocardial revascularization — recognition and management. N Engl J Med 304:1249–1253, 1981
4. Kopf GS, Riba A, Zito R: Intraoperative use of nifedipine for hemodynamic collapse due to coronary artery spasm following myocardial revascularization. Ann Thorac Surg 34:457–460, 1982
5. Zeff RH, Iannone LA, Kongtahworn C et al: Coronary artery spasm following coronary artery revascularization. Ann Thorac Surg 34:196–200, 1982
6. Cohen DJ, Foley RW, Ryan JM: Intraoperative coronary artery spasm successfully treated with nitroglycerin and nifedipine. Ann Thorac Surg 36:97–100, 1983
7. Zingone B, Salvi A, Branchini B: Perioperative coronary artery spasm leading to myocardial ischaemia after vein graft surgery. Br Heart J 49:280–283, 1983
8. Buxton AE, Hirshfeld JW, Jr, Untereker WJ et al: Perioperative coronary arterial spasm: Long-term follow-up. Am J Cardiol 50:444–451, 1982
9. Bashour T: Cardiac rhythm disorders complicating coronary artery spasm. Clin Cardiol 7:510–512, 1984
10. Oliva PB, Breckinridge JC: Arteriographic evidence of coronary artery spasm in acute myocardial infarction. Circulation 56:366–374, 1977
11. Maseri A, L'Abbate A, Baroldi G et al: Coronary vasospasm as a possible cause of myocardial infarction: A conclusion derived from the study of "preinfarction" angina. N Engl J Med 299:1271–1277, 1978
12. Benacerraf A, Scholl JM, Achard F et al: Coronary spasm and thrombosis associated with myocardial infarction in a patient with nearly normal coronary arteries. Circulation 67:1147–1150, 1983
13. Vincent GM, Anderson JL, Marshall HW: Coronary spasm producing coronary thrombosis and myocardial infarction. N Engl J Med 309:220–223, 1983
14. Levi GF, Proto C: Ventricular fibrillation in the course of Prinzmetal's angina pectoris — a report of two cases. Br Heart J 35:601–603, 1973
15. Sheehan FH, Epstein SE: Determinants of arrhythmic death due to coronary spasm: Effect of preexisting coronary artery stenosis on the incidence of reperfusion arrhythmia. Circulation 65:259–264, 1982
16. Previtali M, Klersy C, Salerno JA et al: Ventricular tachyarrhythmias in Prinzmetal's variant angina: Clinical significance and relation to the degree and time course of S-T segment elevation. Am J Cardiol 52:19–25, 1983
17. Endo M, Kanda I, Hosoda S et al: Prinzmetal's variant form of angina pectoris — re-evaluation of mechanisms. Circulation 52:33–37, 1975
18. Ricci DR, Orlick AE, Cipriano PR et al. Altered adrenergic activity in coronary artery spasm: Insight into mechanism based on study of coronary hemodynamics and the electrocardiogram. Am J Cardiol 43:1073–1079, 1979
19. Yasue H, Touyama M, Shimamoto M et al: Role of autonomic nervous system in the pathogenesis of Prinzmetal's variant form of angina. Circulation 50:534–539, 1974
20. Yasue H, Touyama M, Kata H et al: Prinzmetal's variant form of angina as a manifestation of alpha-adrenergic receptor-mediated coronary artery spasm: Documentation by coronary arteriography. Am Heart J 91:148–155, 1976
21. Schroeder JS, Bolen JL, Quint RA et al: Provocation of coronary spasm with ergonovine maleate — new test with results in 57 patients undergoing coronary arteriography. Am J Cardiol 40:487–491, 1977
22. Heupler FA, Jr, Proudfit WL, Razavi et al: Ergonovine maleate provocative test for coronary arterial spasm. Am J Cardiol 631–640, 1978
23. Robertson RM, Bernard YD, Carr RK, Robertson D: Alpha-adrenergic blockade in vasotonic angina: Lack of efficacy of specific alpha-receptor blockade with prazosin. J Am Coll Cardiol 2:1146–1150, 1983
24. Tzivoni D, Keren A, Benhorin J et al: Prazosin therapy for refractory variant angina. Am Heart J 105:262–265, 1983
25. Winniford MD, Filipchuk N, Hillis LD: Alpha-adrenergic blockade for variant angina: A long-term, double-blind, randomized trial. Circulation 67:1185–1188, 1983
26. Robertson D, Robertson RM, Nies AS et al: Variant an-

gina pectoris: Investigation of indexes of sympathetic nervous system function. Am J Cardiol 43:1080–1085, 1979

27. Betriu A, Pomar JL, Bourassa MG, Grondin CM: Influence of partial sympathetic denervation on the results of myocardial revascularization in variant angina. Am J Cardiol 51:661–667, 1983

28. Buda AJ, Fowles RE, Schroeder JS et al: Coronary artery spasm in the denervated transplanted human heart—A clue to underlying mechanisms. Am J Med 70:1144–1149, 1981

29. Yasue H, Nagao M, Omote S et al: Coronary arterial spasm and Prinzmetal's variant form of angina induced by hyperventilation and tris-buffer infusion. Circulation 58:56–62, 1978

30. Girotti LA, Crosatto JR, Messuti H et al: The hyperventilation test as a method for developing successful therapy in Prinzmetal's angina. Am J Cardiol 49:834–841, 1982

31. Mudge GH, Jr, Grossman W, Mills RM, Jr et al: Reflex increase in coronary vascular resistance in patients with ischemic heart disease. N Engl J Med 295:1333–1337, 1976

32. MacAlpin RN, Kattus AA, Alvaro AB: Angina pectoris at rest with preservation of exercise capacity— Prinzmetal's variant angina. Circulation 47:946–958, 1973

33. Ellis EF, Oelz O, Roberts IG et al: Coronary arterial smooth muscle contraction by a substance released from platelets: Evidence that it is thromboxane A_2. Science 193:1135, 1977

34. Cheirchia S, Patrono C, Crea F et al: Effects of intravenous prostacyclin in variant angina. Circulation 65:470–477, 1982

35. Shepherd JT, Vanhoutte PM: Spasm of the coronary arteries: Causes and consequences (the scientist's viewpoint). Mayo Clin Proc 60:33–46, 1985

36. Fouad FM, Estafanous FG, Bravo EL et al: Possible role of cardioaortic reflexes in postcoronary bypass hypertension. Am J. Cardiol 44:866, 1979

37. Uchida Y, Murao S: Excitation of afferent cardiac sympathetic nerve fibers during coronary occlusion. Am J Physiol 226:1094–1099, 1974

38. Longhurst JC: Cardiac receptors: Their function in health and disease. Prog Cardiovasc Dis 32:201–22, 1984

39. Gaasch WH, Lufschanowski R, Leachman RD, Alexander JK: Surgical management of Prinzmetal's variant angina. Chest 66:614–621, 1974

40. Betriu A, Solignac A, Bourassa MG: The variant form of angina: Diagnostic and therapeutic implications. Am Heart J 87:272–278, 1974

41. Wiener L, Kasparian H, Duca PR et al: Spectrum of coronary arterial spasm. Clinical, angiographic and myocardial metabolic experience in 29 cases. Am J Cardiol 38:945–955, 1976

42. Johnson AD, Stroud HA, Vieweg WVR, Ross J, Jr: Variant angina pectoris—clinical presentations, coronary angiographic patterns, and the results of medical and surgical management in 42 consecutive patients. Chest 73:786–794, 1978

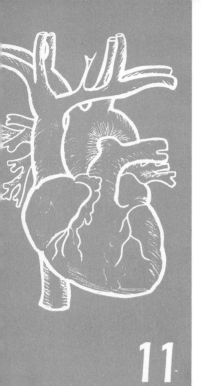

11

SURGERY FOR VENTRICULAR TACHYARRHYTHMIAS

Lewis Wetstein

John M. Herre

William J. Welch

Robert A. Bauernfeind

Approximately 400,000 Americans die suddenly each year.[1] Recent studies utilizing ambulatory monitoring have demonstrated that, in most cases, increasingly frequent and complex ventricular ectopy precedes the development of ventricular tachycardia and fibrillation.[2,3] Pathologic studies suggest that about 25% of these deaths are the result of acute myocardial infarction, whereas most of the remaining 75% occur in the setting of remote myocardial infarction.[4] In the past, the vast majority of patients with out-of-hospital ventricular fibrillation died. However, recent improvements in cardiopulmonary resuscitation have improved survival to about 30% in some cities.[5,6] Although patients who are resuscitated from ventricular fibrillation in the setting of acute myocardial infarction have a prognosis similar to other patients with acute myocardial infarction, the group with ventricular fibrillation remote from myocardial infarction has a very high rate of recurrence if not treated appropriately.[5]

Recurrent, sustained ventricular tachycardia is a potentially life-threatening arrhythmia now recognized with increasing frequency in patients with ischematic heart disease. In many patients, these arrhythmias are refractory to all medical therapy; that is, all antiarrhythmic agents, administered either singly or in combination, have failed to control the spontaneous occurrence of the tachycardia, or the arrhythmia remains easily inducible in the clinical electrophysiology laboratory with programmed electrical stimulation. Among those patients with medically refractory ventricular arrhythmias that are not treated by operation, the mortality is approximately 78% to 80%.[7,8]

Surgical therapy has recently become a viable alternative for patients with medically refractory arrhythmias as well as for patients with aborted sudden death.[9,10] This chapter reviews the rationale, management, and results of surgical therapy for ventricular tachyarrhythmias.

ELECTROPHYSIOLOGY

Cardiac tachyarrhythmias are generally ascribed to either abnormal impulse formation (automaticity) or reentrant mechanisms. Cardiac cells, including those of the sinus node, certain areas of the atria (i.e., coronary sinus), atrioventricular (AV) node, and His–Purkinje system, have the potential to become pacemakers through spontaneous diastolic depolarization.[11-13] In contrast, the remaining myocardial cells maintain a steady membrane potential of approximately −90 millivolts until activated. The rate of impulse formation in automatic cells varies and determines which cells will control the underlying heart rhythm. Depolarization of automatic cells results in a wave of depolarization that stimulates adjacent myocardium. Usually, the sinus node has the highest rate of diastolic depolarization and, therefore, dominates the cardiac rhythm-suppressing subsidiary pacemakers.[14,15] However, when the rate of impulse formation of the sinus node is slower than that of any other automatic cells, subsidiary pacemakers take over and control the heart rate.

AUTOMATIC ARRHYTHMIAS

Tachycardias may result from an increase in the rate of depolarization of pacemaker cells. Several factors, including hypoxemia, hyperkalemia, hypercalcemia, increased catecholamines, and drugs, can increase automaticity.[12,16-21] In the setting of an acute myocardial infarction, accelerated idioventricular rhythms are common and may be the result of enhanced automaticity in injured Purkinje fibers.[22-25] Automatic rhythms are often characterized by an initial "warm-up" (gradual increase in rate) as opposed to reentrant tachycardias, which start abruptly at a relatively constant rate. Arrhythmias that occur as the result of enhanced automaticity are not readily provoked or terminated by programmed electrical stimulation.

Tachycardias may also result from triggered automaticity. Some myocardial cells demonstrate spontaneous delayed after-potentials, which can reach threshold and initiate a train of depolarizations.[26] Although a number of factors, including myocardial infarction and digitalis intoxication, have been associated with the development of after-depolarizations in the animal laboratory, the role of triggered activity in clinical arrhythmias is unknown. Rapid heart rates and premature depolarizations can increase the amplitude of the delayed after-potentials and, if the threshold potential is reached, initiate a series of triggered depolarizations. Differentiating such triggered arrhythmias from reentrant arrhythmias using the clinical techniques of programmed electrical stimulation is problematic at the present time.

REENTRANT ARRHYTHMIAS

The majority of spontaneous, recurrent, sustained tachyarrhythmias associated with chronic heart disease or previous myocardial infarction are due to reentry,[27,28] an abnormality of impulse propagation. Ischemia alters both conduction and refractoriness.[27,29] Thus, during electrical depolarization, a wavefront may block one pathway of a potential reentrant circuit and conduct exclusively along the other limb. If conduction is sufficiently slow, or the pathway sufficiently circuitous, the wavefront may activate the previously refractory pathway retrogradely. After successful retrograde penetration and conduction, the wavefront may reenter and activate the original antegrade pathway and set up a circus movement. Therefore, the electrophysiologic substrate for reentry is unidirectional block, slow conduction over an alternate pathway, and recovery of excitability in the pathway (Fig. 11-1).

Although the vast majority of ventricular tachyarrhythmias occur in the setting of previous myocardial infarction, not all patients with previous myocardial infarction are susceptible to the development of recurrent ventricular tachycardia. Factors such as morphology and the size of the infarct[30] seem to play a significant role in the occurrence of reentrant tachycardias.

EXPERIMENTAL BACKGROUND

Reentrant tachycardias originate in the peri-ischemic region surrounding an infarction.[27,31] The border zone between healthy, oxygenated myocardium, infarcted muscle, and ischemic myocardium contains the electroanatomical substrate necessary for the initiation of ventricular arrhythmias.[32-36] Adjacent cells in the milieu of interdigitating normal, infarcted, and jeopardized myocardium have markedly different refractory periods and conduction properties.[37,38] A propagated impulse may, therefore, be blocked in one direction but conducted in another. In the chronic situation, cells that appear normal and well perfused but that adjoin the ischemic and infarcted tissue may behave abnormally, similarly satisfying the conditions for reentry.[39-41]

Work in our laboratory has demonstrated that

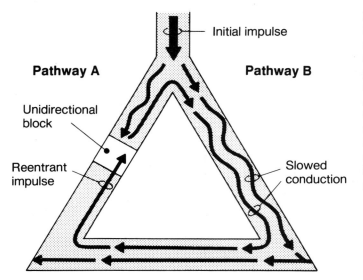

Pathway A

Pathway B

Initial impulse

Unidirectional block

Reentrant impulse

Slowed conduction

FIG. 11–1. An electrical impulse is conducted through myocardial tissue, encounters an area of block **(A)** because of prolonged refractoriness, and is conducted exclusively along another pathway **(B)**. After the alternate pathway is traversed with sufficient delay, it may reexcite, or reenter, the original pathway, which is no longer refractory, inducing a reentrant pathway.

the microanatomy of the peri-ischemic zone surrounding an infarction plays a significant role in the generation of reentrant ventricular tachycardia.[30] Experimental heterogeneous infarcts in the canine model were highly susceptible to the initiation of ventricular tachyarrhythmias (Fig. 11–2).[42,43] Induction of sustained ventricular tachycardia occurred when programmed electrical stimulation was performed in viable myocardial sites in close proximity to the previous infarction.[42–44] In contrast, dogs with homogeneous infarcts were no more susceptible to the initiation of these arrhythmias than were noninfarcted or sham-operated controls (Fig. 11–3).[45–46]

The presence of heterogeneity in myocardial tissues surrounding an infarction provides the electroanatomical substrate for the generation of reentrant tachyarrhythmias.[40,45] Because all tissue may not have been damaged uniformly, adjacent cells may exhibit varying properties of excitability, conduction, and refractoriness. Local anatomical and electrophysiologic derangements dictate whether or not a wave front will be

slowed or blocked. This disorganized pattern of impulse conduction results in the "asynchronization" of adjacent muscle fibers. Neighboring tissue will recover at significantly disparate rates. Finally, as the depressed myocardium recovers, it may be prematurely excited by impulses from the adjacent muscle, resulting in a reentrant tachycardia. It is not clear what cellular alterations are necessary in one animal (or human) to increase susceptibility to sustained ventricular tachycardia while another animal develops nonsustained ventricular tachycardia.

In comparison, the homogeneous infarct has a distinct border zone between irreversibly damaged muscle and adjacent uniformly viable myocardium.[38,47] Although a border zone abutting the damaged muscle exists, this zone has been demonstrated to be less than 100 microns in width in the normothermic working heart.[48] An impulse, therefore, that encounters this uniform scar appears to be uniformly propagated or blocked and rarely satisfies the conditions necessary for sustained ventricular tachycardia. Only in a relatively large homogeneous infarction do

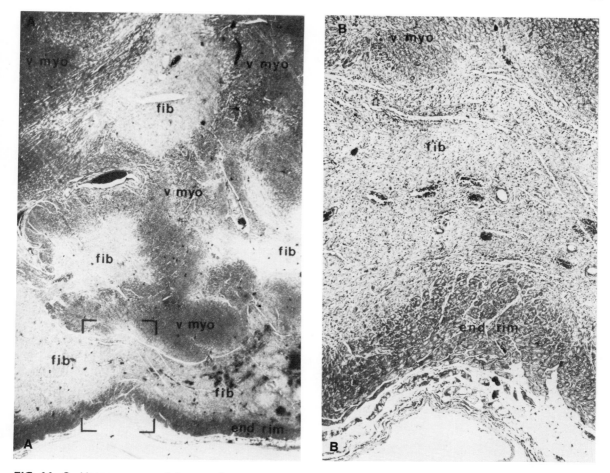

FIG. 11–2. Heterogeneous infarct at 2 weeks. **(A)** This subendocardial infarct has a variegated histologic appearance. Necrotic myocardium has been resorbed and subsequently replaced by young fibrous tissue **(fib)**. Irregularly shaped fingers of viable myocardium **(v myo)** interdigitate between the scar tissue in a "jigsaw puzzle" pattern. A subendocardial rim **(end rim)** of viable myocardium remains. (Hematoxylin-eosin × 10) **(B)** The field bracketed in Figure 11–1A is seen to better advantage at higher magnification. The subendocardial rim of viable myocardium **(end rim)** is separated from deeper islands of viable myocardium **(v myo)** by young fibrous tissue **(fib)**. (Hematoxylin-eosin × 10)

the conditions appear to be satisfied for inducible, sustained reentrant arrhythmias.[30]

It appears that there are other parameters that also play significant roles in the inducibility of these arrhythmias. For example, infarct size was a significant factor in the inducibility of ventricular arrhythmias in a recent canine study.[49] In fact, infarct pattern (heterogeneous versus homogeneous myocardial infarction) in combination with infarct size was the most significant factor in

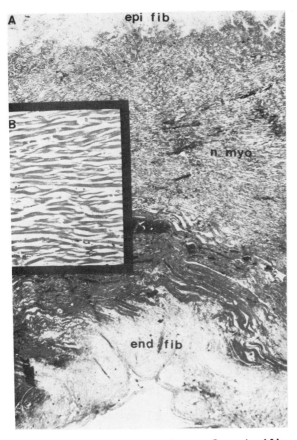

FIG. 11–3. Homogeneous infarct at 2 weeks. **(A)** This infarct is transmural. The necrotic subendocardial and subepicardial myocardium have been resorbed and replaced by young fibrous tissue **(end fib; epi fib).** The intervening myocardium **(n myo)** has undergone coagulative necrosis but has yet to be resorbed. (Hematoxylin-eosin × 10) **(B, inset)** The necrotic myocardium **(n myo)** is shown at higher magnification. Although the myofiber cell bodies are preserved, the fibers are necrotic, as indicated by the loss of sarcolemmal nuclei. (Hematoxylin-eosin × 100)

sustained ventricular tachycardia demonstrated in another animal investigation.[30] Therefore, it is believed that a critical mass and/or pattern of infarcted tissue may be necessary for arrhythmias initiation (*i.e.,* "border zone interface" area).[30] Also, the presence of a viable epicardial rim was important for the induction of sustained ventricular tachycardia in animals subjected to chronic myocardial infarction, and it has recently been postulated that this may be important by acting as the fast retrograde loop of the reentrant circuit.

ELECTROPHYSIOLOGIC TESTING

Programmed Ventricular Stimulation. The recognition and evaluation of reentrant tachyarrhythmias have been enhanced considerably by the development of programmed ventricular stimulation.[35,50,51] Using this technique, the mechanisms of ventricular tachycardia can be studied; wide-complex tachycardias can be differentiated into supraventricular and ventricular arrhythmias; rational drug selection for effective treatment can be made; and pacemaker, automatic defibrillator, or surgical therapy can be selected in cases refractory to medical management.

Indications for electrophysiologic testing in patients with documented or suspected ventricular tachycardia include diagnosis of wide-complex tachycardia; evaluation of unexplained syncope; drug testing for treatment of sustained ventricular tachycardia; and endocardial mapping before cardiac surgery.[52]

Most patients with recurrent, sustained (>1 minute or requiring termination because of hemodynamic compromise), wide-complex tachycardia or ventricular fibrillation should undergo electrophysiologic study for delineation of mechanism and determination of optimal treatment. Patients with incessant or extremely frequent episodes of ventricular tachycardia may undergo drug trials based on long-term, continuous monitoring. However, this method should be used with caution because spontaneous variation in arrhythmia is common.[53] Many patients have infrequent episodes of sustained ventricular tachycadia or fibrillation, and a reduction in ventricular premature complexes may not reflect a reduction in susceptibility to sustained ventricular tachycardia or fibrillation.[54] In addition, determination of patients suitable for surgical or pacemaker therapy requires electrophysiologic study.

In our laboratory, patients are studied in the nonsedated, postabsorptive state at least five half-lives after the discontinuation of all antiarrhythmic agents. Using local anesthesia, multiple quadripolar electrode catheters are introduced through the right or left femoral vein and advanced under fluoroscopic guidance to the regions of the high right atrium and tricuspid valve. Basic intervals are recorded, and sinus and AV node function is determined by standard techniques.[55] One electrode from the arm is advanced to the right ventricular apex. The ventricular effective refractory period is determined during sinus rhythm and after eight paced beats (S_1) at cycle lengths of 600 msec and 500 msec by scanning diastole with single premature extrastimuli (S_2) at 10-msec to 20-msec intervals until ventricular tachycardia is induced or the extrastimulus fails to elicit a ventricular response (Fig. 11 – 4). If a single extrastimulus fails to reproduce the patient's spontaneously occurring ventricular tachycardia or fibrillation, a second premature extrastimulus (S_3) is employed. The coupling interval for S_2 is increased to 50 msec over the refractory period, and S_3 is introduced with an S_2S_3 coupling interval equal to the S_1S_2 interval. The S_2S_3 coupling interval is decreased in 10-msec to 20-msec steps until S_3 fails to capture the ventricle. The S_1S_2 interval is then shortened until S_3 again captures the ventricle. The sequence is repeated until the minimum intervals

for both S_1S_2 and S_2S_3 are achieved. If these techniques fail to reproduce the spontaneously occurring arrhythmia, then a third estrastimulus (S_4) is introduced in a similar manner. Finally, short bursts of ventricular pacing (6 to 8 beats) are delivered at cycle lengths between 400 msec and 240 msec.

If programmed stimulation performed at the right ventricular apex fails to reproduce the spontaneously occurring arrhythmia, then the entire sequence may be repeated at another site, usually the right ventricular septum or outflow tract. If right ventricular stimulation has not been successful, a similar protocol is employed at one or more left ventricular sites.

Similar protocols are employed currently in most laboratories. With these techniques, ventricular tachycardia can be induced in approximately 80% of patients with right ventricular stimulation alone and in approximately 90% of patients when both right and left ventricular stimulations are employed.[54,56]

If decisions regarding pharmacologic, surgical, or pacemaker treatment are to be based on the results of programmed electrical stimulation, then it is important that the induced arrhythmia represent the spontaneous arrhythmia.[54,57] While the induction of nonclinical arrhythmias is a problem with all extrastimulation protocols, it occurs more commonly with more rigorous techniques.[57-59] Thus, when a spontaneous arrhythmia has been documented electrocardiographically, aggressive techniques are useful because one can separate clinical from nonclinical arrhythmias. However, when no documented arrhythmia is available for comparison, as for example when a patient is being studied because of syncope, the use of more than two extrastimuli may lack sufficient specificity to be of value.[60]

Pharmacologic therapy for ventricular tachycardia may be tested by performing programmed electrical stimulation during drug therapy. On subsequent days, individual drugs are tested by

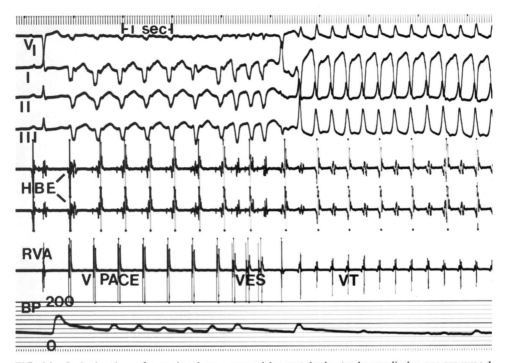

FIG. 11–4. Induction of sustained monomorphic ventricular tachycardia by programmed ventricular stimulation during electrophysiologic study. (**V₁, I, II, III,** surface ECG leads V₁, I, II, and III, respectively; **HBE,** His bundle electrograms; **RVA,** right ventricular apex electrogram; **BP,** arterial blood pressure, scale 0 to 200 mm Hg; **V PACE,** ventricular drive pacing at cycle length 500 msec [120 beats per minute]; **VES,** three ventricular extrastimuli [S_2, S_3, S_4]; **VT,** induced ventricular tachycardia)

programmed electrical stimulation by way of a single indwelling temporary electrode after oral or intravenous dosing. Therapy with standard agents is frequently successful when the drug prevents induction of the sustained clinical arrhythmia.[50,61,62]

INDICATIONS FOR SURGICAL THERAPY

Patients should be considered for surgical treatment for recurrent, sustained ventricular tachycardia when conventional therapy has failed or when they have recurrent, sustained ventricular tachycardia and require open-heart surgery for other reasons. In addition, sustained ventricular tachycardia must be induced reproducibly by programmed electrical stimulation. The process of drug testing is difficult and may require weeks of hospitalization. A dilemma facing the clinician is how to predict the success of medical therapy by using a variety of invasive and noninvasive parameters. Spielman and colleagues[63] have evaluated multiple invasive and noninvasive variables in 84 patients with sustained ventricular tachycardia to predict the response to serial testing with programmed electrical stimulation.

A "positive response" to drugs is correlated with age of greater than 45 years, an ejection fraction of greater than 50%, hypokinesis as the only contraction abnormality, or the absence of structural heart disease. Drug failures were predicted by the induction of ventricular tachycardia with only one extrastimulus, a His bundle electrogram to QRS complex (HV) interval of more than 60 msec, pathologic Q waves, or the presence of a left ventricular aneurysm. No single variable adequately predicted the outcome of programmed electrical stimulation, but by employing multivariant analysis, 20 patients were prospectively correctly classified as drug failures and pharmacologic responses were correctly predicted in four of five patients. Similarly, Swerdlow and colleagues[64] used multivariant analysis to predict responses during programmed electrical stimulation for ventricular tachycardia. Again, no single variable predicted the therapeutic outcome. However, a higher probability of drug response was associated with the absence of structural heart disease, lower New York Heart Association functional class, fewer coronary artery stenoses, the absence of left ventricular aneurysms, female sex, and fewer episodes of ventricular tachycardia prior to presentation.

The response to procainamide in the electrophysiologic laboratory may predict the response to other conventional agents. Waxman and associates[65] found that 60 of 69 patients whose tachycardia remained inducible after procainamide therapy also had inducible ventricular tachycardia after all other conventional agents. Thus, patients who fail to respond to procainamide should be considered for investigational drugs or surgical intervention.

Further refinement of programmed stimulation techniques may permit more accurate identification of patients who will fail medical therapy and who should be referred directly for surgical management. Finally, noninvasive computerized electrocardiography, using signal-averaging techniques, is now under investigation.[66]

Preliminary work suggests that patients who are highly susceptible to recurrent ventricular tachyarrhythmias can be identified by such methods and perhaps the success or failure of medical or surgical therapy predicted.

SURGICAL INTERVENTION FOR MEDICALLY REFRACTORY VENTRICULAR TACHYCARDIA

EVALUATION OF THE PATIENT PRIOR TO SURGICAL THERAPY FOR VENTRICULAR TACHYCARDIA

When the decision is made to approach the ventricular tachycardia surgically, precise localization of the focus becomes desirable. This is best accomplished by preoperative catheter electrode mapping and intraoperative direct endocardial mapping. Preoperative mapping is performed in the cardiac catheterization laboratory with biplane fluoroscopy. Catheter electrodes are placed in the right ventricle, left ventricle, and coronary sinus (Fig. 11–5). Sustained ventricular tachycardia is then induced using the techniques described above. Ventricular electrograms are recorded from multiple sites, identified fluoroscopically, within both ventricles and along the coronary sinus.[67] Using the onset of the QRS complex on the surface ECG as a reference point, the site of earliest activation is determined. This site will often demonstrate activation before the onset of the QRS complex. It is critical that the tachycardia induced and mapped represent the patient's clinical arrhythmia. If multiple morphologies of of ventricular tachycardia are either induced or observed spontaneously, then each must be individually mapped. If they originate from different areas within the ventricle, then the contemplated operative procedure must include all sites. The greater the number of distinct sites located, the less the likelihood of the procedure's success.

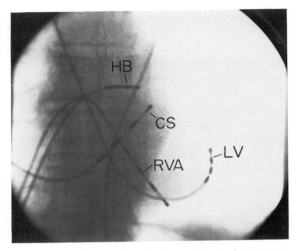

FIG. 11–5. Electrode catheter positions in antero-posterior projection during endocardial mapping. (**CS,** coronary sinus; **HB,** His bundle recording position; **LV,** left ventricle; **RV,** right ventricle)

INTRAOPERATIVE MAPPING

More precise localization of the site of origin of tachycardia is possible if mapping can be performed under direct vision in the operating room.[68] With the patient on normothermic partial or total cardiopulmonary bypass, ventricular tachycardia is induced by the techniques described above. Epicardial mapping may be performed prior to ventriculotomy. However, epicardial breakthrough of the wavefront may not accurately reflect the location of the endocardial origin of the tachycardia. Because the focus generally lies on the endocardial surface, mapping should be performed with the ventricle opened during ventricular tachycardia. Ventricular electrograms are recorded from multiple sites by moving a bipolar electrode probe over the endocardial surface of the ventricle and recording electrograms.[69] As with catheter mapping, the site of origin of the ventricular tachycardia is identified by the earliest activation relative to the QRS complex. Again, if multiple morphologies of ventricular tachycardia have been observed, then each must be individually mapped.

Techniques are being developed currently for computer-assisted, simultaneous, multiple-site acquisition of data to allow a map to be generated on the basis of fewer beats. This will allow intraoperative mapping to be performed rapidly and will make the technique applicable to patients with less stable tachycardias.

SURGICAL INTERVENTIONS

Because the pathologic basis for the majority of sustained ventricular tachycardias is related to the presence of occlusive coronary artery disease and the formation of a post-myocardial infarction aneurysm, the earliest surgical interventions focused on resection of the aneurysm and restoration of coronary blood flow. However, despite successful myocardial revascularization and left ventricular aneurysmectomy, ventricular tachycardia recurred in the majority of patients.[70-73] In all probability, the failure rate of these earlier surgical procedures was related to two main factors: either the procedures were carried out without the benefit of electrophysiologic investigation and, therefore, failed to identify the ventricular site (border zone area) that was responsible for the reentrant tachyarrhythmia;[68,74] or sustained ventricular tachyarrhythmias that frequently originate from the left ventricular septum were untouched by standard left ventricular aneurysmectomy.

DIRECTED SURGICAL PROCEDURES

Endocardial Resection. Electrophysiologic investigations have demonstrated that the origin of earliest activation in patients with sustained ventricular tachycardia lies in close proximity to the edge of the endocardial scar.[75] These data ultimately led to the development of the localized endocardial resection procedure described in 1979 by Harken and associates.[31] Intraoperative endocardial electrophysiologic mapping was performed during induced or spontaneous ventricular tachycardia with a finger-held ring electrode through the opened aneurysm or infarction scar (Fig. 11-6).[75,76] Intraoperative mapping identifies the area of earliest activation, thus localizing the focus responsible for initiation of the tachycardia. A well-defined plane is then developed between the scarred endocardium and underlying muscle, and the endocardium is excised in the region of earliest activation (Fig. 11–7). Localized endocardial resection has resulted in the ablation of reentrant ventricular tachycardia

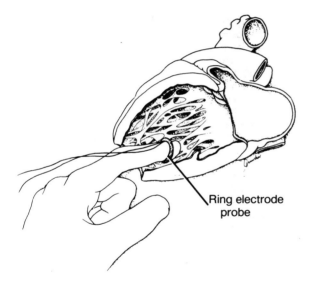

Ring electrode probe

FIG. 11–6. "Mapping" ventricular tachycardia. *Because the ventricle has been entered through the aneurysm or infarcted tissue, the earliest activation during induced ventricular tachycardia is identified by recording circumferentially and at 1-cm levels from the aneurysmal edge using a ring electrode. (Wetstein L, Landymore RW, Herre JM: Current status of surgery for ventricular tachyarrhythmias. Surg Clin North Am 65:571, 1985; with permission)*

in the majority of patients previously refractory to medical management.[75,77] Clinical as well as experimental results suggest that the endocardial excision technique is not arrhythmogenic; perhaps the resulting cicatrix in the endocardium produces uniform slowing or total cessation of a provoked reentrant wave front that encounters this area.[45,78,79]

Harken and associates reported results in 107 patients who had undergone limited resection for medically refractory ventricular tachycardia.[80] Mortality within 30 days of operation was 9%. In 70 patients (67%), the ventricular tachycardia was no longer inducible by programmed electrical stimulation following endocardial resection. In 20 patients (18%), the arrhythmia occurred either spontaneously or was inducible in the electrophysiologic laboratory, but these patients responded to medical therapy. There were two late sudden deaths, presumably from recurrent arrhythmias. Seven patients remained inducible postoperatively despite medication, but five of these had no clinical recurrence. The overall success rate was 85% (*i.e.,* surgery was partially or completely successful in abolishing clinical ventricular tachycardia). More recently, the results of Harken and colleagues have been confirmed by Kienzle and associates, who reported outcomes in 36 patients who survived endocardial resection.[81] Ventricular tachycardia remained inducible without medication in 11 (30%), but was not inducible with medication in four of these patients. Ventricular tachycardia recurred in 2 of 29 patients without inducible ventricular tachycardia at the time of discharge, and 1 of 7 patients with inducible ventricular tachycardia. Thus, inducible ventricular tachycardia did not preclude a successful outcome. Similar results have been reported by Brodman and associates from Albert Einstein College of Medicine in New York.[82] Twenty-two patients underwent electrophysiologically guided endocardial resection with a 30-day operative mortal-

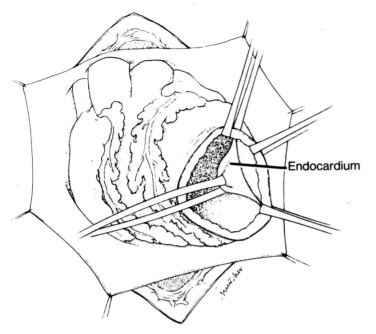

FIG. 11–7. The endocardial resection procedure. The left ventricle has been entered through the aneurysm or previously infarcted tissue. The endocardium at the earliest site of activation is removed, encompassing a 2-cm to 3-cm margin (Wetstein L, Landymore RW, Herre JM: Current status of surgery for ventricular tachyarrhythmias. Surg Clin North Am 65:571, 1985; with permission)

ity of 14%. Ventricular tachycardia was controlled with endocardial resection or medication of 68% of the survivors. Ventricular tachycardia was induced postoperatively in six patients with programmed electrical stimulation. Only three of these patients developed sustained, spontaneous ventricular tachycardia, and one patient died suddenly.

Moran and colleagues from Northwestern University in Chicago reported 40 patients who underwent complete endocardial resection with removal of all visible endocardial scarring.[83] With a combination of endocardial resection and antiarrhythmics, all patients are free of ventricular arrhythmias. Ninety-two percent of these patients were noninducible following complete endocardial resection, while the remaining patients were controlled with conventional antiarrhythmics following surgery. Intraoperative mapping was not possible in 30% of patients because the

arrhythmia was noninducible or rapidly degenerated into ventricular fibrillation. The authors concluded from this experience that complete endocardial resection satisfactorily ablates drug-resistant ventricular arrhythmias, regardless of whether or not mapping was possible during surgery.

Landymore has described a similar technique of encircling endocardial resection and has recently reported his experience with encircling endocardial resection without intraoperative mapping in ten patients.[84,85] All ten patients had failed conventional medical therapy and had reproducible, sustained ventricular tachycardia during electrophysiologic testing. There were no early deaths, but there were two late deaths that were unrelated to recurrence of ventricular arrhythmias. The remaining eight patients are alive and well with a mean follow-up of 17.3 months. Although there were no spontaneous clinical arrhythmias, ventricular tachycardia was induced in one patient with programmed electrical stimulation following complete endocardial resection but not after loading with procainamide. This patient remains free of arrhythmias at 17 months. The results of these two studies[83,85] suggest that encircling endocardial resection with complete removal of endocardial scarring may yield superior results when compared with the localized endocardial resection procedure. The success of encircling endocardial resection may be related to the fact that many patients may have multiple reentrant pathways and that complete endocardial resection effectively removes all ventricular sites that have the potential for ventricular reentry.

Cryosurgery. Cryosurgery, with freezing of myocardial tissue to $-60°C$, has been used to ablate ventricular foci responsible for the initiation of ventricular tachycardia.[46,86,87] Experimental investigations have revealed that this procedure results in a uniform infarct that in and of itself is not arrhythmogenic.[46] The most appealing aspect of this technique is the ability to interrupt reentrant pathways that otherwise might be relatively inaccessible, for example, pathways in close proximity to the conduction system or papillary muscles of the mitral valve (Fig. 11–8). Endocardial excision in these regions might result in heart block or mitral valve dysfunction. Unfortunately, there has been limited experience with this technique, and further experimental work is necessary in this field before cryosurgery becomes a reliable procedure or adjunct for the management of patients with drug-resistant ventricular tachycardia.

Electrode Catheter Ablation. Some patients with recurrent, sustained ventricular tachycardia refractory to medical management are not candidates for endocardial resection because of poor operative risk due to severely compromised left ventricular function or coexisting, noncardiac

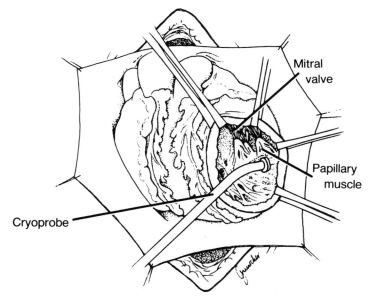

Mitral valve

Papillary muscle

Cryoprobe

FIG. 11–8. An example of cryosurgery. After the left ventricle is entered and the endocardium "mapped," the cryoprobe is applied to the endocardium. Here, the earliest site of activation was the base of the papillary muscle. (Wetstein L, Landymore RW, Herre JM: Current status of surgery for ventricular tachyarrhythmias. Surg Clin North Am 65:571, 1985; with permission)

disease. Recent evidence suggests that if an electrode catheter can be positioned adjacent to the focus of the tachycardia, one or several high-energy, direct current shocks delivered through the catheter may ablate the focus. Catheter endocardial mapping is performed using standard techniques; when the site of earliest endocardial activation is identified, the patient is anesthetized with a short-acting barbiturate, and one or more 200- to 300-joule shocks are delivered using the catheter as the cathode and an external paddle as the anode. The paddle may be placed anteriorly, posteriorly, or laterally.[88,89] Alternatively, for septal foci the discharge may be delivered between two electrode catheters placed on opposite sides of the septum.[90]

NONDIRECTED SURGICAL PROCEDURES

Encircling Endocardial Ventriculotomy. Encircling endocardial ventriculotomy (EEV) was the first operation specifically designed for the management of medically refractory ventricular tachycardia and was described by Guiraudon and colleagues in 1978.[91] Theoretically, this technique was supposed to transect reentrant pathways located in the border zone surrounding the infarction and to interrupt the electrical continuity of these pathways from the remaining normal myocardium.[91,92] EEV was performed by way of a perpendicular ventricular incision, sparing only the epicardial surface and coronary vessels (Fig. 11–9). Unfortunately, the EEV follows the edge of the endocardial scar recognized only by visual inspection. The resultant near-transmural incision should interrupt the reentrant pathway or contain the arrhythmia within its boundaries. Thus, if the tachycardia were to be initiated, the depolarization wave front issuing from the origin of the tachycardia would be unable to exit into normal myocardium. Guiraudon and associates reported a successful outcome in 17 of 23 patients who had undergone EEV.[93] Two patients

(9%) died, and four of the twenty-one surviving patients (19%) had spontaneous recurrence of ventricular tachycardia following operative intervention with a follow-up of 1 to 55 months.

Subsequent procedures have shown that EEV significantly impairs left ventricular function but is effective because the encircling ventriculotomy incision either interrupts the ventricular pathway, isolates the reentrant pathway from normal viable myocardium, or extends the infarction into the region of the border zone surrounding the aneurysm.[94-96] The recurrence rate of ventricular tachyarrhythmias, the unfortunate and severe hemodynamic consequences of this radical procedure, and the significant operative mortality have cast doubt on the likelihood that this technique will become an accepted method for managing medically refractory ventricular tachycardia.

Antitachycardia Pacemakers. In addition to pacing for complete heart block to prevent the ventricular tachycardia that occurs in a setting of bradycardia, rapid ventricular pacing can terminate some forms of ventricular tachycardia.[97-99] Patients in whom bursts of right ventricular pacing reproducibly terminate ventricular tachycardia during exhaustive evaluation in the electrophysiologic laboratory may be candidates for permanently implanted devices that deliver burst pacing at the signal of the patient or physician.[99,100] Patients can trigger these pacemakers externally to institute burst pacing, which may terminate the arrhythmia at the first signs or symptoms of ventricular tachycardia (Fig. 11–10). An alternative device can be programmed to terminate ventricular tachycardia automatically following detection based on rate criteria.[97]

Although burst pacing often interrupts ventricular tachycardia, it may accelerate the tachycardia or cause ventricular fibrillation in approximately 7% of patients.[101] Patients with intrinsically slower ventricular tachycardia or

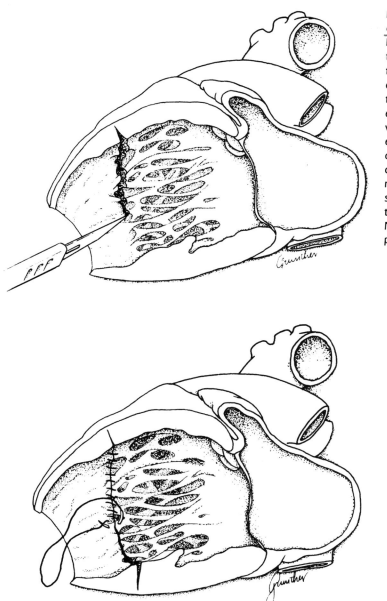

FIG. 11–9. <u>Encircling endo-cardial ventriculotomy.</u> **(A)** The left ventricle is entered and the endocardium proximal to the diseased zone is incised completely and circumferentially, sparing only the epicardial surface and coronary vessels. **(B)** The incision for the encircling endocardial ventriculotomy is subsequently closed. (Wetstein L, Landymore RW, Herre JM: Current status of surgery for ventricular tachyarrhythmias. Surg Clin North Am 65:571, 1985; with permission)

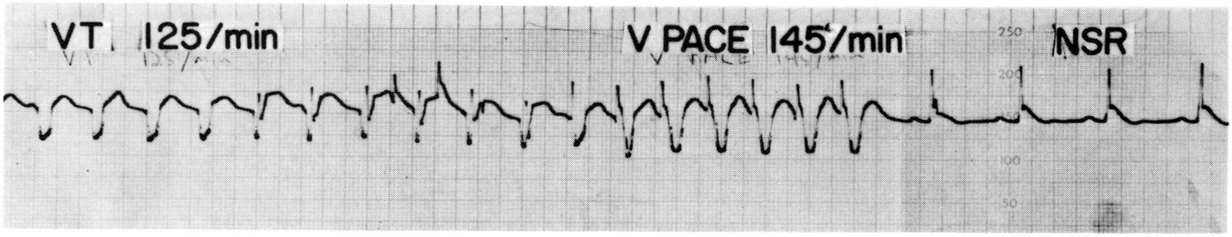

FIG. 11–10. Termination of ventricular tachycardia by burst pacing using an implanted device. (**VT,** ventricular tachycardia; **V PACE,** ventricular pacing; **NSR,** normal sinus rhythm)

whose ventricular tachycardia is slowed by drugs may be candidates for devices capable of burst pacing. A decreased likelihood of acceleration results from application of critically timed single or double extrastimuli rather than burst pacing. Thus, devices have been designed to detect ventricular tachycardia and to deliver decrementally applied extrastimuli until the critical coupling interval that results in termination of the ventricular tachycardia is achieved. Timing must be programmable because the critical coupling intervals change with time and with drug therapy. Implantable devices currently under investigation contain computer algorithms[102] that can detect ventricular tachycardia, attempt decremental sequences of extrastimuli until ventricular tachycardia is interrupted, and remember the successful treatment for more rapid cardioversion of future episodes, all without reliance on patient cooperation.

Permanently implanted devices capable of both burst pacing for termination of ventricular tachycardia and performance of noninvasive programmed electrical stimulation have been developed. These devices are useful for long-term serial evaluation of drugs and for termination of spontaneously occurring ventricular tachycardia.[103]

Implantable Transvenous Cardioverter. The termination of sustained ventricular tachycardia using synchronized, transthoracic, direct current cardioversion can be accomplished with substantially less energy than is required for the termination of ventricular fibrillation. The development of the implantable transvenous cardioverter was based on the assumption that even lower currents might be effective if delivered directly to the endocardium. Using a canine model of myocardial infarction created by a Harris two-staged procedure, Jackman and Zipes were able to induce sustained ventricular tachycardia in 14 animals.[104,105] Single shocks of ≤ 1 joule reproducibly terminated 25 of 30 morphologies or induced ventricular tachycardia with cycle lengths ≥ 200 msec. No acceleration of ventricular tachycardia or induction of ventricular fibrillation was seen in these tachycardias.

The first human studies of transvenous cardioversion were performed using temporary electrodes (Medtronic) and an external cardioverter (Medtronic 2326). Zipes and associates reported the termination of recurrent, sustained ventricular tachycardia in five of seven patients using 0.75 to 2 joules.[106] In addition, ventricular fibrillation in one patient was terminated repeatedly with asynchronous shocks of 25 joules. These observations now have been extended in a multicenter trial.

More recently, Zipes and colleagues have reported the use of a totally implantable system for electrical cardioversion of ventricular tachycardia in seven patients.[102] This first-generation device (Medtronic) detects sustained ventricular tachycardia based on a programmable cycle length, a programmable number of complexes (in order not to attempt to cardiovert nonsustained ventricular tachycardia), and an abrupt increase in cycle length from normal sinus rhythm (in order not to attempt to cardiovert sinus tachycardia, which would be expected to increase in rate over a period). The device then attempts to cardiovert three times at a programmed energy before attempting twice at 2 joules. Programmable backup pacing is provided. In addition, the device can be programmed temporarily to deliver rapid asynchronous pacing for pace-termination of ventricular tachycardia and can be used to deliver one or more programmed extrastimulus to induce ventricular tachycardia for testing purposes.

Implantation is accomplished by the same techniques as are employed for a standard VVI single-chamber demand pacemaker. Although still in the early phases of development, this device offers several advantages over antitachycardia pacemakers and automatic defibrillators. Synchronized transvenous cardioversion is less likely to accelerate ventricular tachycardia than burst pacing and, in some cases, may be more efficacious in the termination of ventricular tachycardia. Its implantation does not require a thoracotomy and thus will be less expensive and better tolerated. Careful patient selection and extensive preoperative testing will be required if long-term results are to match these early observations.

Automatic Implantable Cardioverter/Defibrillator. Despite advances in pharmacologic, pacemaker, and surgical therapy for malignant ventricular arrhythmias, these modalities are not successful in all patients. Direct current cardioversion has proven to be useful in the vast majority of patients when applied early after the onset of ventricular tachycardia or fibrillation. This led to the development during the 1970s of a totally

automatic implantable defibrillator and, later, an automatic implantable cardioverter/defibrillator (AICD).[107]

The device currently available senses ventricular tachycardia on the basis of a preprogrammed rate and a probability density function that identifies the width and sinusoidal nature of the QRS complex. Ventricular fibrillation is identified by a probability density function that detects the absence of a baseline and regular electrical activity.

Defibrillation or cardioversion is accomplished by discharge either between two electrode patches on the left and right ventricles (Fig. 11–11), or between one electrode patch on the left ventricular apex and an electrode catheter in the superior vena cava. These electrodes also serve as sensing electrodes for the probability density

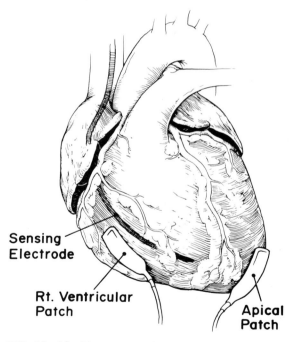

Sensing Electrode

Rt. Ventricular Patch

Apical Patch

FIG. 11–11. Placement of left apical patch, right ventricular patch, and sensing electrode for the automatic implantable defibrillator.

function. Rate sensing is accomplished either by a single bipolar electrode placed in the right ventricular apex or by two epicardial screw-in electrodes. Energy output settings for defibrillation range from 25 to 42 joules.

The techniques for implantation of the AICD may vary depending upon concomitant surgical procedures and the overall condition of the patient. AICD implantation may be performed as an isolated procedure, or it may be combined with coronary artery bypass surgery, valve replacement, or arrhythmia surgery. When a median sternotomy is performed, all electrodes and patches can be attached epicardially. This approach will obviously be chosen when concomitant cardiac surgery is performed. In addition, electrodes and patches may be implanted at the time of arrhythmia surgery for later attachment to an AICD. A subxiphoid thoracotomy may be performed in patients who are not undergoing other cardiac procedures. The superior vena cava and right ventricular apex electrodes are placed under fluoroscopic control and are tunneled under the skin to the pocket. The patch electrodes are placed by way of the anterior pericardiotomy. A left anterolateral thoracotomy may be employed in a patient who has had a previous median sternotomy and who may have residual scar tissue preventing access from the subxiphoid region. A separate incision is made in the left periumbilical region for placement of the AICD. The device and leads are tunneled subcutaneously.[108] A left subcostal approach may be used for both access to the pericardium superiorly and creation of a pocket inferiorly. Two sutureless myocardial electrodes as well as two electrode patches can be inserted using this approach, obviating the need for fluoroscopy and tunneling of electrodes.[109]

Patient Selection and Preoperative Testing. All patients being considered for AICD implantation undergo complete electrophysiologic study to determine inducibility of ventricular tachycardia and to assess the potential effectiveness of pharmacologic, pacemaker, or surgical therapy. Only if these methods fail clinically, or are predicted to fail electrophysiologically, should implantation of the AICD be contemplated.

Intraoperative Testing. Measurement of defibrillation threshold or minimum energy required to terminate ventricular fibrillation is the most important aspect of intraoperative testing. The defibrillation threshold should be at least 5 joules below the initial defibrillator energy. Sensing of both induced ventricular tachycardia and fibrillation is also tested (Fig. 11 – 12).[110]

Postoperative Follow-up. Prior to discharge, sensing and discharge of the device may be tested, particularly if medication changes have been made. Patients capable of exercise should undergo an exercise tolerance test to be certain that sinus tachycardia will not meet rate criteria for ventricular tachycardia. Follow-up of patients with automatic implantable defibrillators (AIDs) now exceeds 4 years. One-year mortality from sudden death for patients with early AID models was approximately 10%, whereas the new AID models appear to reduce 1-year mortality to approximately 2%.[107]

VENTRICULAR TACHYARRHYTHMIAS IN THE ABSENCE OF CORONARY HEART DISEASE

Surgical therapy has been employed in patients with intractable ventricular tachycardia devoid of structural heart disease.[111] Here the only cardiac abnormality noted has been global dilation of the heart secondary to functional posttachycardia heart failure.[112] Therefore, intraoperative electrophysiologic mapping during ventricular tachycardias must be done to localize the site of origin of the arrhythmia. Surgical approaches have included simple ventriculotomy exclusion

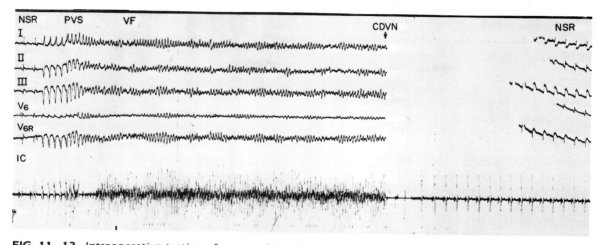

FIG. 11–12. Intraoperative testing of automatic implantable defibrillator. (**NSR,** normal sinus rhythm; **PVS,** programmed ventricular stimulation; **VF,** ventricular fibrillator; **CDVN,** cardioversion [automatic defibrillation]; **I, II, III, V₆, V₆ᵣ,** surface ECG leads I, II, III, V₆, V₆ᵣ, respectively; **IC,** intracardiac electrogram)

procedures and cryoablation, but the results have been poor, perhaps because many of these arrhythmias occur within the ventricular septum.[93]

Some patients with ventricular tachycardia have a nonischemic cardiomyopathy. Angiographic and hemodynamic data indicate abnormal myocardial contractility. Usually, there is diffuse dilation of both ventricles with widespread, patchy myocardial fibrosis at autopsy. Their ventricular tachyarrhythmias frequently occur in the right ventricle, and an approach to such patients has been to employ a combination of cryoablation and surgical isolation of the apparent site of origin of the arrhythmia.[93]

Fontaine and colleagues[113] have described a form of cardiomyopathy affecting primarily the right ventricle, which they have termed "arrhythmogenic right ventricular dysplasia," a congenital transmural infiltration of adipose tissue resulting in weakness and aneurysmal bulging of the infundibulum, apex, and posterior basilar region. Right ventricular dysplasia presents clinically with recurrent ventricular tachycardia of the left bundle branch form.

Uhl's syndrome is a rare congenital cardiomyopathy that may be an extreme form of arrhythmogenic right ventricular dysplasia.[114] The right ventricle is extremely dilated, but the tricuspid valve remains in a normal position, differentiating it from Ebstein's anomaly.

Guiraudon and associates employed simple ventriculotomy and/or aneurysm excision in 12 patients with arrhythmogenic right ventricular dysplasia, and reported one operative death and a 25% recurrence of ventricular tachycardia postoperatively.[93] The current approach to such patients employs a transmural encircling ventriculotomy to isolate the arrhythmogenic myocardium from the remainder of the heart.[111] Because the three pathologically abnormal regions of the right ventricle in arrhythmogenic right ventricular dysplasia may be electrically silent on epicardial mapping, every attempt should be made to isolate each pathologic area.

VENTRICULAR TACHYARRHYTHMIA ASSOCIATED WITH CONGENITALLY PROLONGED Q-T SYNDROME

Polymorphic ventricular tachycardia, or torsades de pointes, is frequently associated with long Q-T syndrome. Torsades de pointes may result from heterogeneous abnormalities of repolarization (dispersion of refractoriness), as opposed to most other ventricular tachycardias, which are believed to be abnormalities in myocardial depolarization.[44,115] The surgical management of torsades de pointes associated with congenital long Q-T syndrome has centered on modification of cardiac autonomic innervation. Yanowitz and colleagues showed that unilateral disruption of sympathetic tone altered the shape of the T wave and the width of the Q-T interval.[116] Right stellate ganglion resection or left stellate ganglion stimulation resulted in Q-T prolongation.[117,118] In fact, right stellate ganglionectomy produces the following changes, which are consistent with long Q-T syndrome: an increase in vulnerability to ventricular fibrillation, a propensity toward episodes of T-wave alternans, and a greater incidence of arrhythmias during exercise as well as during emotional stress.[119-121] In contrast, left stellate ganglion resection has been reported to abolish symptoms in patients with long Q-T syndrome.[120,122] However, at Duke University, other experiences with left stellate ganglion resection have indicated equally early success but late failure.[123]

Because the mortality rate in untreated patients is extremely high (77%) and the therapeutic modalities are still somewhat controversial, an international registry for patients with long Q-T syndrome has been established to address and further define appropriate therapeutic modalities.[122]

CONCLUSION

The optimum surgical technique for the management of medically refractory ventricular tachyarrhythmias has not yet been described. Therefore, each individual case should be assessed and managed differently, depending on the patient's anatomy, overall condition, and the mechanism of his particular arrhythmia. For these reasons, it is incumbent on the surgeon to be familiar with the various approaches and advances, realizing that surgery may correct tachyarrhythmias that cannot be controlled medically.

REFERENCES

1. Lown B: Sudden cardiac death: The major challenge confronting contemporary cardiology. Am J Cardiol 43:313–328, 1979
2. Panadis ID, Margaunth J: Sudden death in hospitalized patients: Cardiac rhythm disturbance detected by ambulatory electrocardiographic monitoring. J Am Coll Cardiol 2:798–805, 1983
3. Pratt CM, Francis MJ, Luck JC et al: Analysis of ambulatory electrocardiograms in 15 patients during spontaneous ventricular fibrillation with special reference to preceding arrhythmic events. J Am Coll Cardiol 2:789–797, 1983
4. Reichenbach DD, Moss NS, Meyer E: Pathology of the heart in sudden cardiac death. Am J Cardiol 39:865–872, 1977
5. Cobb LA, Werner JA, Trobaugh GB: Sudden cardiac death. I. A decade's experience with out-of-hospital resuscitation. II. Outcome of resuscitation, management, and future directions. Modern Concepts in Cardiovascular Disease 49:31–42, 1980
6. Thompson RG, Hallstrom AP, Cobb LA: Bystander-initiated cardiopulmonary resuscitation in the management of ventricular fibrillation. Ann Intern Med 90:737–740, 1979

7. Friedman M, Manwaring JH, Rosenman RH et al: Instantaneous and sudden deaths: Clinical and pathological differentiation in coronary artery disease. JAMA 225:1319–1328, 1973

8. Ruskin JN, MiMarco JP, Garan H: Out-of-hospital cardiac arrest: Electrophysiologic observations and selection of long-term anti-arrhythmic therapy. N Engl J Med 303:607–613, 1980

9. Wetstein L, Engle TR, Kowey PR, Kelliher GJ: Surgical management and mapping of cardiac arrhythmias. Cardiovasc Clin 16(1):151–166, 1985

10. Wetstein L, Michelson EL, Moore RW, Harken AH: Surgical therapy for ventricular tachyarrhythmias. Surg Gynecol Obstet 157:487–496, 1983

11. Bandura JP, Brody DA: Electronic transmission through blocked canine Purkinje tissue: Role of calcium. Circulation 52:11–18, 1978(A)

12. Hoffman BB, Cranefield PF: Electrophysiology of the heart. New York, McGraw–Hill, 1960

13. Hordof AJ, Spotnitz A, Mary–Rabine L et al: The cellular electrophysiology of digitalis of human atrial fibers. Circulation 57:223–229, 1978

14. Vassalle M: Generation and conduction of impulses in the heart under physiological and pathological conditions. Pharmacol Ther 3:1–39, 1977

15. Weidman S: Heart: Electrophysiology. Annual Review of Physiology 36:155–170, 1974

16. Ferrier GR, Moe GK: Effect of calcium on acetylstrophanthidin-induced transient depolarization in canine Purkinje tissue. Circ Res 33:508–515, 1973

17. Carmeliet EE: Chloride and potassium permeability in cardiac Purkinje fibers. Bruxelles Presses Academiques Europeenes, Brussels, 1961

18. Weingart R, Kass RS, Tsien RW: Roles of calcium and sodium ions in the transient inward current induced by strophanthidin in cardiac Purkinje fibers. Biophys J 17:13A, 1977

19. Armour JA, Hageman GR, Randall WC: Arrhythmias induced by local cardiac nerve stimulation. Am J Physiol 233:1068–1075, 1972

20. Tsien RW: Effects of epinephrine on the pacemaker potassium current of cardiac Purkinje fibers. J Gen Physiol 64:293–319, 1974

21. Davis LD: Effect of changes in cycle length on diastolic depolarization produced by ouabain in canine Purkinje fibers. Circ Res 32:206–214, 1973

22. Ferrier GR, Saunders JH, Mendez CA: A cellular mechanism for the generation of ventricular arrhythmias by acetylstrophanthidin. Circ Res 32:600–609, 1973

23. Friedman PL, Stewart JF, Fenoglio JJ, Wit AL: Survival of subendocardial Purkinje fibers after extensive myocardial infarction in dogs. In vitro and in vivo correlations. Circ Res 33:597–661, 1973

24. Hope RR, Scherlag BJ, El-Sherif N, Lazzara R: Hierarchy of ventricular pacemakers. Circ Res 39:883–888, 1976

25. Horowitz LN, Spear JF, Moore EN: Subendocardial origin of ventricular arrhythmias in 24-hour-old experimental myocardial infarction. Circulation 53:56–63, 1975

26. Fisch C, Greenspan K, Anderson GJ: Exit block. Am J Cardiol 28:402, 1971

27. Scherlag BJ, El-Sherif N, Hope R, Lazzara R: Characterization and localization of ventricular arrhythmias resulting from myocardial ischemia and infarction. Circ Res 35:372–383, 1974

28. Wit AL, Cranefield PF: Triggered activity in cardiac muscle fibers of simian mitral valve. Circ Res 38:85–98, 1976

29. Han J: Mechanisms of ventricular arrhythmias associated with myocardial infarction. Am J Cardiol 24:800–813, 1969

30. Wetstein L, Mark R, Kaplinsky E et al: Histopathologic correlates conducive to the initiation of experimental ventricular tachycardia. Am J Med Sci 291:222–231, 1986

31. Harken A, Josephson M, Horowitz LN: Surgical endocardial resection for the treatment of malignant ventricular tachycardia. Ann Surg 190:456, 1979

32. Boineau JP, Cox JL: Slow ventricular activation in acute myocardial infarction: A source of reentrant premature ventricular contractions. Circulation 48:702–713, 1973

33. Janse MJ, Van Capelle FJL, Morsink J et al: Flow of "injury" current and patterns of excitation during early ventricular arrhythmias in acute regional myocardial ischemia in isolated porcine and canine hearts: Evidence for two different arrhythmogenic mechanisms. Circ Res 47:151–165, 1980

34. Simson MB, Harden W, Barlow C, Harken AH: Visualization of the distance between perfusion and anoxia along an ischemic border. Circulation 60:1151–1155, 1979

35. Wellens HJJ: Electrical stimulation of the heart in the study and treatment of tachycardias, pp 14–22. Baltimore, University Park Press, 1971

36. Wetstein L, Nussbaum MS, Barlow CH et al: Decrease in acute myocardial ischemia by hyaluronidase in isolated, perfused rabbit hearts. J Surg Res 30:489–496, 1981

37. Pham TD, Fenoglio JJ, Harken AH et al: Structural basis for recurrent sustained ventricular tachycardia. Circulation (Suppl) 64:87, 1981

38. Wetstein L, Rasteger H, Barlow CH, Harken AH: Delineation of myocardial ischemia in an isolated blood per-

fused rabbit heart preparation. J Surg Res 37:285–289, 1984

39. El-Sherif N, Scherlag BJ, Lazzara R, Hope RR: Reentrant ventricular arrhythmias in the late myocardial infarction period. I. Conduction characteristics in the infarction zone. Circulation 55:689–702, 1977

40. Spear JF, Michelson EL, Moore EN: Excitability of cells within a mottled infarct of dogs susceptible to sustained ventricular tachyarrhythmias. J Am Coll Cardiol 1:1099–1110, 1983

41. Spear JF, Michelson EL, Moore EN: Reduced space constant in slowly conducting regions of chronically infarcted canine myocardium. Circ Res 53:176–185, 1983

42. Michelson EL, Spear JF, Moore EN: Electrophysiological and anatomic correlates of sustained ventricular tachyarrhythmias in a model of chronic myocardial infarction. Am J Cardiol 45:583–590, 1980.

43. Wetstein L, Michelson EL, Euler D et al: Mechanism and surgical therapy of reentrant ventricular tachyarrhythmias. Surg Forum 32:266–268, 1981

44. Krikler DM, Curry PVL: Torsade de pointes: An atypical ventricular tachycardia. Br Heart J 38:117–120, 1976

45. Wetstein L, Michelson EL, Simson MB et al: Evaluation of arrhythmogenicity of surgically induced endocardial vs. ischemic myocardial damage. J Thorac Cardiovasc Surg 87:571–576, 1984

46. Wetstein L, Mitamura H, Mark R et al: Non-arrhythmogenicity of therapeutic cryolesions of the myocardium. J Surg Res 39:543–554, 1985

47. Wetstein L, Simson MB, Feldman P, Harken AH: Pharmacologic modification of myocardial ischemia. Circulation 66:548–554, 1982

48. Harken AH, Simson MB, Haselgrove J, et al: Early ischemia after complete coronary ligation in the rabbit, dog, pig and monkey. Am J Physiol 241:H202–H210, 1981

49. Garan H, Ruskin JN, McGovern B, Grant G: Serial analysis of electrically induced ventricular arrhythmias in a canine model of myocardial infarction. J Am Coll Cardiol 5:1095–1106, 1985

50. Horowitz LN, Josephson ME, Farshidi A et al: Recurrent sustained ventricular tachycardia. III. Role of the electrophysiologic study in selection of anti-arrhythmic regimens. Circulation 58:986–997, 1978

51. Wellens HJJ: Value and limitations of programmed electrical stimulation of the heart in the study and treatment of tachycardia. Circulation 57:845–858, 1978

52. Josephson ME, Horowitz LN: Electrophysiologic approach to therapy of recurrent sustained ventricular tachycardia. Am J Cardiol 43:631–642, 1979

53. Winkle RA: Antiarrhythmic drug effect mimicked by spontaneous variability of ventricular ectopy. Circulation 57:1116–1120, 1978

54. Buxton AE, Josephson ME: Ventricular tachycardia—1983. PACE 7:96–107, 1984

55. Josephson ME, Seides SF: Clinical Cardiac Electrophysiology. Philadelphia, Lea & Febiger, 1979

56. Ruskin JN, Schoenfeld MH, Garan J: Role of electrophysiologic techniques in the selection of antiarrhythmic drug regimens for ventricular arrhythmias. Am J Cardiol 52:41C–46C, 1983

57. Mann DE, Luck JC, Griffin JC et al: Induction of clinical ventricular tachycardia using programmed stimulation: Value of third and fourth extra-stimuli. Am J Cardiol 52:501–506, 1983

58. Brugada P, Abdollah H, Heddle B, Wellens HJJ: Results of a ventricular stimulation protocol using a maximum of premature stimuli in patients without documented or suspected ventricular tachycardia. Am J Cardiol 52:1214–1218, 1983

59. Wetstein L, Michelson EL, Simson MB et al: Initiation of ventricular tachyarrhythmias with programmed stimulation: Sensitivity and specificity in an experimental canine model. Surgery 92:206–211, 1982

60. Akhtar M: Clinical applications of rapid ventricular burst pacing versus extrastimulation for induction of ventricular tachycardia. J Am Coll Cardiol 4:305–307, 1984

61. Mason JW, Winkle RA: Electrode-catheter arrhythmia induction in the selection of antiarrhythmic drug therapy for recurrent ventricular tachycardia. Circulation 58:971–985, 1978

62. Mason JW, Winkle RA: Accuracy of the ventricular tachycardia-induction study for predicting long-term efficacy and inefficacy of antiarrhythmic drugs. N Engl J Med 303:1073–1077, 1980

63. Spielman SR, Schwartz JS, McCarthy DM et al: Predictors of the success or failure of medical therapy in patients with chronic recurrent sustained ventricular tachycardia: A discriminant analysis. J Am Coll Cardiol 1:401–408, 1983

64. Swerdlow DC, Gong G, Echt DS et al: Clinical factors predicting successful electrophysiologic/pharmacologic study in patients with ventricular tachycardia. J Am Coll Cardiol 1:409–416, 1983

65. Waxman HL, Buxton AE, Sadowski BA, Josephson ME: The response to procainamide during electrophysiologic study for sustained ventricular tachyarrhythmias predicts the response to other medications. Circulation 67:30–37, 1983

66. Simson MB, Untereker WJ, Spielman SR et al: Relations between late potentials on the body surface and directly recorded fragmented electrograms in patients with ventricular tachycardia. Am J Cardiol 51:105–112, 1983

67. Mann DE, Laurie GE, Luck JC et al: Importance of pac-

ing site in containment of ventricular tachycardia. J Am Coll Cardiol 5:781–787, 1985

68. Harken AH, Josephson ME: When is myocardial mapping clinically valuable? Am J Surg 145:748–751, 1983

69. Josephson ME, Horowitz LN, Harken AH: Surgery for recurrent sustained ventricular tachycardia associated with coronary artery disease. The role of endocardial resection. Ann NY Acad Sci 77:381–395, 1982

70. DeSoyza N, Murphy ML, Bassett JK et al: Ventricular arrhythmia in chronic stable angina pectoris with surgical or medical treatment. Ann Intern Med 89:10–14, 1979

71. Singer DH, Ten Eick RE, Deboer A: Electrophysical correlates of human atrial tachyarrhythmias. In Dreifus LS, Likoff W (eds): Cardiac Arrhythmias, pp 97–111. New York, Grune & Stratton, 1973

72. Tabry IF, Geha AS, Hammond GL, Baue AE: Effect of surgery on ventricular tachyarrhythmias associated with coronary arterial occlusive disease. Circulation (Suppl) I(58):166–170, 1978

73. Tilkian AG, Pfeifer JF, Barry WH et al: The effect of coronary bypass surgery on exercise-induced ventricular arrhythmias. Am Heart J 92:707–714, 1976

74. Mason JW, Stinson EB, Winkle RA et al: Relative efficacy of blind left ventricular aneurysm resection for the treatment of recurrent ventricular tachycardia. Am J Cardiol 49:241–248, 1982

75. Horowitz LN, Josephson ME, Harken AH: Epicardial and endocardial activation during sustained ventricular tachycardia in man. Circulation 61:1227–1238, 1980

76. Wittig JH, Boineau JP: Surgical treatment of ventricular arrhythmia using epicardial, transmural, and endocardial mapping. Ann Thorac Surg 20:117–126, 1975

77. Horowitz LN, Harken AH, Kastor JA, Josephson ME: Ventricular resection guided by epicardial and endocardial mapping for treatment of recurrent ventricular tachycardia. N Engl J Med 302:589–593, 1980

78. Martin JR, Untereker WS, Harken AH et al: Aneurysmectomy and endocardial resection for ventricular tachycardia: Favorable hemodynamic and antiarrhythmic results in patients with global left ventricular dysfunction. Am Heart J 103:960–965, 1982

79. Wetstein L, Michelson EL, Simson MB et al: Increased interphase between normoxic and ischemic tissue as the cause for reentrant ventricular tachyarrhythmias. J Surg Res 33:526–534, 1982

80. Harken A, Josephson M: Recurrent ventricular tachycardia: How effective is surgical management. Am J Surg 145:718, 1983

81. Kienzle MG, Doherty JV, Roy D et al: Subendocardial resection for refractory ventricular tachycardia: Effects on ambulatory electrocardiogram, programmed stimulation and ejection fraction and relation to outcome. J Am Coll Cardiol 2:853–858, 1983

82. Brodman R, Fisher J, Johnston D et al: Results of electrophysiologically guided operations for drug-resistant recurrent ventricular tachycardia and ventricular fibrillation due to coronary artery disease. J Thorac Cardiovasc Surg 87:431, 1984

83. Moran J, Kehoe R, Loeb J et al: Extended endocardial resection for the treatment of ventricular tachycardia and ventricular fibrillation. Ann Thorac Surg 34:538, 1982

84. Landymore R, Kinley C, Gardner M: Encircling endocardial resection for sustained drug-resistant ventricular tachycardia. Can J Surg 27:24, 1984

85. Landymore R, Kinley C, Gardner M: Encircling endocardial resection with complete removal of endocardial scar without intraoperative mapping for the ablation of drug-resistant ventricular tachycardia. J Thorac Cardiovasc Surg 89:18–24, 1985

86. Gallagher JJ, Anderson RW, Kasell J et al: Cryoablation of drug-resistant ventricular tachycardia in a patient with a variant of scleroderma. Circulation 57:190–197, 1978

87. Klein GJ, Harrison L, Idler RF et al: Reaction of the myocardium to cryosurgery: Electrophysiology and arrhythmogenic potential. Circulation 59:364–372, 1979

88. Hartzler GO: Electrode catheter ablation of refractory focal ventricular tachycardia. J Am Coll Cardiol 2:1107–1113, 1983

89. Winston SA, Morady F, Davis JC et al: Catheter ablation of ventricular tachycardia. Circulation 70:II–412, 1984

90. Winston SA, Davis JC, Morady F et al: A new approach to electrode catheter ablation for ventricular tachycardia originating from the interventricular septum. Circulation 11:412, 1984

91. Guiraudon G, Fontaine G, Frank R et al: Encircling endocardial ventriculotomy: A new surgical treatment for life-threatening ventricular tachycardias resistant to medical treatment following myocardial infarction. Ann Thorac Surg 26:438–444, 1978

92. Fontaine G, Guiraudon G, Frank R et al: The surgical management of ventricular tachycardia. Herz 4:276–284, 1979

93. Guiraudon G, Fontaine G, Frank R et al: Sugical treatment of ventricular tachycardia guided by ventricular mapping in 23 patients without coronary artery disease. Ann Thorac Surg 32:439–450, 1981

94. Ungerleider RM, Holman WL, Calcagno D et al: Encircling endocardial ventriculotomy for refractory ischemic ventricular tachycardia. III. Effects on regional left ventricular function. J Thorac Cardiovasc Surg 83(6):857–864, 1982

95. Ungerleider RM, Holman WL, Stanley TE III et al: Encircling endocardial ventriculotomy for refractory ischemic ventricular tachycardia. I. Electrophysiologic effects. J Thorac Cardiovasc Surg 83:840–849, 1982

96. Ungerleider RM, Holman WL, Stanley TE III et al: Encircling endocardial ventriculotomy for refractory ischemic ventricular tachycardia. II. Effects on regional myocardial blood flow. J Thorac Cardiovasc Surg 83(6):850–856, 1982

97. Fisher JD, Cohen HL, Mehra R et al: Cardiac pacing and pacemakers. II. Serial electrophysiologic-pharmacologic testing for control of recurrent tachyarrhythmias. Am Heart J 93:658–668, 1977

98. Haft JL: Treatment of arrhythmias by intracardiac electrical stimulation. Prog Cardiovasc Dis 16:539–568, 1974

99. Johnson RA, Hutter AM, Desanctis RW et al: Chronic overdrive pacing in the control of refractory ventricular arrhythmias. Ann Intern Med 80:380–383, 1974

100. Cooper TB, Maclean WAH, Waldo Al: Overdrive pacing for supraventricular tachycardia: A review of theoretical implications and therapeutic techniques. PACE 1:196–221, 1978

101. Fisher JD, Mehra R, Furman S: The treatment of ventricular tachycardia with bursts of ventricular pacing. Am J Cardiol 41:94–102, 1978

102. Zipes DP, Festoff B, Schaal SF et al: Treatment of ventricular arrhythmia by permanent atrial pacemaker and cardiac sympathectomy. Ann Intern Med 68:591–597, 1968

103. Herre JM, Griffin JC, Nielson AP et al: Permanent triggered antitachycardia pacemakers in the management of recurrent sustained ventricular tachycardia. J Am Coll Cardiol 6:206–212, 1985

104. Harris AS: Delayed development of ventricular ectopic rhythms following experimental coronary occlusion. Circulation 1:1318, 1950

105. Jackman WM, Zipes DP: Low-energy synchronous cardioversion of ventricular tachycardia using a catheter electrode in a canine model of subacute infarction. Circulation 66:187–195, 1982

106. Zipes DP, Heger JJ, Miles WM, Prystowsky EN: Preliminary experience with the implantable transvenous cardioverter. PACE 7:1325–1330, 1984

107. Echt DS, Armstrong K, Schmidt P et al: Clinical experience, complications, and survival in 70 patients with the automatic implantable cardioverter defibrillator. Circulation 71:289–296, 1985

108. Watkins L, Mower MM, Reid PR et al: Surgical techniques for implanting the automatic implantable defibrillator. PACE 7:1357–1362, 1984

109. Lawrie GM, Griffin JC, Wyndham CRC: Epicardial implantation of the automatic implantable defibrillator by left subcostal thoracotomy. PACE 7:1370–1374, 1984

110. Reid PR, Griffin LSL, Mower MM et al: Implantable cardioverter defibrillator: Patient selection and implantation protocol. PACE 7:1338–1343, 1984

111. Cox JL: Surgery for cardiac arrhythmias. Curr Probl Cardiol July 1983

112. Cox JL: The surgical management of cardiac arrhythmias. In Spender FC (ed): Gibbon's Surgery of the Chest, pp 1552–1584. Philadelphia, WB Saunders, 1983

113. Fontaine G, Guiraudon G, Frank R: Management of chronic ventricular tachycardia. In Narala OA (ed): Innovations in Diagnosis and Management of Cardiac Arrhythmias. Baltimore, Williams & Wilkins, 1979

114. Uhl HSM: A previously undescribed malformation of the heart: Almost total absence of the myocardium of the right ventricle. Bulletin Johns Hopkins Hospital 91:197–205, 1952

115. Wellens HJJ, Durren DR, Liem LL, Lie KI: Effects of digitalis in patients with paroxysmal atrioventricular nodal tachycardia. Circulation 52:779–785, 1975

116. Yanowitz F, Preston JB, Abildskov JA: Functional distribution of right and left stellate innervation to the ventricles. Production of neurogenic electrocardiographic changes by unilateral alteration of sympathetic tone. Cir Res 18:416–428, 1966

117. Malliani A, Schwartz PJ, Zanchetti A: Neural mechanism and life-threatening arrhythmias. Am Heart J 100:705, 1980

118. Moss AJ, McDonald J: Unilateral cervicothoracic sympathetic ganglionectomy for the treatment of long Q-T interval syndrome. N Engl J Med 285:903, 1971

119. Schwartz PJ, Malliani A: Electrical alteration of the T-wave: Clinical and experimental evidence of its relationship with the sympathetic nervous system and with the long Q-T syndrome. Am Heart J 89:45–50, 1975

120. Schwartz PJ, Snebold NG, Brown AM: Effects of unilateral cardiac sympathetic denervation on the ventricular fibrillation threshold. Am J Cardiol 37:1034–1040, 1976

121. Schwartz PJ: Experimental reproduction of the long Q-T syndrome. Am J Cardiol 41:374, 1978

122. Schwartz PJ: The idiopathic long Q-T syndrome. Ann Intern Med 99:561–562, 1983

123. Benson DW, Jr, Cox JL: Surgical treatment of cardiac arrhythmias. In Robert NK, Gelband H (eds): Cardiac Arrhythmias in the Neonate, Infant and Child, 2nd ed. pp 341–366. New York, Appleton–Century–Crofts, 1982

SELECTED READINGS

Grayboys TB, Lown B, Podrid PJ, DeSilva R: Long-term survival of patients with malignant ventricular arrhythmia treated with anti-arrhythmic drugs. Am J Cardiol 50:437–443, 1982

Griffin JC, Mason JW, Calfee RV: The treatment of ventricular tachycardia using an automatic tachycardia terminating pacemaker. PACE 4:582–588, 1981

Josephson ME, Horowitz LN, Farshidi A: Continuous local electrical activity: A mechanism of recurrent ventricular tachycardia. Circulation 57:659–665, 1978

Kowey PR, Mullan DF, Wetstein L: Pacemaker therapy—1985. In Wetstein L, Myerowitz PD (eds): Latest advances in cardiac surgery. Surg Clin North Am 65:595–611, 1985

Mehra R, Zeiler RH, Gouch WB, El-Sherif N: Reentrant ventricular arrhythmias in the late myocardial infarction period. 9. Electrophysiologic/anatomic correlation of reentrant circuits. Circulation 67:11–24, 1983

Michelson EL, Spear JF, Moore EN: Initiation of sustained ventricular tachyarrhythmias in a canine model of chronic myocardial infarction: Importance of the site of stimulation. Circulation 63:776–784, 1981

Mirowski M, Reid PR, Mower MM et al: Termination of malignant ventricular arrhythmias with an implanted automatic defibrillator in human beings. N Engl J Med 303:322–324, 1980

Wetstein L, Engle TR, Kowey PR, Kellihar GJ: Surgical management and mapping of cardiac arrhythmias. Cardiovasc Clin 16(1): 151–166, 1985

Mirowski M, Reid PR, Watkins L et al: Treatment of life-threatening ventricular arrhythmias with automatic implantable defibrillators. Am Heart J 102:265–270, 1981

Mirowski M, Reid PR, Winkle RA et al: Mortality in patients with implanted automatic defibrillators. Ann Intern Med 98:585–588, 1983

Myerburg RJ, Conde CA, Sung RJ et al: Clinical, electrophysiologic and hemodynamic profile of patients resuscitated from prehospital cardiac arrest. Am J Med 68:568–576, 1980

Reddy CP, Sartini JC: Nonclinical polymorphic ventricular tachycardia induced by programmed cardiac stimulation: Incidence, mechanisms and clinical significance. Circulation 62:988–995, 1980

Robertson JF, Cain ME, Horowitz LN et al: Anatomic and electrophysiologic correlates of ventricular tachycardia requiring left ventricular stimulation. Am J Cardiol 48:263–268, 1981

Schwartz PJ, Stone HL: Effects of unilateral stellectomy upon cardiac performance during exercise in dogs. Circ Res 44:637–645, 1979

Spear JF, Horowitz LN, Hodess AB et al: Cellular electrophysiology of human myocardial infarction. I. Abnormalities of cellular activities. Circulation 59:247–256, 1979

Spear JF, Michelson EL, Spielman SR, Moore EN: The origin of ventricular arrhythmias 24 hours following experimental anterior septal coronary artery occlusion. Circulation 55:844–852, 1977

Watkins L, Morowski M, Mower MM et al: Automatic defibrillation in man: The initial surgical experience. J Thorac Cardiovasc Surg 82:492–500, 1981

Zipes DP, Jackman WM, Heger JJ et al: Clinical transvenous cardioversion of recurrent life-threatening ventricular tachyarrhythmias: Low energy synchronized cardioversion of ventricular tachycardia and termination of ventricular fibrillation in patients using a catheter electrode. Am Heart J 103:789–794, 1982

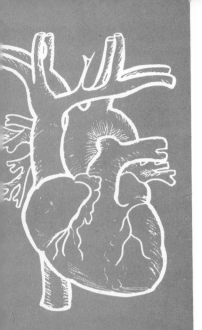

12

USE OF SOMATOSENSORY EVOKED POTENTIALS DURING THORACIC ANEURYSM SURGERY

John C. Laschinger

Eugene A. Grossi

Joseph N. Cunningham, Jr.

Paraplegia remains an all too frequent and devastating complication of surgical procedures on the descending thoracic and thoracoabdominal aorta. The incidence of this complication remains high and has been largely unaffected despite numerous alterations in surgical and anesthetic techniques. As a result, significant controversies persist concerning both the cause of paraplegia and the efficacy of various adjuncts (*i.e.*, shunt/bypass) employed in the hope of preventing spinal cord ischemia and paraplegia.

The failure to significantly reduce the incidence of paraplegia over the last three decades stems from several factors. First, these aortic lesions are relatively infrequent. As a result, only three centers have accumulated sufficient experience to publish reports describing studies of more than 50 patients.[1-7] In addition, the majority of these and other clinical series in the literature suffer from being retrospective reviews.[1-6,8-12] Prospective studies in this area have been hindered by the prior inability to determine intraoperatively the effect of specific variables on the adequacy of spinal cord blood flow.

In an effort to determine the causes of paraplegia and the effects of specific variables on the adequacy of spinal cord blood flow during surgical procedures on the descending thoracic and thoracoabdominal aorta, we adapted the technique of monitoring somatosensory evoked potentials (SEP) in a series of experimental and clinical studies.

TECHNIQUE OF SEP MONITORING

The techniques for both clinical and experimental use of SEP monitoring are similar and are shown schematically for clinical use in Figure 12–1. Somatosensory evoked potentials are measured by means of a clinical evoked potential system (TM 3000, TRACOR Analytic Inc., Oak Grove Village, IL). SEP traces are generated by stimulation of the right posterior tibial nerve with a bipolar input channel. After conduction of the impulse by way of the dorsal spinal column, the cortical response to 200 consecutive stimuli is recorded from needle electrodes placed in the midline of the scalp at the nasion and 55% of the distance between the nasion to the inion. A separate grounding electrode is placed on the left shoulder. Potentials are then amplified 10,000 times and processed with a 10-H low-pass and a 250-H high-pass filter. To improve the signal-to-noise ratio of these small potentials, 200 consecutive responses activated by supermaximal stimuli to the nerve (4 × the motor twitch threshold, 20 mA; 0.4 msec duration pulse; 2.3/sec) are averaged for each SEP trace. In addition, a no-stimulus control tracing is recorded to establish background noise levels.

A typical SEP tracing is shown in Figure 12–2. Two parameters are serially monitored: latency of onset and amplitude of the generated response. Increases in latency and/or decreases in amplitude of the SEP tracing indicate spinal cord ischemia.[13-15] Generation of new tracings every

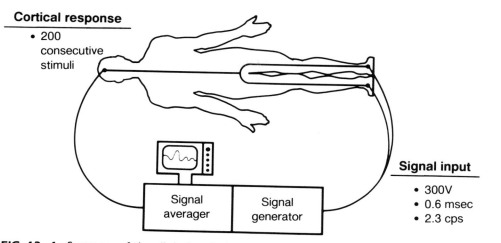

Cortical response

- 200 consecutive stimuli

Signal input

- 300V
- 0.6 msec
- 2.3 cps

Signal averager

Signal generator

FIG. 12–1. Summary of the clinical technique of SEP monitoring. See text for details.

2 minutes for comparison to baseline data demonstrates changes in these parameters caused by ischemia. All SEP data are stored in a computer to allow subsequent retrieval and comparison of traces as needed.

The entire monitoring system, which is compact, portable, and easily positioned in a convenient location within the surgical theater, is shown in Figure 12–3. Halogenated anesthetic agents are strictly avoided because their use modifies the cortical response to peripheral nerve stimulation and renders SEP monitoring useless. Care must also be taken to avoid misinterpretation of evoked potentials occurring as a result of electrical artifacts secondary to the use of electrocautery.

EVIDENCE FOR SPINAL CORD ISCHEMIA FOLLOWING AORTIC CROSS-CLAMPING

The effect of simple aortic cross-clamping (AXC) on spinal cord blood flow (SCBF) has been well studied.[13–19] Simple proximal AXC without shunt or bypass has been shown experimentally to result in significant decreases in SCBF distal to the midthoracic (T6) spinal cord. Similar distal spinal cord ischemia is believed to occur clinically in response to proximal AXC, although the means to document this have been unavailable previously. This inability to detect the presence of spinal cord ischemia clinicaly has fostered much controversy about the relationship between AXC duration and the incidence of paraplegia. The importance of this relationship has been stressed by some and refuted by others, notably Crawford.[1,2,6,7,19]

To examine this relationship more closely, we first performed a series of experiments designed to determine whether changes in SEP occurred in response to significant decreases in SCBF and could thus serve as a barometer of the severity of spinal cord ischemia. Secondly, we sought to determine what relationship, if any, existed between the duration of spinal cord ischemia and the subsequent incidence of paraplegia. The results of these studies clearly showed that following proximal AXC, blood flow to the distal spinal cord falls significantly (Fig. 12–4). Furthermore,

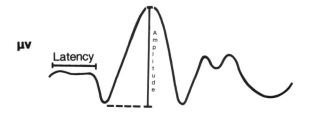

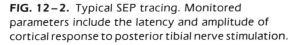

FIG. 12-2. Typical SEP tracing. Monitored parameters include the latency and amplitude of cortical response to posterior tibial nerve stimulation.

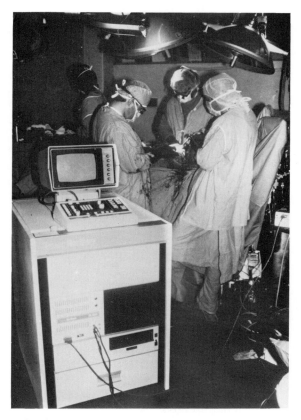

FIG. 12-3. Complete SEP monitoring system.

such changes are associated with ischemic dysfunction of the cord severe enough to produce loss of conduction of SEP signals by posterior spinal cord columns.[13,15] These changes in animals are progressive and time dependent, resulting in SEP loss approximately 8 minutes after proximal AXC (Fig. 12-5). Upon reperfusion of the distal aorta, a reactive hyperemic response is seen in previously ischemic spinal cord segments (see Fig. 12-4) that is accompanied by return of SEP (see Fig. 12-5) toward normal.[13,15]

Subsequent studies in our laboratory have shown that the duration of SEP loss during the cross-clamp interval is a significant determinant of the subsequent incidence of paraplegia.[20] In these studies, animals underwent proximal AXC, after which SEP was observed until a complete loss occurred. Animals were then randomly assigned to two groups undergoing distal reperfusion either 5 or 10 minutes after SEP loss was noted. Once again, complete SEP loss was associated with significant distal (below T6) spinal cord ischemia, confirming the relationship between these two events. No differences were observed between the two groups when comparing either the time to SEP loss or the magnitude of SCBF changes resulting from proximal AXC. However, a significant difference in the incidence of paraplegia was observed. In animals undergoing distal reperfusion 5 minutes after SEP loss, no paraplegia was seen (Table 12-1). In animals in whom the AXC interval was extended by 10 minutes after SEP loss, 66% of animals (p < .005) suffered severe neurologic injury.

In this same study, we investigated the possibility of pharmacologically modifying this relationship between duration of SEP loss and paraplegia.[20] Methylprednisolone (30 mg/kg) was administered intravenously to a third group of animals immediately prior to AXC and 4 hours postoperatively. The administration of steroids in this fashion produced dramatic results (Table

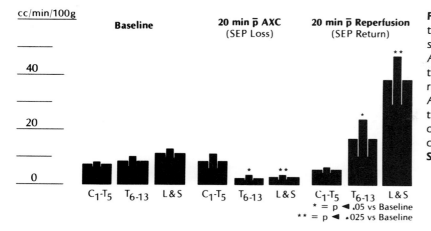

FIG. 12–4. Results of segmental spinal cord blood flow studies following proximal AXC. Note the significant distal (**T6–13, L&S**) ischemia and reactive hyperemia following AXC and reperfusion, respectively. SEP status at the time of SCBF studies is noted. (**C**, cervical; **T**, thoracic; **L**, lumbar; **S**, sacral)

12–1). In these animals, despite extension of the AXC interval by 10 minutes after SEP loss, no paraplegia was observed. This was significant (p = .02) when compared to control animals, in whom a similar duration of SEP loss resulted in a 66% incidence of neurologic injury. Because the administration of steroids did not affect either the magnitude of SCBF changes following AXC or the time course of SEP changes due to ischemia when compared to group I and II animals, we have concluded that the observed differences in the incidence of paraplegia between these groups must have resulted from the ability of steroids to increase the tolerance of spinal cord tissues to ischemia.[20] The exact mechanism of this protective effect remains to be fully elucidated.

In summary, we have shown experimentally that the presence of significant spinal cord ischemia causes ischemic dysfunction of the spinal cord severe enough to result in loss of SEP conduction. Furthermore, the duration of this ischemic state (as measured by the duration of SEP loss during the AXC interval) is related to the subsequent incidence of paraplegia. Therefore *loss* of SEP is now regarded as a sensitive indicator of the presence of severe spinal cord ischemia.

TABLE 12–1

RELATIONSHIP OF DURATION OF SEP LOSS DURING THE CROSS-CLAMP INTERVAL TO POSTOPERATIVE ISCHEMIC SPINAL CORD INJURY

| Group | N | AXC Duration (min) | | Postoperative Neurologic Status | | |
		Prior to SEP Loss	Total	Normal	Ataxia	Paraplegia
I	6	7.66 ± 0.62	12.66	6	—	—
II	9	7.56 ± 0.60	17.56	3*	1	5†
III (Methylprednisolone 30 mg/kg)	6	8.33 ± 1.80	18.33	6	—	—

* p = .02 versus Group I or III

† p = .04 versus Group I or III

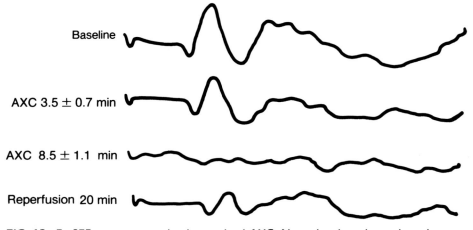

FIG. 12–5. SEP response to simple proximal AXC. Note the time-dependent decay in both latency and amplitude, which progresses to SEP loss 8 to 10 minutes after AXC.

The duration of such ischemia is related to the subsequent incidence of paraplegia. The possibility that pharmacologic interventions may favorably influence the relationship between the duration of SEP loss and the subsequent incidence of paraplegia is exciting and deserves more intensive experimental study.[20,21]

INTERVENTIONS TO AVOID OR REVERSE SPINAL CORD ISCHEMIA

Next we sought to determine experimentally whether adjuncts such as shunt or bypass play any role in preventing spinal cord ischemia after proximal AXC. Clinical data are contradictory, and conclusive evidence showing that the use of such adjuncts results in significant protection from paraplegia is lacking.[1–12] However, these studies again suffer numerous deficiencies in that all were performed prior to our ability to determine intraoperatively the adequacy of SCBF by SEP measurements. In addition, the majority of these studies were retrospective, used historical controls, and mentioned no attempts to

confirm the adequacy of distal perfusion as ascertained by measurements of distal aortic perfusion pressure.

Our initial animal studies have clearly shown that maintenance of normal distal aortic perfusion pressure (mean 100 mm Hg) results in preservation of normal levels of SCBF (Fig. 12–6) with no observed changes in SEP.[13] Subsequent studies have shown (Fig. 12–7) that similar preservation of SCBF is achieved with mean distal perfusion pressures of 70 mm Hg. However, with mean distal pressures of 40 mm Hg, 83% of animals exhibit SEP changes consistent with ischemic dysfunction (significant decreases in amplitude of SEP tracing) and 17% (1 of 6) progressed to complete SEP loss and associated severe distal spinal cord ischemia.[14]

Data suggest that for such adjuncts to be truly effective they *must* be properly employed. Distal perfusion pressures must be measured routinely and maintained at adequate levels if the efficacy of such devices is to be ensured. Inadequacies in distal perfusion pressures have been shown to result experimentally in ischemic SEP changes

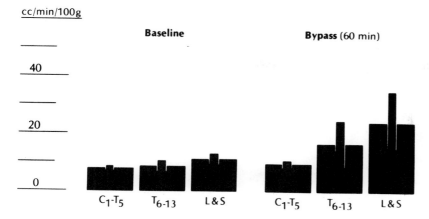

cc/min/100g

Baseline   **Bypass** (60 min)

40

20

0

C_1-T_5 T_{6-13} L & S C_1-T_5 T_{6-13} L & S

FIG. 12–6. Results of segmental SCBF studies in animals undergoing partial bypass. Note the prevention of distal spinal cord blood flow changes when the normal (mean 100 mm Hg) distal perfusion pressure is maintained following AXC. (**C,** cervical; **T,** thoracic; **L,** lumbar; **S,** sacral)

and/or severe spinal cord ischemia with SEP loss.

IMPORTANCE OF IDENTIFICATION OF CRITICAL INTERCOSTALS— ROLE OF SEP

One of the limitations of all operative techniques and adjuncts employed in surgery on thoracic aortic lesions is that paraplegia is likely to result in a large number of patients secondary to interruption of blood flow to vessels critical to spinal cord blood supply.[1,2,8,9,22–25] The location of these vessels is highly variable and may occur anywhere from T5 to the aortic bifurcation.[24,25] Previous attempts to localize these vessels preoperatively using angiographic techniques have failed. As a result, it is argued that although this is an unfortunate circumstance, interruption of such vessels is largely unpreventable and is a function of both the patient's particular anatomy and the location of the lesion.[1,2,4,6,8] Specifically, this would readily explain the continued significant incidence of paraplegia previously observed in patients in whom shunt/bypass was employed with documentation of adequate distal perfusion pressure. Although localization of such vessels

has not been previously possible using preoperative angiography, the addition of intraoperative SEP monitoring offers significant promise for the intraoperative localization of these vessels when adequate distal shunt/bypass is employed.

As previously demonstrated, maintenance of adequate distal aortic perfusion pressure (approximately 70 mm Hg in dogs) prevents spinal ischemia following proximal AXC.[13,14] Animal studies performed subsequently have shown that through the combined use of *adequate* distal aortic perfusion and SEP monitoring, consistent and reliable intraoperative localization of vessels critical to SCBF could be achieved.[26] In these studies it was shown that when multiple intercostal vessels that were not critical to spinal cord blood supply (left subclavian–T7) were excluded from the proximal systemic and distal bypass circulations, no changes in SCBF (Fig. 12–8) or SEP (Fig. 12–9) were observed. Progressive exclusion of lower aortic segments (T7–10, T10–13, L1–3, L3–6, L6–7) resulted in SEP loss in all animals at varying levels. Such SEP loss in the face of adequate distal perfusion pressure was interpreted as a signal that vessels critical to spinal cord blood supply had been excluded from the systemic and bypass circulations, resulting in spinal cord ischemia. Radioactive microsphere determinations

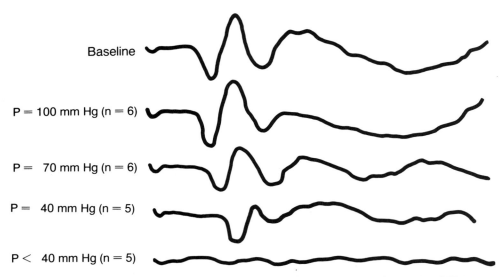

FIG. 12–7. SEP response to varying distal aortic perfusion pressure. Note that SEP is unchanged when the distal perfusion pressure is 70 mm Hg. With distal pressures of 40 mm Hg, SEP loss was seen in one animal (17%; 1/6), and significant changes in amplitude of the SEP response were seen in the remaining five (83%). SEP loss occurred in all animals with perfusion pressures <40 mm Hg.

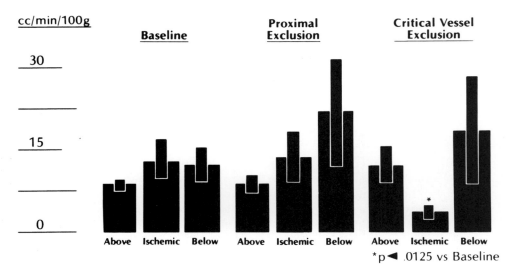

FIG. 12–8. SCBF studies showing the use of SEP for intraoperative localization of critical vessels to spinal cord blood supply. Proximal exclusion of multiple vessels that are not critical to spinal cord blood supply has no effect on SCBF. When vessels critical to cord blood supply are excluded from systemic and bypass circulations, segmental spinal cord ischemia is seen.

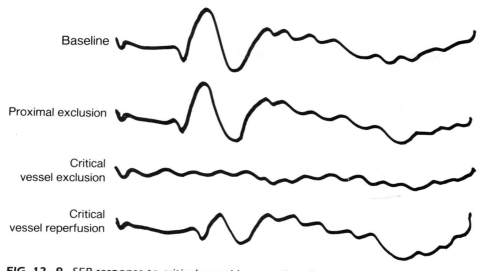

FIG. 12−9. *SEP response to critical vessel interruption. Exclusion of multiple proximal vessels that are not critical to SCBF has no effect on SEP. When "critical vessels" are excluded, SEP loss results because of spinal cord ischemia. When these critical vessels are reperfused, SEP returns toward normal.*

of SCBF performed at the time of SEP loss confirmed the presence of severe segmental spinal cord ischemia. Subsequent selective reperfusion of these "critical vessels" excluded at the time of SEP loss resulted in a reactive hyperemic response in the previously ischemic spinal cord segments and return of the SEP tracing toward normal. The observations that SEP loss and spinal cord ischemia occurred at different levels of aortic exclusion in each animal highlights the variability in location of these critical vessels. Most importantly, the consistent ability to reliably localize these vessels using combined adequate distal perfusion and SEP monitoring further suggests the utility of these techniques in the future to prevent paraplegia.

Several key points are highlighted by these experimental studies. First, we have clearly shown that maintenance of *adequate* distal perfusion

pressure following AXC by adjunctive partial bypass results in prevention of spinal cord ischemia. Preservation of normal spinal cord perfusion by such adjuncts following AXC is confirmed by maintenance of normal SEP. Use of adjuncts to provide distal perfusion, however, does not guarantee prevention of paraplegia. Severe neurologic injury may result despite the use of adjuncts if distal perfusion pressure is not maintained at adequate levels or if the location and extent of the lesion necessitates interruption of flow to vessels critical to spinal cord blood supply. Use of combined adequate distal perfusion and intraoperative SEP monitoring offers the best hope for paraplegia prevention as spinal cord ischemia secondary to distal hypotension is prevented and the ability to intraoperatively recognize interruption of blood flow to "critical vessels" is achieved.

RESULTS OF CLINICAL STUDIES

To date we have prospectively studied 33 patients to determine if SEP monitoring offers similar clinical benefits for detection and prevention of spinal cord ischemia following cross-clamping of the descending thoracic aorta. Intraoperative SEP changes and the duration of any such changes were analyzed with respect to postoperative neurologic status in an attempt to confirm our experimental findings clinically. For the purposes of our clinical study, only complete SEP loss was used to define the presence of significant spinal cord ischemia. The decision to use shunt/bypass devices as adjuncts to the surgical procedure was made preoperatively on the basis of the individual surgeon's preference, and the conduct of the operation (except in two cases) was not altered based on intraoperative SEP findings. In addition, all patients underwent thorough pre- and postoperative neurologic exams by the same neurologist. A summary of preoperative patient data is shown in Table 12–2. Results of our clini-

TABLE 12–2
SUMMARY OF PREOPERATIVE PATIENT DATA

Patient Data	No. of Patients
Age	
58.5 (range 2 to 83 years)	33
Sex	
Male	23
Female	10
Cause	
Atherosclerotic	22
Traumatic	3
Coarctation	3
Dissection	3
Mycotic	1
False aneurysm	1
Distal Extent of Aneurysm	
T8 and above	10
T9 to bifurcation	23

cal studies have mirrored those found experimentally, allowing definition of four SEP response types.

Failure to use shunt or bypass devices (simple AXC) uniformly resulted in spinal cord ischemia and SEP loss in all patients in whom this technique was used. This has been defined as an SEP type-I response (Fig. 12–10). In this situation SEP loss occurs shortly after AXC because of severe distal aortic hypotension and spinal cord ischemia. Furthermore, SEP monitoring offers no benefit for localization of critical spinal cord vessels in this situation. As a result, a high incidence (37%) of paraplegia was observed in this group of patients.

When distal shunt or bypass was used, three different response types were observed depending on the adequacy of distal aortic perfusion. Maintenance of adequate distal perfusion (defined as mean pressure > 60 mm Hg) and the absence of any significant change in SEP (type-II SEP response) were taken as evidence of the adequacy of distal aortic perfusion by either a shunt or bypass device or by physiologic collaterals in patients with congenital coarctation (Fig. 12–11). Preservation of a normal SEP tracing in this setting also allowed the surgeon to surmise that vessels critical to spinal cord blood supply were being perfused by either the systemic or the bypass circulation and therefore did not originate from the aortic segment excluded by cross-clamp placement. Therefore, all vessels in the excluded segment could be routinely ligated without fear of paraplegia occurring postoperatively. As was expected, no postoperative neurologic deficits were seen in any patient exhibiting this SEP response type.

In contrast, loss of SEP despite maintenance of adequate distal perfusion pressure by a shunt or bypass device provided the surgeon with a warning that vessels critical to spinal cord blood supply must originate in the aortic segment that is excluded from the sytemic and bypass circula-

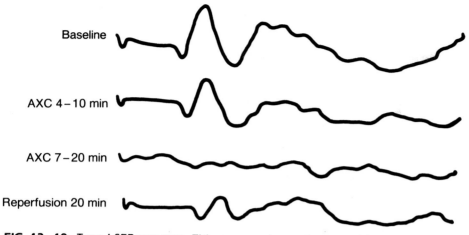

FIG. 12-10. Type-I SEP response. This response is usually seen with simple proximal AXC and no distal perfusion. Note the time-dependent decay in SEP, progressing to complete loss.

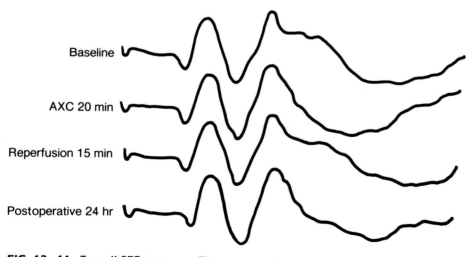

FIG. 12-11. Type-II SEP response. This response is seen when adequate (>60 mm Hg) distal perfusion is maintained following AXC and no "critical intercostals" lie in the aortic segment, which is excluded from the systemic and bypass circulations.

tions (type-III SEP response, Fig. 12–12). This response was observed in two patients and indicated to the surgeon that reimplantation of intercostal vessels from within the excluded aortic segment was necessary if paraplegia was to be prevented. These were the only two patients in whom intraoperative SEP findings were allowed to alter the conduct of the surgical procedure. Successful reimplantation of specific pairs of intercostal vessels within the excluded aortic segment was achieved in both patients, and paraplegia was prevented.

Finally, provision of inadequate distal perfusion pressure (mean pressure <40 mm Hg) despite the use of shunt and/or bypass devices again resulted in significant spinal cord ischemia and SEP loss (type-IV SEP response, Fig. 12–13). This occurred despite the provision of what had previously been considered "adequate" flow rates (3 to 5 liters/minute) to the distal aorta, and it underscores the importance of routinely measuring distal perfusion pressure. It is important to note that when distal perfusion is inadequate (mean pressure <40 mm Hg), spinal cord ischemia occurs, and the ability to utilize SEP for localization of vessels critical to spinal cord blood supply is also sacrificed because SEP loss results. As a result, use of distal perfusion devices without ensuring their adequacy produces an unacceptably high paraplegia rate (33%). The adequacy of distal perfusion can only be assessed by combined monitoring of SEP and distal perfusion pressure, and the notion of adequate flow rates based on any parameters other than these should be abandoned.

OTHER VARIABLES AFFECTING POSTOPERATIVE INCIDENCE OF PARAPLEGIA

Five clinical variables were also analyzed to determine their role in the production of postoperative paraplegia. The results are summarized in

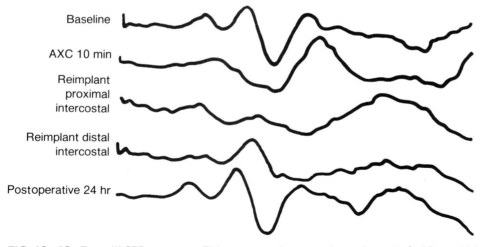

Baseline

AXC 10 min

Reimplant proximal intercostal

Reimplant distal intercostal

Postoperative 24 hr

FIG. 12–12. Type-III SEP response. This response is seen when adequate (>60 mm Hg) distal perfusion is maintained but vessels critical to SCBF lie within the aortic segment and are excluded from the systemic and bypass circulations. Successful reimplantation of such critical vessels results in SEP return toward normal and prevention of paraplegia.

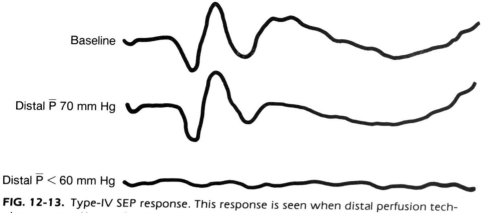

FIG. 12-13. Type-IV SEP response. This response is seen when distal perfusion techniques are used but perfusion pressures are not maintained at adequate (> 60 mm Hg) levels.

Table 12–3. The incidence of postoperative paraplegia in this series was not significantly affected by either the distal extent of aneurysm or the insertion of a peripheral perfusion device per se. Maintenance of adequate distal perfusion pressure (mean distal pressure of ≥60 mm Hg) throughout the AXC interval resulted in paraplegia prevention in all patients in whom it was achieved. It is important to note that this includes the two patients in whom maintenance of adequate distal perfusion and SEP monitoring (type-III response) allowed recognition of critical-vessel interruption and appropriate reimplantation with prevention of paraplegia. In contrast, in those patients in whom distal perfusion was either inadequate (pressure <60 mm Hg) or not employed, the incidence of postoperative paraplegia was significantly higher (35.7%, p = .01 versus adequate perfusion).

When spinal cord ischemia (SEP loss) was observed at any time during the AXC interval, a significant increase in the incidence of postoperative paraplegia was seen (31.2%, p = .02 versus no SEP loss). Further analysis of these data revealed that the duration of such ischemia (duration of SEP loss) during the AXC interval was the most sensitive predictor of postoperative neurologic status. When SEP loss was either prevented or limited in duration to less than 30 minutes, paraplegia did not occur. In contrast, when the duration of SEP loss following AXC exceeded 30 minutes, 71% of patients developed paraplegia postoperatively (p <.001).

IMPLICATIONS

The implications of these experimental and clinical studies are numerous. First, the use of intraoperative SEP monitoring has allowed us to clearly identify spinal cord ischemia as the common factor in the production of paraplegia. The results of these studies have clearly shown that spinal cord ischemia is reliably detected by intraoperative SEP monitoring. Causes of spinal cord ischemia confirmed by both clinical and experimental observations include proximal AXC without shunt or bypass, failure to maintain adequate distal perfusion pressure despite use of shunt or bypass, and interruption of flow to vessels critical to spinal cord blood supply. Such ischemia results in SEP loss, and the duration of

TABLE 12-3
RELATIONSHIP OF SELECTED VARIABLES TO INCIDENCE OF
POSTOPERATIVE PARAPLEGIA

Variable	Incidence of Postoperative Paraplegia	p Value*
Distal Extent of Aneurysm		
Group a. Above T8	10% (1/10)	NS
Group b. T9 to Bifurcation	17.4% (4/23)	
Use of Shunt/Bypass		
Group a. Yes	8% (2/25)	NS
Group b. No	37.5% (3/8)	
Distal Perfusion Pressure Following AXC		
Group a. ≥60 mm Hg	0 0/19)	.01
Group b. <60 mm Hg	35.7% (5/14)	
Spinal Cord Ischemia (SEP loss) After AXC		
Group a. No	0 (0/17)	.02
Group b. Yes	31.2% (5/16)	
Duration of Spinal Cord Ischemia		
Group a. 0-30 min	0 (0/26)	.001
Group b. >30 min	71.2% (5/7)	

* p value for incidence of paraplegia for group a versus group b for each variable. Significance of differences calculated by Fisher's Exact test. NS = p > .05.

such loss has been shown to be related to the subsequent incidence of paraplegia. The demonstrated ability to alter this relationship experimentally by pharmacologic intervention is exciting and warrants further study.

Ischemia of the spinal cord can be prevented only if adequate distal perfusion is achieved following proximal AXC. Use of shunt/bypass per se, without *ensuring* the adequacy of such perfusion by both SEP and distal pressure monitoring, offers no protection from paraplegia. Adequate distal perfusion pressure has been clinically defined as 60 mm Hg, although individual patients may require even higher distal perfusion pressures to prevent ischemia as determined by SEP. Finally, the combined use of SEP and adequate distal perfusion has, for the first time, allowed intraoperative detection of the interruption of flow to vessels critical to spinal cord blood supply.

Interpretation of these results has led us to de-

vise a clinical operative protocol that is now under prospective evaluation. The goal of this study is significant paraplegia prevention through the combined use of intraoperative SEP monitoring and partial bypass to maintain adequate distal perfusion pressure. The benefits of achieving adequate distal perfusion so that SEP monitoring can be effectively employed can be readily discerned from Fig. 12-14. One can see that failure to either employ (type-I SEP response) or achieve (type-IV SEP response) adequate distal perfusion following proximal AXC results in severe spinal cord ischemia and SEP loss. Placement of the spinal cord in a precarious state of severe ischemia unnecessarily exposes the patient to the risk of severe neurologic injury while preventing the surgeon from gaining any useful information about the location of critical vessels or the need for reimplantation of such vessels. Therefore, a high incidence of paraplegia can be expected to result depending on the duration of this ischemic state and the frequency of critical intercostal interruption.

In contrast, it becomes clear that maintenance of adequate distal perfusion allows SEP monitoring to be used as an effective adjunct in paraplegia prevention (see Fig. 12–14). In the vast majority of cases, adequate distal perfusion (type-II SEP response) will prevent spinal cord ischemia and signal the surgeon that no vessels critical to spinal cord blood supply lie in the excluded aortic segment. When SEP is lost despite adequate distal perfusion (type-III SEP response), the surgeon is alerted *intraoperatively* that attempts at reimplantation of vessels from the excluded aortic segment are indicated if paraplegia is to be prevented.

It is hoped that by adoption of this protocol, paraplegia prevention can be achieved. Ob-

viously, however, the problem of paraplegia is difficult because *multiple factors* are involved. Furthermore, in a significant number of patients, unfavorable anatomy (aortoiliac occlusion, extensive thoracoabdominal aneurysm, distal aortic dissection, and so forth) often results in an inability to provide adequate distal perfusion following proximal AXC. Under these circumstances, effective clinical use of SEP monitoring cannot be achieved and the incidence of paraplegia will vary with the duration of spinal cord ischemia and the effectiveness of blind reimplantation of critical intercostal arteries.

Obviously, further large prospective studies are needed. SEP monitoring, however, has provided valuable information about the causes of paraplegia. Hopefully, continued and more widespread application of this technique will

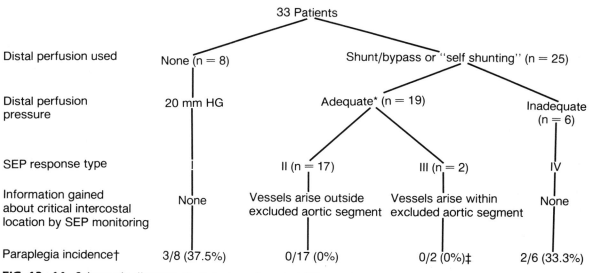

FIG. 12–14. Schematic diagram of clinical results using SEP monitoring. Note that SEP monitoring, when combined with maintenance of adequate distal perfusion pressure, allowed information to be gained about the location of critical intercostals, resulting in complete paraplegia prevention. (* adequate, ≥60 mm Hg, † p = .01 for incidence of paraplegia with adequate distal perfusion versus none or inadequate distal perfusion, ‡ paraplegia prevented by successful intercostal reimplantation)

allow significant progress to be made in decreasing the incidence of this catastrophic complication.

REFERENCES

1. Crawford ES, Fenstermacher JM, Richardson W, Sandiford F: Reappraisal of adjuncts to avoid ischemia in the treatment of thoracic aneurysms. Surgery 67:187–196, 1970
2. Crawford ES, Waler HS, Saleh SA, Normann NA: Graft replacement of aneurysms in descending thoracic aorta: Results without bypass or shunting. Surgery 89:73–85, 1981
3. DeBakey ME, McCollum CH, Graham JM: Surgical treatment of aneurysms of the descending thoracic aorta. Long-term results in 500 patients. J Cardiovasc Surg 19:571–576, 1978
4. Crawford ES, Snyder DM, Gwen CC, Roethan JOF, Jr: Progress in treatment of thoracoabdominal and abdominal aortic aneurysms involving celiac, superior mesenteric and renal arteries. Ann Surg 188:404–422, 1978
5. Reul GJ, Cooley DA, Hallman GL et al: Dissecting aneurysms of the descending aorta. Improved surgical results in 91 patients. Arch Surg 110:632, 1975
6. Livesay JJ, Cooley DA, Ventimiglia RA et al: Surgical experience in descending thoracic aneurysmectomy without adjuncts to avoid ischemia. Ann Thorac Surg 39:37–46, 1985
7. Carlson DE, Karp RB, Kouchoukos NT: Surgical treatment of aneurysms of the descending thoracic aorta: An analysis of 85 patients. Ann Thorac Surg 35:58–69, 1983
8. Najafi H, Javid H, Hunter J et al: Descending aortic aneurysmectomy without adjuncts to avoid ischemia. Ann Thorac Surg 30:326–335, 1980
9. Adams HD, Van Geertruyden HH: Neurologic complications of aortic surgery. Ann Surg 144:574–610, 1956
10. Lawrence GH, Hessel EA, Sauvage LR, Krause AH: Results of use of the TDMAC–heparin shunt in surgery of aneurysms of the descending thoracic aorta. J Thorac Cardiovasc Surg 73:393–398, 1977
11. Donahoo JS, Brawley RK, Gott VL: The heparin-coated vascular shunt for thoracic aortic and great vessel procedures: A ten-year experience. Ann Thorac Surg 23:507–513, 1977
12. Connors JP, Ferguson TB, Roper CL, Weldon CS: The use of the TDMAC–heparin shunt in replacement of the descending thoracic aorta. Ann Surg 181:735–741, 1975
13. Laschinger JC, Cunningham JN, Jr, Catinella FP et al: Detection and prevention of intraoperative spinal cord ischemia after crossclamping of the thoracic aorta. Use of somatosensory evoked potentials. Surgery 92:1109–1117, 1982
14. Laschinger JC, Cunningham JN, Jr, Nathan IM et al: Experimental and clinical assessment of the adequacy of partial bypass in maintenance of spinal cord blood flow during operations on the thoracic aorta. Ann Thorac Surg 36:417–426, 1983
15. Coles JG, Wilson GJ, Sima AF et al: Intraoperative detection of spinal cord ischemia using somatosensory cortical evoked potentials. Ann Thorac Surg 34:299–308, 1982
16. Gelman S, Reves JG, Fowler K et al: Regional blood flow during crossclamping of the thoracic aorta and infusion of nitroprusside. J Thorac Cardiovasc Surg 85:287–291, 1983
17. Fried LC, Aparicio O: Experimental ischemia of the spinal cord. Histologic studies after anterior spinal artery occlusion. Neurology 23:289–293, 1973
18. Wadough F, Arndt CF, Metzger H et al: Direct measurements of oxygen tension on the spinal cord surface of pigs after occlusion of the descending thoracic aorta. J Thorac Cardiovasc Surg 89:787–794, 1985
19. Van Harreveld A, Schade JP: Nerve cell destruction by asphyxiation of the spinal cord. J Neuropathol Exp Neurol 21:410–423, 1962
20. Laschinger JC, Cunningham JN, Jr, Cooper MM et al: Prevention of ischemic spinal cord injury following aortic crossclamping. Use of corticosteroids. Ann Thorac Surg 38:500–507, 1984
21. Nylander WA, Plunkett RJ, Hammon JW et al: The opental modification of ischemic spinal cord injury in the dog. Ann Thorac Surg 33:64–68, 1982
22. Fried LD, DiChiro G, Doppman JL: Ligation of major thoraco-lumbar spinal cord arteries in monkeys. J Neurosurg 13:608–614, 1969
23. Spencer FC, Zimmerman JM: The influence of ligation of intercostal arteries on paraplegia in dogs. Surg Forum 9:340–342, 1958
24. Adamkiewicz A: Die blutfegasse des menschlichen rukenmarkesoer flache sitz. Acad Urss Wein Math Natur Klass 85:101, 1882
25. Djinjian R, Hurth M, Houdart M et al: Arterial supply of the spinal cord. In Djinjian R (ed): Angiography of the Spinal Cord, pp 3–13. Baltimore, University Park Press, 1970
26. Laschinger JC, Cunningham JN, Jr, Nathan IM, Krieger KH, Spencer FC: Intraoperative identification of vessels critical to spinal cord blood supply. Use of somatosensory evoked potentials. Curr Surg 41:107–109, 1984

13

NONINVASIVE TECHNIQUES TO EVALUATE RESULTS IN CARDIAC SURGERY

Harold L. Lazar
Arthur J. Roberts

Improved methods of myocardial protection have significantly reduced the operative mortality for cardiac surgery. These advances have been the result of extensive laboratory research in myocardial metabolism, ultrastructure, and contractility. Unfortunately, many of the techniques used to evaluate these parameters are invasive and cannot be safely used in clinical practice. These invasive methods may distort and manipulate the myocardium, thus prohibiting accurate serial measurements. In addition, observations made in animal preparations may not reflect clinical conditions. Because of these limitations, clinicians have sought noninvasive methods to accurately determine changes in cardiac function following surgery. This chapter will discuss the various noninvasive techniques currently available to assess myocardial function in the postoperative period.

ELECTROCARDIOGRAPHY

Traditionally, the ECG has been the standard for determining perioperative myocardial damage. Following coronary artery bypass graft (CABG) surgery, an infarction is very likely if there are new and persistent Q waves of at least 0.04 second duration, which are associated with ST–T wave changes.[1] A myocardial infarction (MI) may also be suspected if there is ST-segment depression greater than 2 mm for more than 48 hours and if there is deep T-wave inversion for more than 48 hours. Transient, nonspecific T-wave changes, ST-segment depression less than

2 mm, and isolated premature ventricular contractions (PVCs) may reflect transient ischemia, but they are unreliable predictors of permanent myocardial damage.

Not all new Q waves seen following cardiac surgery are synonymous with acute myocardial necrosis. Transient Q waves can be produced by ischemia without infarction and by temporary alterations in ventricular metabolism and temperature.[2-4] New Q waves have been seen in patients with patent bypass grafts and improved postoperative ventriculograms.[5] It has also been suggested that Q waves can be "unmasked" by the improved postoperative contraction of a contralateral ventricular segment.[6] Roberts has estimated that approximately 20% of new Q waves developing after CABG surgery may be associated with little or no readily detectable perioperative myocardial damage.[7]

The specificity of postoperative ECG changes has been enhanced when they have been associated with enzyme elevations, stress testing, and radionuclide imaging.[1,8-10] However, in the absence of enzyme changes and alterations in radionuclide ventriculography, ECG changes alone are poor predictors of changes in postoperative global or regional function.

SERUM ENZYMES AND ISOENZYMES

The specificity and sensitivity of routine cardiac enzymes to diagnose myocardial damage following cardiac surgery has been disappointing because so many factors can lead to increased enzyme release. Right-sided heart failure, passive hepatic congestion or necrosis, and transfusion reactions can falsely elevate postoperative serum glutamic-oxaloacetic transaminase (SGOT) levels.[11] Lactate dehydrogenase (LDH) levels can be increased by pulmonary infarction, renal cortical damage, and hemolysis whereas muscle trauma increases creatine phosphokinase (CPK).[12,13]

In an attempt to increase the sensitivity and specificity of postoperative enzymes, the MB fraction of CPK has been measured. However, it has been shown that CPK–MB is also increased following surgical trauma, global ischemia without infarction, hemodilution, hypothermia, and intraoperative defibrillation.[14,15] In addition, the rate of clearance of CPK–MB may also be affected by the anesthetic technique used.[14] Because the CPK–MB fraction may be elevated in as many as 90% of patients undergoing CABG, the shape of the postoperative serum CPK–MB curve, rather than the total absolute level may be a better guide to the degree of myocardial damage.[16] Roberts has shown that a prolonged plateau or a second peak in postoperative CPK–MB is a more sensitive indicator of ischemic damage.[17] In addition, he found that CPK–MB values that fell outside the range of the mean plus two standard deviations from a previously determined cohort of selected, uncomplicated CABG surgical patients is also a sensitive indicator of perioperative myocardial damage. This guideline is especially important because normal enzyme values vary from institution to institution, and one should be cautious in comparing absolute values in a multicenter study.

Although CPK–MB may be a sensitive method to rule out an infarction in unstable patients prior to CABG, its role in the postoperative period remains to be defined. Even abnormal postoperative elevations may not be associated with depressed postoperative ejection fractions.[7] A more sensitive indicator of ischemic damage in the postoperative period may ultimately be the reversal of the normal $LDH_1 : LDH_2$ ratio.[18] At the present time, however, elevated serum isoenzymes in the absence of definitive ECG or radionuclide studies remain a poor indicator of postoperative myocardial damage.

MYOCARDIAL "HOT SPOT" IMAGING

Myocardial "hot spot" imaging is a noninvasive technique used to visualize areas of myocardial necrosis directly by the uptake of specific radiopharmaceutical agents. The most common agent currently used is technetium 99m pyrophosphate (^{99m}Tc – PYP). Jennings has shown that calcium is deposited in crystalline form in irreversibly damaged myocardial cells.[19] Pyrophosphate will complex with calcium, and its uptake in the myocardium can be detected by a gamma camera.[20] It has been shown that at least 3 grams of myocardial necrosis must be present to scintigraphically identify an acute infarct.[21] In addition, coronary blood flow must be reduced by at least 20% to 40% to obtain the greatest uptake of ^{99m}Tc – PYP.[22]

The time interval between the onset of an infarct and the acquisition of the scan is also important. Scans become positive 12 hours after an infarct and fade or become negative 6 to 10 days later.[23,24] Roberts has shown, however, that if ^{99m}Tc – glucoheptonate is used, an infarct may be identified as early as 6 hours following surgery.[25]

There are several factors that limit the usefulness of "hot spot" scanning following surgery. Experimental studies have shown that although the size of anterior infarcts can be accurately predicted, this technique is much less reliable for inferior wall or subendocardial infarcts.[26] Increased uptake of ^{99m}Tc – PYP can be seen in conditions other than acute myocardial necrosis. These include remote infarcts, ventricular aneurysms, and subsequent cardioversions. Because as many as 30% of patients may have abnormal scans postoperatively, it is important to have both pre- and postoperative scans before a postoperative infarct can be accurately diagnosed.[27] These scans are also limited by their ability to differentiate "hot spots" because of actual necrosis and those areas that represent potentially reversible reperfusion injuries. Roberts has shown that when the only evidence for a perioperative MI is a positive ^{99m}Tc–PYP scan, no corresponding depression is seen in left ventricular ejection fraction either in the early or late postoperative periods.[7]

MYOCARDIAL "COLD SPOT" IMAGING

Myocardial "cold spot" imaging is based on the properties of the monovalent cationic radionuclide thallium–201(Tl^{201}), which has biologic properties, similar to potassium, over a wide range of myocardial blood flows. Because the uptake of Tl^{201} is proportional to myocardial blood flow, this scan can be performed at rest and following exercise. "Cold spot" imaging has helped to predict graft patency following CABG. Ritchie has shown that patients with no new perfusion defects during rest and exercise postoperatively have a graft patency approaching 86%.[28] Patients with new perfusion defects at rest or upon exercise have a diminished graft patency, which approaches 50%.

RADIONUCLIDE VENTRICULOGRAPHY

This method involves an *in vivo* autologous erythrocyte-labeling technique.[29] A computer-based time–activity curve is generated, and ventricular contractions are observed in video format. This technique allows either first-pass or equilibrium multigated scans, which permit serial studies to be obtained over a 6-hour period. Global ejection fraction, left ventricular volume, and regional wall motion can be measured at rest

and during exercise. The correlation between contrast ventriculography and radionuclide ventriculography is excellent.[17]

Serial radionuclide ventriculograms permit the accurate assessment of changes in left ventricular performance following CABG surgery and correlate well with the clinical status of the patients.[30] Successful results from CABG surgery have been associated with an increased ejection fraction (EF) following exercise, regardless of whether the resting EF is increased or unchanged from the preoperative rate.[31] Roberts has found this technique to be a sensitive indicator of the effectiveness of various methods of myocardial protection.[32]

ECHOCARDIOGRAPHY

M-Mode echocardiography provides information about ventricular volumes, wall thickness, EF, and shortening velocities. The usefulness of this technique is limited, however, because it provides a smaller view of the left ventricle for analysis. In contrast, two-dimensional echocardiography allows the clinician to obtain a wider dimension of the ventricle. The technique utilizes a series of ultrasound beams that are transmitted from a transducer such that long and cross-sectional views are visualized. Two-dimensional echocardiography has been used in the open- and closed-chest models, and provides accurate data regarding global and regional function.[33–36] It has been especially helpful in showing changes in left ventricular (LV) compliance following global and regional ischemia.[37,38] Spotnitz has shown that LV mass changes detected by two-dimensional echocardiography relate to LV water content, and he has studied these mass changes experimentally and during clinical cardiac surgery.[39,40] In preliminary studies in the operating room, we have shown a close correlation between EF and regional wall motion changes using intraoperative two-dimensional echocardiography and gated blood pool scans obtained on the seventh postoperative day. Recently, we have also employed a retroesophageal two-dimensional echo probe during cardiac surgery. This probe is positioned in the esophagus and can continuously monitor changes in ventricular volume and wall motion throughout the procedure. This eliminates the hand-held views in the operative field, which are necessary with conventional two-dimensional echocardiography.

Recently, intraoperative contrast two-dimensional echocardiography has been used to evaluate aortic and mitral insufficiency following operative repair and to determine the presence of residual shunts following atrial septal defect (ASD) and ventricular septal defect (VSD) closure.*[41] The accuracy with which two-dimensional echocardiography can detect changes in intraoperative regional and global venticular function and its ability to assess the results of valve repairs will alow the surgeon to initiate therapy intraoperatively before permanent myocardial damage occurs.

CONCLUSIONS

The development of accurate noninvasive technology such as two-dimensional echocardiography and radionuclide ventriculography has allowed the clinician to better evaluate the results of clinical cardiac surgery. Intraoperative echocardiography and Doppler flow studies will be able to warn the surgeon of LV dysfunction and prosthetic valve leaks. The surgeon may then be able to institute a plan of therapy to reverse these problems in the operating room. In addition, accurate noninvasive technology will better define the results of surgery in certain subgroups of pa-

* Takamato S: Personal communication.

tients so that indications and timing for certain procedures are better established. Finally, the effects of various cardioplegic techniques to preserve LV function in the human heart will be more accurately assessed.

REFERENCES

1. Hultgren HN, Shettigar VR, Pfeifer JR et al: Acute myocardial infarction and ischemic injury during surgery for coronary artery disease. Am Heart J 94:146, 1977
2. Oldham HN, Roe CR, Young WG et al: Intraoperative detection of myocardial infarction during coronary artery surgery by plasma creatine phosphokinase isoenzyme analysis. Surgery 74:917, 1973
3. Gross, H, Rubin IL, Laufer H et al: Transient abnormal Q waves in the dog without myocardial infarction. Am J Cardiol 14:669, 1964
4. Klein HO, Gross H, Rubin IL: Transient electrocardiographic changes simulating myocardial infarction during open-heart surgery. Am Heart J 79:463, 1968
5. Aintablan A, Hamby RI, Hoffman I et al: Significance of new Q waves after bypass grafting: Correlations between graft patency, ventriculogram, and surgical venting technique. Am Heart J 95:429, 1978
6. Bassan MD, Oatfield R, Hoffman I et al: New Q waves after aortocoronary bypass surgery. N Engl J Med 290:349, 1974
7. Roberts AJ, Spies SM, Lichtenthal PR et al: Changes in left ventricular performance related to perioperative myocardial infarction in coronary artery bypass graft surgery. Ann Thorac Surg 33:516, 1983
8. Blomquist CG: Use of exercise testing for diagnostic and functional evaluation of patients with arteriosclerotic heart disease. Circulation 44:1120, 1971
9. Bartel AG, Behar VS, Peter RH et al: Exercise stress testing in evaluation of aorto-coronary bypass surgery: Report of 123 patients. Circulation 48:141, 1973
10. Ritchie JL, Trobaugh GB, Hamilton GW et al: Myocardial imaging with thallium-201 at rest and during exercise: Comparison with coronary arteriography and resting and stress electrocardiography. Circulation 56:66, 1977
11. Assad–Morell JL, Frye RL, Connolly DC et al: Relation of intraoperative or early postoperative transmural myocardial infarction to patency of aorto-coronary bypass grafts and to diseased ungrafted coronary arteries. Am J Cardiol 35:767, 1975
12. Roe CR, Limbird LL, Wagner GS et al: Combined isoenzymes analysis in the diagnosis of myocardial injury. J Lab Clin Med 80:577, 1972

13. Bolooki H, Sommer L, Faraldo A et al: The significance of serum enzyme studies in patients undergoing direct coronary artery surgery. J Thorac Cardiovasc Surg 65:863, 1973

14. Roberts R, Sober BE: Effect of selected drugs and myocardial infarction on the disappearance of creatine kinase from the circulation in conscious dogs. Cadiovasc Res 11:103, 1977

15. Strom S: Myocardial enzyme release in coronary bypass and valve replacement surgery. Acta Med Scand (Suppl) 633:1, 1979

16. Klein MS, Coleman E, Weldon CS et al: Concordance of electrocardiographic and scintigraphic criteria of myocardial injury after cardiac surgery. J Thorac Cardiovasc Surg 71:934, 1976

17. Roberts AJ, Spies SM, Sanders JR et al: Serial assessment of left ventricular performance following coronary bypass graft surgery: Early postoperative results using myocardial protection afforded by multidose hypothermic potassium crystalloid cardioplegia. J Thorac Cardiovasc Surg 81:69, 1981

18. Papadopoulas NM, Hufnagel CA: Evaluation of lactate dehydrogenase isoenzyme patterns in serum of patients undergoing cardiac surgery. J Thorac Cardiovasc Surg 76:173, 1978

19. Shen AC, Jennings RB: Myocardial calcium and magnesium in acture ischemic injury. Am J Pathol 67:417, 1972

20. Bonte FJ, Parkey RW, Graham KD et al: A new method for radionuclide imaging of acute myocardial infarcts. Radiology 110:473, 1974

21. Stokely EM, Buja LM, Tenis SE et al: Measurement of acute myocardial infarcts in dogs with technetium-99 stannous pyrophosphate scintigrams. J Nucl Med 17:1, 1976

22. Buja LM, Parkey RW, Stokely EM et al: Pathophysiology of technetium-99m stannous pyrophosphate and thallium-201 scintigraphy of actue anterior myocardial infarcts in dogs. J Clin Invest 57:1508, 1976

23. Buja LM, Parkey RW, Dees JH et al: Morphologic correlates of technetium-99m stannous pyrophosphate imaging of acute myocardial infarcts in dogs. Circulation 52:596, 1975

24. Parkey RW, Bonte FJ, Meyer SL et al: A new method for radionuclide imaging of acute myocardial infarction in humans. Circulation 50:540, 1974

25. Roberts AJ, Combes JR, Jacobstein JG et al: Perioperative myocardial infarction associated with coronary artery bypass graft surgery: Improved sensitivity in the diagnosis within 6 hours after operation with 99m Tc-glucoheptonate myocardial imaging and myocardial-specific isoenzymes. Ann Thorac Surg 27:42, 1979

26. Willerson TJ, Parkey RW, Stokey EM et al: Infarct sizing with technetium-99m stannous pyrophosphate scintigraphy in dogs and man, the relationship between scintigraphic and precordial mapping estimates of infarct size in patients. Cardiovasc Res 11:291, 1977

27. Hung J, Kelley DT, McLaughlin AF et al: Preoperative and postoperative technetium-99m pyrophosphate myocardial scintigraphy in the assessment of operative infarction in coronary artery surgery. J Thorac Cardiovasc Surg 78:68, 1979

28. Ritchie JL, Narahara KA, Trobough GB et al: Thallium-201 myocardial imaging before and after coronary revascularization: Assessment of regional myocardial blood flow and graft patency. Circulation 56:830, 1977

29. Zimmer AM, Pavel DG, Patterson UN: In vivo red blood cell labeling using consecutive injections of stannous pyrophosphate and technetium-99m pertechnetate (abstr). J Nucl Med 17:566, 1976

30. Newman GE, Rerych SK, Jones RH, Sabiston DC: Noninvasive assessment of the effects of aorto-coronary bypass grating on ventricular function during rest and exercise. J Thorac Cardiovasc Surg 70:617, 1980

31. Kamath ML, Hellman CK, Schmidt DH et al: Improvement of left ventricular function after myocardial revascularization. J Thorac Cardiovasc Surg 79:645, 1980

32. Roberts AJ, Spies SM, Meyers SN et al: Early and long term improvement in left ventricular performance following coronary bypass surgery. Surgery 88:467, 1980

33. Moynihan PF, Panai AF, Feldman CI: Quantitative detection of regional left ventricular contraction abnormalities by two dimensional echocardiography. I. Analysis of methods. Circulation 63:752, 1981

34. Wyatt HL, Ming KH, Meerbaum S et al: Cross-sectional echocardiography. I. Analysis of mathematical models for quantifying mass of the left ventricle in dogs. Circulation 60:1104, 1979

35. Eaton LW, Maughan WL, Shoukas AA et al: Accurate volume determination in the isolated ejecting canine left ventricle by two-dimensional echocardiography. Circulation 60:320, 1979

36. Collins RH, Haasler GB, Krug JH et al: Canine left ventricular volume and mass during thoracotomy by two-dimensional echocardiography. J Surg Res 33:294, 1982

37. Lazar HL, Haasler GB, Collins RH et al: Mechanisms of altered ventricular compliance following ischemia using two dimensional echocardiography. Current Surg 39:253, 1982

38. Lazar HL, Spotnitz HM: Ventricular compliance, shape and mass during regional ischemia and reperfusion analyzed by two-dimensional echocardiography. J Am Coll Cardiol 1(2):616, 1983

39. Rosenblum HM, Haasler GB, Spotnitz WD et al: Effects of simulated clinical cardiopulmonary bypass and car-

dioplegia on mass of the canine left ventricle. Ann Thorac Surg 39:139, 1985

40. Spotnitz WD, Clark MB, Rosenblum HM et al: Effect of cardiopulmonary bypass and global ischemia on human and canine left ventricular mass: Evidence for inter-species differences. Surgery 96:230, 1984

41. Eguaras MG, Pasalodos J, Gonzalez V et al: Intraoperative contrast two-dimensional echocardiography: Evolution of the presence and severity of aortic and mitral regurgitation during cardiac operations. J Thorac Cardiovasc Surg 89:573, 1985

14

SELECTION OF PATIENTS FOR MYOCARDIAL REVASCULARIZATION

David P. Faxon

Myocardial revascularization by reversed saphenous vein coronary artery bypass grafting (CABG) was popularized by Favaloro and colleagues at the Cleveland Clinic in 1968.[1] Its potential for improving blood supply to the heart and for relieving symptoms was quickly realized, and the technique is now widely applied to symptomatic patients with obstructed coronary artery disease.[2] In addition to saphenous vein bypass surgery, internal mammary artery bypass grafting and percutaneous transluminal coronary angioplasty (PTCA) have emerged as procedures that also may have advantages in selected patients.[3,4] Advances in the technical aspects of these procedures have improved overall success rates and have decreased the number of complications, resulting in broader clinical application. In part as a result of these advances, a consensus on who should undergo myocardial revascularization is still unclear. Some of the current dilemmas are related to whether coronary bypass grafting prolongs life. It is also unclear whether it reduces subsequent myocardial infarction and whether it is best performed early or late in the course of the disease. Some of these questions have been addressed by three large multicenter randomized trials of medical versus surgical therapy in patients with coronary artery disease. However, neither the role of angioplasty nor the impact of internal mammary artery grafting on long-term success has yet been assessed adequately. Unfortunately, we have only limited information about these newer techniques, and their proper place in a treatment strategy for patients with coronary artery disease remains speculative.

SELECTION OF PATIENTS WITH STABLE ANGINA FOR MYOCARDIAL REVASCULARIZATION

ANGINA INADEQUATELY CONTROLLED ON MEDICAL THERAPY

In the past the development of techniques to relieve angina were spurred by the inability to adequately control patients' symptoms despite the use of aggressive medical therapy. Although therapy has changed considerably over the past two decades with the development of numerous beta-blocking agents, calcium antagonists, and long-acting nitrates, a sizable portion of patients continue to have significant angina requiring revascularization (Table 14–1). In patients undergoing cardiac catheterization in the CASS study, more than 40% were referred for revascularization because of severe and uncontrolled symptoms.[5]

Numerous studies have shown that bypass surgery is effective in relieving angina in 76% to 90% of patients, with only 5% to 6% showing clinical deterioration.[2] For this reason, bypass surgery has been generally accepted as the treatment of choice for patients with angina that is inadequately controlled on medical therapy.

TABLE 14–1
CRITERIA FOR SELECTION OF PATIENTS FOR
MYOCARDIAL REVASCULARIZATION

Indications for Revascularization
Angina inadequately controlled on medical therapy
Unstable angina despite medical therapy
Mildly symptomatic patients
  Left main coronary artery disease (> 50%)
  Three-vessel disease and poor LV function
  Three-vessel disease and inducible ischemia on exercise tolerance test

Less Certain Indications
Proximal left anterior descending disease and two-vessel coronary disease and mild symptoms

Medical Therapy
Unstable angina that rapidly responds to medical therapy
Single- and double-vessel disease with mild symptoms
Asymptomatic patients

Long-term follow-up studies have shown that CABG may have a significant incidence of closure after 7 years, with as many as 45% of bypass grafts closed at 11 years.[6,7] In addition, the ability to perform a second bypass on the patient at this stage is limited, with 42% of patients unrevascularizable in some series.[8] Recognition of this fact has promoted the use of internal mammary artery grafting, a technique shown to have excellent short-term and now long-term patency.[3] These grafts appear to be remarkably free of significant atherosclerosis. Large series of long-term follow-up, however, are still not sufficient to allow firm conclusions about the role of internal mammary grafting on long-term patency.

Angioplasty has also been applied with increasing frequency to patients with single-vessel disease as well as to selected patients with multivessel disease.[9,10] Although bypass surgery has been proven to be efficacious in these patients, angioplasty may offer a stalling technique to allow bypass surgery to be reserved for the patient with more severe disease or to be used when a patient develops the anatomy that would make him unsuitable for angioplasty. The potential yet unproven advantages of angioplasty over bypass surgery include a lower morbidity and cost and a greater likelihood of returning the patient to meaningful employment.[10]

Due to improvements in surgical technique, most patients with severe angina are candidates for bypass surgery. This was not always the case. In the early 1970s, more than 20% of patients were not considered candidates because of either small or poorly visualized distal vessels or poor left ventricular (LV) function (e.g., ejection fraction [EF] < 35%).[11] Today the incidence of rejection for inoperable anatomy is less than 5%, with many patients having successful bypass surgery despite diffuse coronary disease or poor LV function.[12]

Although the primary goal of bypass surgery is to improve symptoms, increasing evidence has also suggested that survival may be prolonged. Kaiser and associates, using the registry of the coronary artery surgery study (CASS), compared surgically treated patients with severe angina with medically treated patients with severe angina.[13] The groups were matched for baseline variables and closely resembled the randomized group of patients with mild angina. In this observational study, the surgically treated patients had a significantly better survival rate than did the medically treated patients. These results are consistent with other nonrandomized comparisons and support the concept that the presence of severe angina or inducible ischemia on exercise testing are important risk factors for long-term survival and that bypass surgery may have an important impact on the reduction of this risk.

UNSTABLE ANGINA

The treatment of patients with unstable angina is generally hospitalization and the institution of maximal drug therapy. Today, this includes beta blockers, calcium antagonists, and long-acting nitrates. Patients who continue to have symptoms are at high risk for subsequent myocardial infarction and death.[14] Although intravenous nitroglycerin, nifedipine, aspirin, and heparin have been shown to reduce these complications, many patients continue to need urgent revascularization.[15,16] Both bypass surgery and angioplasty have been shown to significantly reduce angina as well as complications in patients with unstable angina.[17,18] Patients whose condition stabilizes on medical therapy and who can be discharged from the hospital are unlikely to need urgent bypass surgery, based upon the results of the National Heart, Lung, and Blood Institute (NHLBI) randomized trial.[19] In this multicenter study, there was no survival benefit from CABG when it was done shortly after hospitalization (91% was 90% at 2 years, $P = $ NS). However, 36% of patients treated medically had recurrence of angina

that was severe enough to warrant later bypass grafting. Because the mortality for this crossover group was not increased, it is generally accepted that revascularization with angioplasty or bypass surgery can be postponed until the recurrence of symptoms dictates the need for revascularization.

MILDLY SYMPTOMATIC OR ASYMPTOMATIC PATIENTS REQUIRING REVASCULARIZATION

MILD ANGINA

Three major randomized trials have addressed the role of bypass surgery in patients with mild to moderate angina.[20-23] All three trials were consistent in a number of areas, despite differences

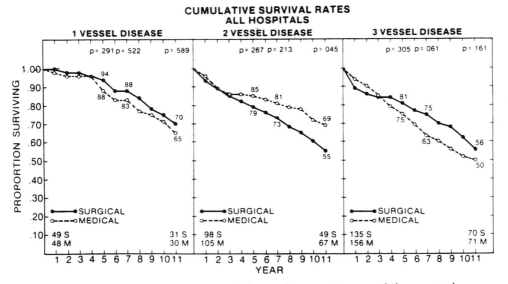

FIG. 14–1. The cumulative 11-year survival rates for one-, two-, and three-vessel disease from the VA Cooperative Study of coronary artery bypass surgery. (Detre KM, Takaro T, Hultgren H et al: Long-term mortality and morbidity results of the Veterans Administration randomized trial of coronary artery bypass surgery. Circulation (Suppl V) 72:84–89, 1985; by permission of the American Heart Association, Inc)

in selection criteria, surgical mortality, and the years of study. Both the Veterans Administration (VA) and the European Coronary Surgery Study (ECSS) trial randomized patients with left main coronary artery disease.[23-25] The VA trial demonstrated a significant survival advantage with surgery for patients with left main coronary artery disease while the ECSS did not. However, only left main coronary artery disease of 50% to 70% was randomized in the ECSS trial, and the number of patients was small, precluding definite conclusions. The CASS trial did demonstrate a survival advantage for patients with significant left main coronary disease in the registry portion of the study.[26] In patients without left main coronary artery disease, the VA and

CASS studies showed no overall advantage for bypass surgery in patients with mild angina, while the ECSS study did (Figs. 14–1 and 14–2).[23,24,27] Subset analysis disclosed that all three studies could identify patient groups that benefited from surgery. The VA trial patients with three-vessel disease and impaired LV function (angiographic high risk) had a significantly better survival rate at 5, 7, and 11 years (50% versus 62%, $P < 0.0026$) than did patients who were treated medically.[25] Also, a clinical high-risk tercile that benefited from surgery was identified. The ECSS trial demonstrated a benefit in patients with three-vessel disease as well as in patients with two-vessel disease with proximal left anterior descending lesions.[27] Since all pa-

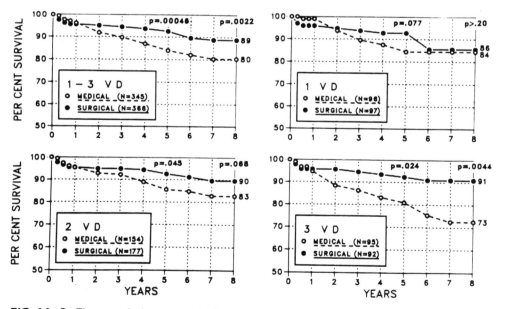

FIG. 14–2. The cumulative survival of patients with one-, two-, and three-vessel disease (> 75%) from the European Coronary Surgery Study group. (Varnauskas E, The European Coronary Surgery Study Group: Survival, myocardial infarction, and employment status in a prospective randomized study of coronary bypass surgery. Circulation (Suppl V) 72(90):101, 1985; by permission of the American Heart Association, Inc)

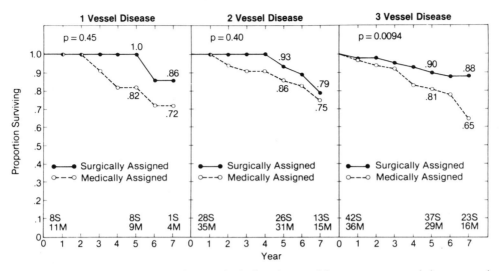

FIG. 14–3. The 7-year cumulative survival of patients with one-, two-, and three-vessel disease and poor left ventricular function from the NHLBI coronary artery surgery study (CASS). (Passamani E, Davis KB, Gillespie MJ et al: A randomized trial of coronary artery bypass surgery: Survival of patients with a low ejection fraction. N Engl J Med 312:1665–1671, 1985; reprinted by permission)

tients had good LV function, the influence of this variable on survival could not be assessed. The CASS trial was also consistent with these two earlier trials in that patients with three-vessel disease and poor LV function ($35 < EF < 50$) had improved survival after 7 years of follow-up (84% versus 70%, $P = 0.01$).[28] Thus the major difference among the three studies was that the ECSS trial showed improved survival in patients with three-vessel disease and good ventricular function as well as in those with two-vessel disease, good ventricular function, and a proximal left anterior descending lesion.

It is important to recognize that the three studies have a number of significant differences that might help to explain the lack of agreement. Although the survival following surgery was nearly identical in all three studies, medical survival was significantly different, rising from 76% at 6 years in the VA trial, to 82% in the ECSS trial, and to

90% in the CASS trial (see Figs. 14–1, 14–2, and 14–3). Although changes in medical therapy over this 10-year period may have been responsible for this improvement, a more plausible explanation may be related to the degree of myocardial ischemia prior to randomization. The VA Cooperative trial identified a high-risk clinical subgroup that comprised patients with severe symptoms, hypertension, prior myocardial infarction, and resting ST-segment abnormalities on the electrocardiogram. In this subgroup, surgery significantly improved survival.[29] Also, 30% of the patients in the VA trial were high risk while only 22% of those in the CASS trial were. In the ECSS trial, 42% of the patients had class-3 angina. As previously mentioned, observational data from the CASS registry have suggested that patients with severe angina survived longer after surgical therapy.[13] In the ECSS trial, patients who exhibited ischemic ST-segment depression greater than 1.5 mm fared better with surgery than with medical therapy (92% versus 79%, $P < 0.001$).[24] The CASS trial also confirmed this with a 94% survival in patients who had angina on their exercise test compared to 89% of those who did not (Fig. 14–4).[30] Examination of the exercise response also showed that the highest risk patients were patients with three-vessel disease and poor LV function and a positive exercise test. Other nonrandomized studies have also suggested that

exercise-induced ischemia or changes in radionuclide EF are important prognostic factors in patients with mild as well as moderate angina.[31,32]

Relief of angina and improvement in quality of life are major objectives in the treatment of coronary artery disease. Although these three major studies differ in mortality, they all have demonstrated a significant reduction in angina and improvement in exercise testing and quality of life.[27,33,34] However, a reduction in myocardial infarction following surgery has not been demonstrated by any of these three major studies.[23,24,35]

Despite criticism of these studies due to either high surgical mortality (the VA trial), potential patient selection bias (ECSS and CASS), small number of patients in subset analysis (CASS), or crossovers (ECSS and CASS), guidelines for patient selection can be identified.[36–38] As described above, surgery appears to be indicated for patients with mild angina in the presence of significant left main coronary artery disease, three-vessel disease and poor LV function, or three-vessel disease with normal LV function and inducible myocardial ischemia. The indications for surgery are less clearly defined among patients with mild symptoms and two-vessel disease with a proximal left anterior descending lesion. In asymptomatic patients adequately treated with medical therapy, patients with single- or double-vessel coronary disease and mild symptoms, and some patients with unstable angina who respond rapidly to medical therapy, surgery should be postponed until worsening of symptoms dictates the need for revascularization.

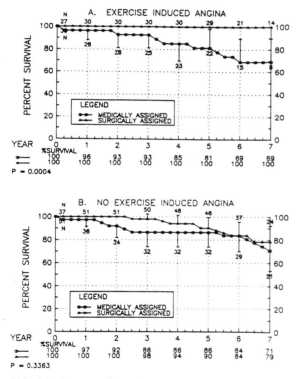

FIG. 14–4. The effect of exercise-induced angina on subsequent survival in medically and surgically assigned patients from the CASS randomized study. (Ryan TJ, Weiner DA, McCabe CH et al: Exercise testing in the coronary artery surgery study randomized population. Circulation (Suppl V) 72:31–38, 1985; by permission of the American Heart Association, Inc)

REFERENCES

1. Favaloro RG: Saphenous vein autograft replacement of severe segmental coronary artery occlusion: Operative technique. Ann Thorac Surg 5:334–339, 1968

2. Rahimtoola SH: Coronary bypass surgery for chronic angina—1981. A perspective. Circulation 65:225–241, 1982

3. Lytle BW, Cosgrove DM, Saltus GL et al: Multivessel coronary revascularization without saphenous vein: Long-term results of bilateral internal mammary artery grafting. Ann Thorac Surg 36:540, 1983

4. Hall D, Gruentzig AR: Percutaneous transluminal coronary angioplasty: Current technique and perspective. Heart Transplantation 3:206–209, 1984

5. Principal Investigators of the CASS and their associates, Killip T, (ed): National Heart, Lung, and Blood Institute Coronary Artery Surgery Study (CASS). Circulation (Suppl I) 63:1, 1981

6. Bourassa MG, Enjalbert M, Campeau L et al: Progression of atherosclerosis in coronary arteries and bypass grafts: Ten years later. Am J Cardiol 53:102C–107C, 1984

7. Loop FD, Lytle BW, Gill CC et al: Trends in selection and results of coronary reoperations. Ann Thorac Surg 36:380, 1983

8. de Feyter PJ, Serruys PW, Brower RW et al: Comparison of preoperative, operative, and postoperative variables in asymptomatic or minimally symptomatic patients to severely symptomatic patients three years after coronary artery bypass grafting: Analysis of 423 patients. Am J Cardiol 55:362–366, 1985

9. Baim D, Faxon DP: Coronary angioplasty. In Grossman (ed): Cardiac Catheterization and Angiography, pp 473–492. Philadelphia, Lea, & Febiger, 1986

10. Proceedings of the National Heart, Lung, and Blood Institute Workshop on the outcome of percutaneous transluminal coronary angioplasty. Am J Cardiol 53:1C–146C, 1984

11. Cohn PF: Clinical, angiographic, and hemodynamic factors influencing selection of patients for coronary artery bypass surgery. Prog Cardiovasc Dis 18:223, 1975

12. Kaiser GC: CABG 1984: Technical aspects of bypass surgery. Circulation 72:V46–V58, 1985

13. Kaiser GC, Davis KB, Fisher LD et al: Survival following coronary artery bypass grafting in patients with severe angina pectoris (CASS). J Thorac Cardiovasc Surg 89:513–524, 1985

14. Mulcahy R, Daly L, Graham I et al: Unstable angina: Natural history and determinants of prognosis. Am J Cardiol 48:525–528, 1981

15. Rahimtoola SH: Unstable angina: Current status. Mod Conc Cardiovas Dis 54:19–23, 1985

16. Ouyang P, Brinker JA, Mellits ED et al: Variables predictive of successful medical therapy in patients with unstable angina: Selection by multivariant analysis from clinical, electrocardiographic, and angiographic evaluations. Circulation 70:367–376, 1984

17. Rahimtoola S: Coronary bypass surgery for unstable angina. Circulation 69:842–848, 1984

18. Faxon DP, Detre KM, McCabe CH et al: Role of percutaneous transluminal coronary angioplasty in the treatment of unstable angina. Report from the National Heart, Lung and Blood Institure, Percutaneous Transluminal Coronary Angioplasty, and Coronary Artery Surgery Study Registries. Am J Cardiol 53:131C–135C, 1984

19. Unstable angina pectoris: National Cooperative Study Group to compare medical and surgical therapy. II. In-hospital experience and initial follow-up results in patients with one, two and three vessel disease. Am J Cardiol 42:839, 1978

20. Murphy ML, Hultgren HN, Detre K et al: Treatment of chronic stable angina. A preliminary report of survival data of the randomized Veterans Administration Cooperative Study. N Engl J Med 297:621–627, 1977

21. European Coronary Surgery Study Group: Coronary bypass surgery in stable angina pectoris: Survival at two years. Lancet 1:889, 1979

22. CASS Principal Investigators and Their Associates: Coronary Artery Surgery Study (CASS): A randomized trial of coronary artery bypass surgery. Survival data. Circulation 68:939–950, 1983

23. Takaro T, Hultgren H, Lipton M et al: VA Cooperative Randomized Study for coronary arterial occlusive disease. II. Left main disease. Circulation (Suppl III) 54:107–117, 1976

24. European Coronary Surgery Study Group: Long-term results of prospective randomized study of coronary artery bypass surgery in stable angina pectoris. Lancet 2:1173–1180, 1982

25. Detre KM, Takaro T, Hultgren H et al: Long-term mortality and morbidity results of the Veterans Administration randomized trial of coronary artery bypass surgery. Circulation (Suppl V) 72:84–89, 1985

26. Chaitman BR, Bourassa MG, Davis K et al: Effect of coronary bypass surgery on survival patterns in subsets of patients with left main coronary artery disease. Report of the Collaborative Study in Coronary Artery Surgery (CASS). Am J Cardiol 48:765–777, 1981

27. Varnauskas E, the European Coronary Surgery Study Group: Survival, myocardial infarction, and employment status in a prospective randomized study of coronary bypass surgery. Circulation (Suppl V) 72:90–101, 1985

28. Passamani E, Davis KB, Gillespie MJ et al: A randomized trial of coronary artery bypass surgery: Survival of patients with a low ejection fraction. N Engl J Med 312:1665–1671, 1985

29. Veterans Administration Coronary Artery Bypass Surgery Cooperative Study Group: Eleven year survival in the Veterans Administration randomized trial of coro-

nary bypass surgery for stable angina. N Engl J Med 311:1333, 1984

30. Ryan TJ, Weiner DA, McCabe CH et al: Exercise testing in the coronary artery surgery study randomized population. Circulation (Suppl V) 72:31–38, 1985

31. Bonow RO, Kent KM, Rosing DR et al: Exercise-induced ischemia in mildly symptomatic patients with coronary artery disease and preserved left ventricular function: Identification of subgroups at risk of death during medical therapy. N Engl J Med 311:1339, 1984

32. Bonow RO, Epstein SE: Indications for coronary artery bypass surgery in patients with chronic angina pectoris: Implications of the multicenter randomized trials. Circulation (Suppl V) 72:23–30, 1985

33. CASS Principal Investigators and Their Associates. Coronary Artery Surgery Study (CASS): A randomized trial of coronary artery bypass surgery. Quality of life in patients randomly assigned to treatment groups. Circulation 68:951–960, 1983

34. Hultgren HN, Peduzzi P, Detre K et al: The 5 year effect of bypass surgery on relief of angina and exercise performance. Circulation 72:V79–V83, 1985

35. CASS Principal Investigators and Their Associates: Myocardial infarction and mortality in the Coronary Artery Surgery Study (CASS) randomized trial. N Engl J Med 310:750–758, 1984

36. Lawrie GM, DeBakey ME: The coronary artery surgery study. JAMA 252:2609–2611, 1984

37. Gunnar RM, Loeb HS: An alternate interpretation of the CASS study. Circulation 71:193–194, 1985

38. Julian DG: The practical implications of the coronary artery surgery trials. Br Heart J 54:343–350, 1985

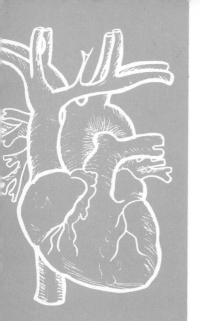

15

RIGHT VENTRICULAR SUPPORT BY PULMONARY ARTERY COUNTERPULSATION

John M. Moran

Historically, cardiac assist devices have been used primarily to aid the failing left ventricle, because of the overriding importance of left ventricular function to overall cardiac performance. Since the first experimental work was described in 1962, intra-aortic balloon counterpulsation (IABC) for support of the left ventricle has been the subject of intensive laboratory and clinical investigation.[1] The first clinical application in 1968 was rapidly followed by widespread clinical use, which proved the usefulness of IABC beyond doubt by providing highly significant salvage in patients requiring a partial form of left ventricular assist on a temporary basis.[2] The idea of applying the same principle of counterpulsation to the right ventricle is not a new one, but pulmonary artery balloon counterpulsation (PABC) has received relatively little attention, and that only in the past few years, although experimental evidence that PABC indeed is a potent modality for the treatment of right ventricular failure was provided in 1970.[3] Pulmonary artery balloon counterpulsation has been utilized sporadically in the clinical setting over the past 5 years and, under certain circumstances, has proven to be effective, providing survival in situations that clearly had lethal potential. This chapter will summarize experimental work in this area and the clinical experience to date, and will attempt to place PABC in perspective vis-à-vis other methods of right ventricular support available at the present time.

EXPERIMENTAL STUDIES

The first demonstration of the effectiveness of PABC, provided by Kralios and associates, utilized a model in which pulmonary hypertension was produced by embolization of the pulmonary circulation with homologous blood thrombi or cornstarch.[3] These researchers showed that counterpulsation using a 25-ml balloon within the pulmonary artery did not provide any substantial hemodynamic changes under normal circulatory conditions, but after induction of right ventricular failure with pulmonary embolization, there was dramatic hemodynamic improvement. This improvement was characterized by significant reduction in right atrial pressure and pulmonary vascular resistance, and improvement in arterial pressure, cardiac output, right ventricular systolic pressure, arterial oxygen saturation, and arterial pH. Spotnitz and colleagues further investigated the principles of counterpulsation applied to the pulmonary artery by ligating the right pulmonary artery in dogs and moving blood in and out of the proximal pulmonary artery with a piston pump in a counterpulsation mode.[4] They reported diminution in preload in both the normal and failing right ventricle and improvement in the cardiac output when counterpulsation was employed in a setting of right ventricular failure. Jett and coworkers demonstrated significant unloading of the failing right ventricle in a model of canine chronic right ventricular hypertrophy.[5] Balloon counterpulsation was provided with an intra-aortic balloon within a graft sewn to the pulmonary artery. PABC significantly reduced right ventricular preloading and afterload, and increased cardiac output and arterial pressure. Opravil and associates created right ventricular failure in dogs using a combination of pulmonary microembolization with glass beads and an infusion of serotonin to further increase pulmonary vascular resistance.[6] Using balloons specifically designed to fit the canine pulmonary artery, they demonstrated hemodynamically effective counterpulsation following production of progressive cardiogenic shock; its reversal was consistently successful using PABC. It was concluded that PABC effectively improved the function of the failing right ventricle caused by acute pulmonary hypertension. Gaines and coworkers produced profound right ventricular failure in goats by inducing ventricular fibrillation while the systemic circulation was supported with a left atrial–aortic bypass pump.[7] They did a comparative study of the various methods available for right ventricular support: (1) passive flow through the pulmonary artery, (2) pulmonary artery counterpulsation using an intra-aortic–type balloon within a prosthetic graft sewn to the pulmonary artery, (3) pulmonary artery pulsation using a single-port, sac-type pulsatile device, and (4) right atrial–pulmonary arterial bypass using a valved pneumatic pulsatile pump. Gaines and associates found that the cardiac index was improved 43% above passive pulmonary flow utilizing PABC. The sac-type pulsatile support device provided a 106% increase in cardiac index above passive flow, and the valved atrial-to-pulmonary-artery bypass pump improved the cardiac index by 128%. In evaluating these results, it must be recognized that the rather unphysiologic condition of ventricular fibrillation existed; any benefits to right ventricular performance that may be

achieved by diminution of right ventricular afterload in the beating heart with PABC are not available. Spence and associates produced global myocardial depression using a propranolol infusion and provided left ventricular support by total left ventricular bypass.[8] PABC was instituted when right ventricular failure supervened and caused limited cardiac output. They were able to demonstrate doubling of the cardiac output and right ventricular stroke work under these circumstances using PABC.

CLINICAL EXPERIENCE WITH PABC

Perioperative right ventricular dysfunction is a threat to patient survival and occurs in several clinical settings: pulmonary hypertension, either primary or secondary, the latter often due to mitral valvular disease; right ventricular infarction; inadequate myocardial protection of the right ventricle; and right ventricular trauma incident to ventriculotomy, usually for congenital heart disease. The diagnosis is readily made by visual observation of a distended, noncontracting right ventricle, together with hemodynamic evaluation, which includes demonstration of elevated right atrial mean pressure in conjunction with low left atrial mean pressure and a low cardiac index. However, biventricular failure occurs more commonly than does isolated right ventricular failure. If a patient cannot be weaned from cardiopulmonary bypass, IABC is promptly instituted after all the usual supportive measures have failed to improve the situation. With subsequent improvement in left ventricular function, right ventricular failure may continue, again manifested by acceptable left ventricular filling pressures and excessively high right atrial pressure. Once the overall assessment has resulted in diagnosis of right ventricular failure, all of the usual methods of support must be tried. These include adequate volume loading, correction of any metabolic problem such as acidosis and hypoxia, use of pulmonary vasodilators, and, of course, continuing inotropic support with appropriate β-adrenergic stimulating agents. With persistent failure of all of these methods to correct right ventricular failure, it is logical to turn to mechanical assist methods.

The least invasive method of right ventricular assistance is pulmonary artery balloon counterpulsation (PABC). This method was first used clinically and reported by Miller and associates.[9] In a setting of biventricular failure following surgery for ischemic heart disease, and with satisfactory response of left ventricular function to IABC, these researchers described the use of an intra-aortic balloon placed within a graft sewn to the pulmonary artery as a reservoir for blood and the functioning balloon. This allowed survival and transfer of the patient from the operating room, although death from arrhythmia occurred after 30 hours when preparations were being made for removal of the pulmonary artery balloon. The first long-term survival with PABC, and that for isolated right ventricular failure as well, was reported by Flege and associates.[10] This occurred in a setting of postoperative right ventricular dysfunction caused by pulmonary hypertension and mitral valvular disease. Dramatically effective hemodynamic improvement followed the institution of PABC in the method described by Miller and coworkers and applied by Flege's group. Subsequently, we reported two cases of secondary right ventricular failure in which IABC was insufficient to allow weaning from cardiopulmonary bypass.[11] Impressive improvement in right ventricular performance and cardiac output was achieved in both patients, although neither became a long-term survivor. In the first patient, the profound dependency of cardiac output on PABC was documented by a diminution in cardiac output from 4 to 2.5 liters/minute when the pulmonary artery balloon con-

sole failed. Although it was replaced within 15 minutes, a downhill course could not be reversed and the patient died within 2 hours. Symbas and associates have reported effective PABC in three patients with biventricular failure, all of whom were able to be transferred from the operating room because this modality was used.[12] In one patient, rapid right ventricular recovery following PABC insertion allowed removal of the right ventricular balloon prior to transfer from the operating room. That patient survived, but the other two succumbed, at 16 hours and 15 days, respectively.

PABC IN PERSPECTIVE

The increasing interest in the treatment of perioperative right ventricular dysfunction that has developed represents a logical progression in the history of cardiac surgery. This appears to be the result, at least in part, of the following factors: (1) with the overall improvement in the results of cardiac surgery in recent years, right ventricular failure has become more clearly identifiable as a cause of operative mortality; (2) a growing appreciation of the interdependence of right and left ventricles in overall cardiac importance has developed; (3) the increasing use of left ventricular assist devices has been found to "unmask" right ventricular failure as a cause of mortality and morbidity; and (4) the balloon counterpulsation principle, which is so firmly established in the treatment of left ventricular dysfunction, has been found to be applicable to the right ventricle.[13] In addition, ischemic heart disease, which constitutes the primary pathologic condition for which corrective cardiac surgery is performed today, affects the right ventricle in the following important ways: primary right ventricular infarction is not uncommon; postinfarction ventricular septal defect often causes profound right ventricular failure; and the right ventricle is less amenable to myocardial protection at operation because of its anterior position under the operative lights, which makes topical hypothermia more difficult to achieve, and because of the frequency of right coronary occlusion, which may not allow adequate distribution of cardioplegia solution.

During attempts to wean patients from cardiopulmonary bypass for right ventricular failure in high-risk situations, the surgeon must be aware of the possibility of either isolated right ventricular failure or isolated right ventricular failure secondary to left ventricular dysfunction. Exquisite judgment must be used in the decision of whether to supply mechanical assistance or to continue cardiopulmonary bypass for a period. Past experience has amply demonstrated that the sooner a device is utilized, the better the end result will be, largely by virtue of minimizing the time on cardiopulmonary bypass. The only situation in which isolated right ventricular support is appropriate is that in which there is clear demonstration of low or normal left atrial pressure and a normal or near-normal quality of left ventricular contraction. In most poor pump-weaning situations, however, biventricular failure will first require left ventricular assist, most often in the form of IABC. If poor or nonexistent right ventricular contractions and/or right atrial pressure in excess of 25 mm Hg persists in either primary or secondary right ventricular failure, consideration must be given to the method of choice for right ventricular support. If, in the weaning process, the right ventricle appears to do well until bypass flow is reduced to 1 to 2 liters/minute and only then demonstrates a degree of failure that obviates further weaning, insertion of a 40-ml PABC within a 20-mm Dacron graft sewn end-to-side in the pulmonary artery is a logical maneuver because it is the least invasive of support methods available. In most such instances, assuming adequate left ventricular function, sufficient hemodynamic improvement should occur

to allow final weaning from the pump and conclusion of the operation.

If right ventricular failure is more profound than indicated above, more potent modalities of assistance should be considered. The use of any extraordinary means of cardiac support must take into consideration the overall salvageability of the patient to avoid inappropriate and futile efforts that may unduly tax operative and postoperative teams and represent economic drain as well. The decision to provide mechanical assistance may be obvious and straightforward in the case of a child with congenital heart disease or a middle-aged patient with ischemic heart disease who was not expected to die at operation. In many instances, the decision will not be clear-cut and will tax the best compassionate judgment of the surgeon.

The method of right ventricular assistance that is available in all cardiac operating suites is right atrial–pulmonary artery (RA–PA) bypass. When the decision is made to provide it, all that needs to be done is to place a pulmonary artery cannula, to revise the cardiopulmonary bypass circuit to exclude the oxygenator, and to adjust venous drainage, if necessary, to drain the right atrium only. As total cardiopulmonary bypass is gradually withdrawn, the RA–PA circuit is activated. Flow rate will be guided by right and left ventricular filling pressures and the appearance of the right ventricle. Thermodilution cardiac output measurements are not reliable because an unmeasurable amount of injectate will enter the bypass circuit. An alternative pumping system is available to replace the relatively blood-traumatic roller pump. It is the centrifugal vortex pump,* which minimizes the need for heparin anticoagulation, is less traumatic to blood, cannot pump air, cannot pump against high resistance, and is therefore more suitable for prolonged partial support than the roller pump.

* Biomedicus, Minneapolis, MN

Experience with this pump has been primarily with left ventricular bypass, but Pennington and associates have utilized it for RA–PA assistance as well.[14] Nearly all reported experience with partial bypass assistance, however, is related to left ventricular bypass, usually left atrial–aortic, and to the use of the roller pump and standard cannulae.[15,16] With this relatively simple approach, which uses universally available equipment, survival of 24% to 50% of patients has been achieved.[16]

There is no question that the most potent modality currently available for uni- or biventricular mechanical assistance is the pneumatically activated sac-type pump. Developed by several investigators in various forms over the past 15 years, both intra- and extracorporeal devices have been used clinically.[17-20] It is beyond the scope of this chapter to provide a complete review of this subject. It is evident, however, that the devices originally developed for left ventricular assistance are perfectly appropriate to use for right ventricular assistance. The largest and most successful of the reported experience to date is that using the Pierce-Donachy–valved, pneumatically powered, angle-port sac-type pump.[7,14] It has a stroke volume of 65 ml and an ejection fraction of approximately 75%. The experience of Pennington and associates dramatically underscores the importance of recognition and treatment of biventricular failure; of 16 patients with biventricular failure who received only left ventricular assistance, none were weaned and none survived.[14] Ten other patients received biventricular support for biventricular failure: seven with predominant right ventricular failure received a right ventricular assist device and an IABP; three were weaned and two are long-term survivors. The remaining three patients with balanced biventricular failure received biventricular assist devices: two were weaned and one is a long-term survivor. Pierce's

group has used RA–PA pumping in two patients with isolated right ventricular failure, both were weaned from the device and discharged from the hospital.[7] They have had no survivors, however, among seven patients requiring biventricular assistance for biventricular failure.

It is evident from a review of the pertinent literature that the role of pulmonary artery pumping in the treatment of perioperative right ventricular failure has not yet been established. Of the few case reports extant, hemodynamic effectiveness and/or survival has been documented; the failure rate is unknown. The experimental evidence suggests that PABC will provide significant support for the failing but beating right ventricle. Jett and colleagues demonstrated an increase in cardiac output of 40% in a model of right ventricular hypertrophy, we demonstrated a 53% improvement in cardiac output in a model of right ventricular failure caused by pulmonary hypertension, and Spence and associates demonstrated an 82% improvement in cardiac output in the pharmacologically depressed right ventricle.[5,6,8] Thus it appears that the lesser degree of improvement afforded by pulmonary artery pumping in the report of Gaines and co-workers may have been due to a totally nonfunctioning right ventricle.[7]

Proper clinical evaluation of PABC awaits the fabrication and testing of a dedicated pulmonary artery balloon such as that used in sheep by Kralios and the one that we designed for use in dogs.[3,6] The currently available methodology, in which a balloon designed for use in the thoracic aorta is placed within a Dacron graft sewn to the pulmonary artery, is somewhat cumbersome and inappropriate. We have designed a balloon for use in humans that is inserted through the pulmonary outflow tract or directly into the pulmonary artery, but clinical investigation has not yet begun. The available experimental and clinical evidence suggests that it will be well tolerated by the pulmonary artery. Whether it will be feasible to insert the device through a peripheral vein is yet another problem awaiting a solution.

REFERENCES

1. Moulopoulos SD, Topaz ST, Kolff WJ: Diastolic balloon pumping (with carbon dioxide) in the aorta: Mechanical assistance to failing circulation. Am Heart J 63:669, 1962
2. Kantrowitz A, Tjonneland S, Freed PS et al: Initial experience with intra-aortic cardiac assistance in cardiogenic shock. JAMA 203:135, 1968
3. Kralios AC, Zwart HHJ, Moulopoulos SD et al: Intrapulmonary artery balloon pumping. J Thorac Cardiovasc Surg 60:215, 1970
4. Spotnitz HM, Berman MA, Reis RL, Epstein SE: The effects of synchronized counterpulsation of the pulmonary artery on right ventricular hemodynamics. J Thorac Cardiovasc Surg 61:167, 1971
5. Jett GK, Siwek LG, Picone AL et al: Pulmonary artery balloon counterpulsation for right ventricular failure: An experimental evaluation. J Thorac Cardiovasc Surg 86:364, 1983
6. Opravil M, Gorman AJ, Krejcie TC et al: Pulmonary artery balloon counterpulsation for right ventricular failure: I. Experimental results. Ann Thorac Surg 38:242, 1984
7. Gaines WE, Pierce WS, Prophet GA, Holtzmann K: Pulmonary circulatory support: A quantitative comparison of four methods. J Thorac Cardiovasc Surg 88:958–964, 1984
8. Spence PA, Weisel RD, Easdown J et al: Pulmonary artery balloon counterpulsation in the management of right heart failure during left heart bypass. J Thorac Cardiovasc Surg 89:264–268, 1985
9. Miller DC, Moreno–Cabral RJ, Stinson EB et al: Pulmonary artery balloon counterpulsation for acute right ventricular failure. J Thorac Cardiovasc Surg 80:760, 1980
10. Flege JB, Jr, Wright CB, Reisinger TJ: Successful balloon counterpulsation for right ventricular failure. Ann Thorac Surg 37:167, 1984
11. Moran JM, Opravil M, Gorman AJ et al: Pulmonary artery balloon counterpulsation for right ventricular failure: II. Clinical experience. Ann Thorac Surg 38:254, 1984
12. Symbas PN, McKeown PP, Santora AH, Vlasis SE: Pulmonary artery balloon counterpulsation for treatment of intraoperative right ventricular failure. Ann Thorac Surg 39:437–440, 1985
13. Pierce WS: Clinical left ventricular bypass: Problems of pump inflow obstruction and right ventricular failure. ASIO J 2:1, 1979
14. Pennington DG, Merjavy JP, Swartz MT et al: The importance of biventricular failure in patients with postoperative cardiogenic shock. Ann Thorac Surg 39:16–26, 1985
15. Rose DM, Colvin SB, Culliford AT et al: Long-term survival with partial left heart bypass following perioperative myocardial infarction and shock. J Thorac Cardiovasc Surg 83:483, 1982
16. Magovern GJ, Park SB, Maher TD: Use of a centrifugal pump without anticoagulants for postoperative left ventricular assist. World J Surg 9:25–36, 1985
17. Donachy JN, Landis DL, Rosenberg G et al: Design and evaluation of a left ventricular assist device: The angle port pump. In Unger F (ed): Assisted Circulation. New York, Academic Press, 1978
18. Bernhard WF, Berger RL, Stetz JP et al: Temporary left ventricular bypass: Factors affecting patient survival. Circulation (Suppl 1)60:131, 1979
19. Norman JC, Duncan JM, Frazier OH et al: Intracorporeal (abdominal) left ventricular assist devices (ALVADs) or partial artificial hearts: A five-year experience. Arch Surg 116:1441, 1981
20. Pierce WS, Parr GVS, Myers JL et al: Ventricular-assist pumping in patients with cardiogenic shock after cardiac operations. N Engl J Med 305:1606, 1981

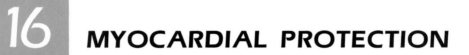

16

MYOCARDIAL PROTECTION

William E. Parks, Jr.

G. Arnaud Painvin

Arthur J. Roberts

Since the advent of cardiac surgery, improved methods have been sought to provide a safe, quiet, and bloodless field in which to operate. In recent years, much effort and expense has been devoted to clinical and experimental research to improve myocardial protection during open-heart surgery. This effort has resulted in a tremendous amount of information on the subject, much of it confusing and somewhat controversial. This chapter will attempt to bring the reader up to date on recent developments in the field while reviewing basic concepts of myocardial protection.

HISTORY OF DEVELOPMENTS IN MYOCARDIAL PROTECTION

Hypothermia was the first technique of myocardial protection to be introduced, and it remains a most important factor in avoiding ischemic injury to the heart.[1-4] Cardioplegia was introduced in Europe by Melrose in 1955, but was subsequently abandoned and then reintroduced in 1964 with a low-sodium, procaine-containing modification by Bretschneider.[5,6] Cross and associates as well as Shumway and associates introduced topical hypothermia as a myocardial protective measure in the late 1950s.[7,8] In 1973 Gay and Ebert reintroduced potassium cardioplegia using a lower concentration of potassium than had been used by Melrose and eliminating the citrate moiety.[9] Subsequently, this method became the most common form of cardioplegia

employed worldwide. Blood cardioplegia was popularized by Follette and Buckberg and associates in 1978.[10] This was followed by the introduction of the concept of secondary cardioplegia by Lazar and Buckberg and colleagues in 1979 and by the concept of warm cardioplegic induction introduced by Rosenkranz and Buckberg and coworkers in 1982.[11-13]

MECHANISMS OF MYOCARDIAL INJURY

ISCHEMIC INJURY

Under normal circumstances, the myocardial energy supply is produced by aerobic metabolism using oxygen delivered by way of coronary blood flow to produce 36 moles of adenosine triphosphate (ATP) per mole of glucose utilized. With ischemia, the heart reverts to anaerobic metabolism, and the amount of ATP produced is reduced to 2 moles per mole of glucose utilized. A small amount of aerobic metabolism continues by way of noncoronary collateral blood flow. With continued ischemia, there is little substrate available for metabolism to meet continued energy needs. The myocardial high-energy phosphate stores are depleted, lactic acid accumulates, producing intracellular acidosis, and enzymes essential for continued anaerobic metabolism are inhibited.[14-18] As a result of the inadequate energy supply, the cell membrane pump fails, producing an influx of sodium with associated intracellular edema and an efflux of potassium with depolarization of the cell membrane. As the membrane systems fail, calcium enters the myocardial cell, which then requires energy to pump this ion back out.[19,20] The myocardial injury that results is termed ischemic contracture. If this process continues and results in widespread irreversible damage, a condition called "stone heart" may develop.[21]

REPERFUSION INJURY

Myocardial injury resulting from reperfusion of an ischemic area of myocardium was first suggested in experimental animal studies and was brought to clinical attention by Bulkley in 1977.[22-27] It is characterized by failure of the heart to take up and utilize oxygen normally. However, the exact cause is uncertain. Some investigators have attributed this injury to influx and subsequent intracellular calcium sequestration, resulting in lowered ATP stores and reduced energy production.[28-30] Other researchers have implicated platelet deposition in the coronary microcirculation or oxygen free-radical–related injury as conditions responsible for reperfusion injury.[31-37] Unquestionably, the finding that oxygen free radicals may play a major role in myocardial injury that occurs during global myocardial ischemia or during the following reperfusion period is a significant observation in the field of myocardial protection. Furthermore, the knowledge that oxygen free-radical scavengers are available to counteract these ill effects opens a new area for therapeutic intervention.[35] Patients with low myocardial energy stores, myocardial hypertrophy, extensive coronary artery disease, or advanced cardiac cachexia, or those who have significant ongoing myocardial ischemia before cardioplegia is given, may be especially susceptible to this injury.[38-43] Inadequate myocardial protection during aortic cross-clamping also predisposes patients to this form of injury.[44]

TECHNICAL FACTORS THAT INFLUENCE MYOCARDIAL PROTECTION

LEFT VENTRICULAR DECOMPRESSION

The routine use of a left ventricular vent during cardiac surgery remains controversial. Some surgeons employ a vent routinely whereas others use this method selectively, and still others never use this technique. The advantages of the vent are reduced left ventricular wall tension, resulting in enhanced preservation of endocardial blood flow; improved visibility, rendering the operative field bloodless; and less rewarming of the left ventricular myocardium. The hazards include air embolism, iatrogenic injury to the mitral valve or to the heart itself, disruption of collateral circulation at the apex of the left ventricle, and the addition of another potential bleeding site.

Results of clinical and experimental studies have been confusing on this issue of left ventricular venting. Buckberg has shown that ventricular fibrillation diverts coronary blood flow away from the subendocardium and that ventricular distention increases this maldistribution.[45] These changes are even more pronounced in hypertrophied ventricles.[46] In clinical studies, Olinger and Bonchek reported improved ventricular function in vented hearts, and more recently, Kanter reported evidence of reduced perfusion injury in hearts vented during this period.[47,48] Other authors, however, have reported no obvious benefit from left ventricular venting in clinical and experimental studies.[49-53] Lucas and associates found no evidence of left ventricular injury with intracavitary left ventricular pressures up to 45 mm Hg during ischemia, whereas Ogilby and Apstein suggested that intermittent left ventricular distention is beneficial during aortic cross-clamping.[54,55]

Several techniques are available to provide left ventricular decompression, the oldest of which is decompression by way of the apex of the left ventricle. This method, however, is associated with interruption of collateral coronary vessels at this site and adds a potential bleeding source in a high-pressure system. Cannulation of the left ventricle by way of the superior pulmonary vein is probably the most commonly used method, but it may create difficulties in insertion and removal. On occasion, postoperative bleeding from this site may be difficult to repair. Venting through the aortic root is easily done but frequently introduces air into the aortic root and coronary arterial system, as may all of the above methods.[52,53] The use of a pulmonary artery catheter to decompress the left ventricle has been shown to be safe and effective and avoids the hazard of air embolism.[55] In addition, this insertion site is easily accessible, which facilitates insertion and removal and is in a low-pressure system that reduces the potential for postoperative bleeding.

The benefits of routine left ventricular venting are not clear-cut and would seem to indicate either selective or routine use of a simple and safe method, such as the pulmonary artery or ascending aortic catheter.[56]

VENOUS CANNULATION TECHNIQUES

The effect of various venous cannulation techniques on the efficiency of venous drainage and on myocardial temperature changes has been investigated by several authors. Arom and associates found that a single atrial cannula provided the most efficient means of draining blood from the right side of the heart.[57] However, when the aorta was cross-clamped, this advantage over the 51F cavoatrial cannula and over bicaval cannulation with two No. 32 USCI catheters without snares was eliminated. The cavoatrial cannula provided the best inferior vena cava drainage, and bicaval cannulation with snares provided the worst right atrial drainage. Bennett and colleagues, in comparing two types of cavoatrial cannulas and bicaval cannulations with and

without snares, found that the Sarns 51F cavoatrial cannula had the most efficient right ventricular decompression and was the only method of venous drainage not affected by displacing the heart out of the pericardium.[58] In another study designed to determine the effect of venous drainage on myocardial protection, Bennett and associates found that cavoatrial cannulation with a 51F Sarns catheter resulted in lower myocardial temperatures and increased endocardial blood flow to the left ventricular and septal regions during reperfusion.[59] The rate of myocardial rewarming was not significantly altered by the method of venous drainage. These animal studies seem to indicate that cavoatrial cannulation provides the most efficient drainage of the right ventricle. Consequently, the level of myocardial protection may be influenced by the pattern of venous drainage. There is some evidence, however, that the cavoatrial method of cannulation may result in a higher incidence of postoperative atrial arrhythmias, and further study is needed to clarify this issue.[60-62]

OXYGENATOR AND FILTRATION METHODS

Cardiopulmonary bypass is associated with trauma to the blood constituents resulting from prolonged exposure to large abnormal surface areas, turbulence, and direct mechanical trauma. This may result in coagulopathy, organ system dysfunction, or reperfusion injury caused by the release of vasoactive substances. Studies comparing membrane and bubble oxygenators are available, and most show no significant difference in hematologic effects unless the period of cardiopulmonary bypass exceeds 3 hours.[63-69] Several studies do show better preservation of platelet counts following use of the membrane oxygenator; however, clinical benefits have not been clearly demonstrated.[63,64,69] At present, both types of oxygenators appear to be satisfactory for most cardiac operations. Robinson, Hearse and colleagues have recently shown that particulate formation related to cardiopulmonary bypass physiology does occur.[70] At least in crystalloid cardioplegic solutions, these investigators have shown that a 0.8-micron filter in the delivery system removes particles. This process of particulate aggregation, when unfiltered, causes a major increase in coronary vascular resistance, coronary arterial "spasm," and, subsequently, decreased coronary blood flow during reperfusion.

PERFUSION TECHNIQUES

Most cardiac operations are performed using moderate hypothermia (25°C to 32°C) and moderately decreased flow rates (2 to 2.2 liters/minute/m²); however, the surgeon may on occasion wish to reduce flow rates even more to minimize myocardial rewarming or to reduce back bleeding from coronary arteries from noncoronary collateral flow. Ellis and associates found no clinically significant cerebral dysfunction when flow rates were reduced below 40 ml/kg and arterial pressure was reduced to less than 60 mm Hg at 28°C.[71] In addition, Hickey and Hoar showed that tissue perfusion was not compromised when flows were reduced from 2.1 to 1.2 liters/minute/m² at 25°C.[72] These studies demonstrate that flow rates can be reduced temporarily, if necessary, without harming the patient.

The value of pulsatile versus nonpulsatile perfusion techniques continues to be debated in the literature. Watkins has demonstrated a higher concentration of prostacyclin (a coronary vasodilator and platelet disaggregant) and reduced elevations in the concentration of thromboxane (a potent platelet aggregant and putative coronary vasoconstrictor) in patients who underwent coronary artery bypass grafting using pulsatile perfusion.[73] Silverman reported evidence of reduced myocardial reperfusion injury in dogs using pulsatile perfusion following 60 minutes of hypothermic, hypokalemic crystalloid cardioplegic arrest.[74] If platelet deposition is a factor in reperfusion injury, as some authors believe, these findings may be related.[31] The benefits of pulsatile versus nonpulsatile perfusion have been described, but these may be related to a failure to accurately define the forms of pulsatile flow that are effective and the circumstances in which they should be used.[75-77] Further investigation in this area is needed before recommending either method as superior. The general characteristics of the systematic perfusate during cardiopulmonary bypass has been shown to influence the adequacy of myocardial protection.[78] In addition, clinically acceptable levels of hemodilution may have important effects on myocardial edema formation and left ventricular mass after cardiopulmonary bypass.[79]

HYPOTHERMIA

SYSTEMIC HYPOTHERMIA

The concept of systemic hypothermia as a means of myocardial protection during intracardiac operations was introduced by Bigelow and associates and Lewis and Taufic.[1-4] As early as 1953, Neptune and Bailey were using deep hypothermia and circulatory arrest to perform lung and heart/lung transplantation in dogs without the aid of cardiopulmonary bypass.[80,81] Sealy subsequently modified this method by adding the use of cardiopulmonary bypass.[82]

Hypothermia protects the myocardium by reducing the heart rate and basal metabolic rate.[83] At 37°C the basal oxygen requirement of the arrested heart is 1 ml/100 g/minute. This value is reduced further at 20°C.[84] Moderate systemic hypothermia has been shown to enhance the effect of myocardial cooling provided by potassium cardioplegia.[85] An additional benefit of moderate systemic hypothermia is some degree of protection of the rest of the body from imperfect tissue perfusion during cardiopulmonary bypass.

TOPICAL HYPOTHERMIA

Topical hypothermia was introduced by Cross in 1957 and then was modified and popularized by Shumway in 1959.[7,8] The administration of cold cardioplegia through the aortic root has been shown to result in uneven myocardial cooling when critical coronary stenoses are present. The addition of topical hypothermia-selective perfusion cooling has resulted in more uniform myocardial cooling.[86,87] Conversely, the use of topical hypothermia alone has been shown to result in temperature gradients and inadequate subendocardial cooling.[88] Myocardial cooling jackets have also been used, but they may not cool the anterior left ventricular wall and septum as effectively as topical cooling.[89,90] Selective intracavitary installation of hypothermic solutions may be a useful adjunct during operations in which a cardiac chamber is entered.[91]

SELECTIVE AORTIC ROOT INFUSION

The primary method of myocardial cooling used clinically is direct infusion of cold cardioplegic solutions through the aortic root. In the presence of aortic insufficiency or when the aorta must be opened, direct infusion into the coronary ostia is used, but ostial stenosis has been reported with this method.[92] As stated previously, nonhomogeneous distribution of cardioplegic solution and uneven cooling may occur in the presence of significant coronary artery stenoses, so topical hypothermia is an important adjunct.[86,93]

The ideal temperature for myocardial protection is uncertain.[94-96] However, most surgeons feel that a myocardial temperature range of 10°C to 20°C is adequate. Tyers and Shragge have reported no benefit in processing myocardial glycogen stores at temperatures below 10°C, and Balderman found that a range of 14°C to 18°C was optimal based on maintenance of ATP levels, left ventricular function and mitochon-

drial function.[96-98] Other investigators disagree about optimal cooling.[99-101] Other variables may also influence this relationship. For example, there is evidence that blood cardioplegia provides no better myocardial protection when given at 10°C than at 20°C, although myocardial cooling is greater at the former temperature.[102] The use of a myocardial temperature probe is a valuable addition to ensure that an adequate amount of cardioplegia has been infused to produce adequate myocardial cooling.[103] It may also be used to determine the sequence of graft placement.[104]

METHOD OF CARDIOPLEGIC DELIVERY

The most commonly used method for delivery of cardioplegic solutions is infusion into the aortic root after aortic cross-clamping. The major disadvantage of this technique is uneven distribution in the presence of critical coronary artery stenoses.[91,93] Several techniques are available to the surgeon to avoid or minimize this problem.

Proximal anastomoses may be placed on the aorta before cross-clamping. This ensures that upon completion of each distal anastomosis, additional areas of myocardium are perfused and protected. This method has been shown experimentally to result in more even distribution of cardioplegia and improved left ventricular function.[105] Clinically, this technique may reduce mortality and incidence of perioperative myocardial infarction.[104,105,106] This method also allows immediate reperfusion of the heart following release of the aortic clamps. An alternate method is placement of the distal anastomoses first, with perfusion of each graft with cardioplegia upon completion of each anastomosis. Roberts and associates and Buckberg and colleagues have shown that this method results in similar degrees of myocardial cooling, postoperative hemodynamic changes, and perioperative myocardial infarction rate.[107] Although the graft perfusion method does not allow immediate reperfusion of the heart after release of the aortic clamp, reperfusion may be partially accomplished by perfusing the grafts with warm blood after release of the cross-clamp and during completion of the proximal anastomoses.[183] A third method used is the performance of all proximal and distal anastomoses in a sequential manner with intervening infusions of cardioplegic solution during a single prolonged period of aortic cross-clamping. Weisel and associates have shown that this method results in more uniform cooling than the method of performing distal anastomoses first.[108,109]

A new alternative to antegrade coronary perfusion is retrograde coronary sinus perfusion, which was first described by Lillihei and colleagues in 1956.[110] Although the oxygen supplied by this method is inadequate to meet the demands of the beating normothermic heart, it appears to be sufficient to protect the hypothermic arrested heart.[111] This method has been shown to improve preservation of the left ventricle during aortic-valve surgery and to provide more uniform cooling of the myocardium in the presence of coronary stenoses.[112–114] Cardioplegia may be infused into the coronary sinus through a balloon-tipped catheter or directly into the right atrium, with the aorta and pulmonary artery cross-clamped and using bicaval venous cannulation with snares.[115] Disadvantages of this method are inadequate right ventricular protection as a result of venous collaterals, and conduction disturbances caused by coronary sinus injury.[112,113] This technique has promise but requires further study before it can gain widespread acceptance. Another retrograde approach to myocardial protection involves pressure-controlled, intermittent coronary sinus occlusion (PICSO).[116] This method involves periodic balloon inflation and deflation, resulting in washout of toxic metabolites and redistribution of coronary blood flow toward ischemic regions.

Very little data are available regarding optimal volumes of cardioplegia or the pressure at which cardioplegia should be administered. Molina and colleagues, in a retrospective analysis, found a reduced need for postoperative inotropic support, lower serum creatine phosphokinase (CPK-MB) levels, and an increased incidence of recovery of spontaneous rhythm in patients who had cardioplegia infused at aortic root pressures of 85 mm Hg to 100 mm Hg in contrast to 35 mm Hg to 40 mm Hg.[117] Johnson and associates, in an experimental study in dogs, found a reduction in left ventricular function when infusion pressures in the coronary arteries exceeded 150 mm Hg.[118] The volume of cardioplegia given by most surgeons is determined by the desired degree of myocardial cooling and the duration of the cross-clamp period. Engleman and associates, in comparing blood cardioplegia and normal-volume crystalloid cardioplegia (1.4 to 3.2 liters) with high-volume crystalloid cardioplegia (3.0 to 7.6 liters), found lower myocardial temperatures and improved myocardial oxygen extraction with the high-volume technique.[119] This study was not randomized and at present the findings have not been confirmed.

COMPOSITION OF CARDIOPLEGIC SOLUTIONS

OXYGENATION

The most controversial issue regarding the composition of cardioplegia has been the optimal vehicle for delivery — blood versus crystalloid solutions. Blood as a vehicle for cardioplegia was originally introduced by Melrose and associates in 1955 and reintroduced by Follette, Buckberg, and associates in 1978.[5,10] The proposed advantages of the blood-based technique are rapid diastolic arrest in an oxygenated environment, thus reducing high-energy phosphate loss, replenishment of oxygen supply during subsequent obstruction of the microcirculation, and the complexity of the apparatus necessary for delivery.

The multiplicity of cardioplegic solutions available, their method of delivery, patient selection, and the methods used to determine myocardial injury have made it difficult to accurately determine which form of cardioplegia is better.[120] There is some clinical evidence, however, that blood cardioplegia provides better myocardial protection in certain subsets of high-risk patients. In experimental studies, Nwaneri and colleagues were unable to demonstrate differences in left ventricular function or better preservation of ATP and creatine phosphate levels when comparing multidose blood cardioplegia with multidose crystalloid cardioplegia; other authors have done so.[10,122,123] Feindel found no evidence of sludging or rouleux formation with blood cardioplegia delivery at 4°C and, using electron microscopy and tetrazolium staining, showed better myocardial tissue preservation with multidose blood cardioplegia.[124] Catinella and Cunningham found no difference in left ventricular function, compliance, or myocardial oxygen consumption using blood cardioplegia during prolonged aortic cross-clamping, but they were able to demonstrate improved regional myocardial blood flow and better preservation of ultrastructure and ATP levels with blood cardioplegia.[125] Robertson found that blood cardioplegia improved delivery beyond obstructed coronary arteries and resulted in better myocardial cooling compared with the crystalloid method.[126]

In clinical studies, Shapira was unable to show improved left ventricular function with blood cardioplegia but demonstrated an increase in rate of spontaneous defibrillation.[127] Roberts and associates, in a nonrandomized matched-pair analysis of patients, were unable to show differences in left ventricular function or in the incidence of perioperative infarction but suggested that cold blood cardioplegia may be advantageous in pa-

tients with preoperatively reduced left ventricular function ejection fraction (40%) or prolonged cross-clamp times (90 minutes).[128] Furthermore, other researchers have shown a reduced incidence of perioperative infarction using cold blood cardioplegia despite an increased ischemic time.[129] Iverson found some improvement in stroke work indices and lower enzyme levels in patients with reduced left ventricular function and increased left ventricular end-diastolic pressure (> 18 mm Hg).[130] In clinical studies other investigators have confirmed improved preservation of ATP levels and mitochondrial integrity.[131,132] There is also evidence that blood cardioplegia improves preservation of the right atrial myocardium.[133] In the first randomized prospective clinical study of blood and crystalloid cardioplegia, Codd and associates have demonstrated a reduced need for inotropic support and a reduction in the incidence of perioperative infarction and in indirect estimates of infarct size.[134] From these clinical and experimental studies, it seems probable that blood cardioplegia may provide better myocardial protection during global ischemia and that this protection may be more evident clinically in high-risk patients.

Oxygenation of crystalloid cardioplegic solutions and the use of fluorocarbon solutions have also been shown to improve oxygen delivery to the myocardium during global myocardial ischemia.[99,135–141] These techniques may prove to be of benefit; however, they have not yet gained widespread clinical application.

BUFFERING

Tissue acidosis is produced during ischemia by the continuous production of hydrogen ions related to the accumulation of toxic metabolites. This process inhibits anaerobic metabolism and results in direct myocardial injury as well. Hypothermia increases pH approximately .15 units per 10°C, but further alkalinization is necessary to provide optimal enzymatic functions at the usual levels of clinical cooling. The buffering solutions most commonly used include bicarbonate, phosphate, tris (hydroxymethyl) aminomethane, glutamate, THAM, or Histidine.[142] Lactate should be not used because it is a poor buffer and it inhibits anaerobic metabolism independent of *p*H. Most investigators recommend alkalinization of cardioplegic solutions. It appears that nonbicarbonate buffers may offer advantages over bicarbonate buffers, if preliminary studies are verified.

OSMOLARITY

Myocardial edema occurs as a result of myocardial ischemia and, therefore, begins to accumulate when the aorta is clamped. Many investigators have suggested that cardioplegic solutions should be slightly hyperosmotic to counteract the propensity for edema formation.[19,84] The ideal osmolarity has not been determined, but the acceptable range of hyperosmolality is from 340 mOsm to 400 mOsm. At 370 mOsm, approximately 2% myocardial dehydration occurs, which does not inhibit myocardial function, and above 540 mOsm,[143] direct myocardial injury may occur and the effectiveness of cardioplegic solutions is inhibited.[144,145]

MEMBRANE STABILIZATION

Stabilization of the myocardial cell membrane by the addition of procaine or steroids has been advocated because of the membrane's susceptibility to ischemic damage. Fey and coworkers have demonstrated that membrane stabilization reduced depression of postischemic myocardial contractility, but they failed to show any reduction in myocardial edema, improved compliance, or more complete recovery of ATP stores.[146] Levinsky and associates, in a clinical study, found that patients treated with steroids had less requirements for inotropic support postoperatively

and showed less ultrastructural damage or myocardial edema formation than a comparable group of patients treated with potassium cardioplegia alone.[147] It is probable, however, that membrane stabilization is not necessary when a properly designed cardioplegic solution is adequately delivered to the myocardium.[84] Further studies are necessary before these drugs can be recommended for clinical usage.

POTASSIUM

Potassium chloride is the agent most commonly used in the United States to achieve rapid diastolic arrest of the heart. Repeat infusions are necessary to maintain arrest and to provide optimal myocardial protection. However, the ideal frequency of administration in patients with ischemic heart disease or myocardial hypertrophy has not yet been determined.[84] Studies in normal dog hearts found the ideal interval to be 20 minutes, but in the clinical circumstances described earlier, a shorter interval may be necessary if noncoronary collateral blood flow is increased.[84] Elevated extracellular potassium concentrations produce asystole by depolarizing the cell membrane, and hypothermia decreases the concentration required to achieve this effect. Nevertheless, the ideal potassium concentration necessary varies with the degree of hypothermia and the amount of noncoronary collateral blood flow. In general clinical usage, ranges of potassium vary from 10 mEq to 40 mEq per liter.[10,148–151] Higher levels of potassium may result in increased myocardial energy demands by allowing calcium influx into the cells.[152] Also, a higher incidence of postoperative heart block is noted clinically with higher potassium infusions.[149]

MAGNESIUM

Magnesium is an essential component of high-energy phosphate molecules and is an important cofactor in cellular enzyme systems. It competes with calcium for receptor sites on the cell membrane and may produce arrest by blocking calcium influx into the cell. Although magnesium is not required to produce cardioplegia, its absence during ischemia or reperfusion may impair ATP synthesis; as a result, the addition of moderate amounts of this substance to cardioplegic solutions is recommended. Although Engleman found that the addition of magnesium was not necessary during 2 hours of aortic cross-clamping in pig hearts using multidose crystalloid potassium cardioplegia, Hearse found that it was an important component and recommended a concentration of 15 mmoles/liter.[153,154] The inclusion of both potassium and magnesium forms the basis of the St. Thomas cardioplegic solution that is popular in Europe.

CALCIUM

Calcium is necessary for myocardial contraction and is required to maintain the integrity of the cell membrane. Cardioplegia is produced by extracellular hypocalcemia by reducing the calcium available for myocardial contraction. Myocardial energy requirements during arrest are also reduced because there is less calcium to sequester. However, extreme hypocalcemia may have adverse ultrastructural and functional effects, so it is advisable to add small amounts of calcium to asanguineous cardioplegic solutions.[155,156] When blood cardioplegia is used, the addition of small amounts of citrate will chelate calcium and produce safe levels of hypocalcemia.[10] Hypocalcemia helps to achieve rapid diastolic arrest and to reduce the damage produced by the use of calcium channel blockers. The most commonly used agents are diltiazem, nifedipine, verapamil, and lidoflazine, and the experimental and clinical results have been encouraging.[157–159, 163, 164, 168–170] However, resumption of electromechanical activity may be somewhat delayed when these agents are used or prolonged heart block may

occur. Consequently, the use of a left ventricular vent during the initial recovery phase may be beneficial.

SUBSTRATE ENHANCEMENT

Patients with ischemic heart disease complicated by left ventricular hypertrophy, reduced left ventricular function, unstable angina, or acute myocardial necrosis may have depleted energy stores that are lowered further by episodes of hypotension or hypertension prior to cardiopulmonary bypass. These energy stores may be partially replenished by substrate that is provided by noncoronary collateral blood flow or blood cardioplegia but not by ordinary asanguineous cardioplegic solutions. The addition of substrate is especially important when the latter solutions are used but may be less important when oxygenated cardioplegic solutions are used.

GLUCOSE

Glucose is provided by noncoronary collateral blood flow and by blood cardioplegia when the systemic perfusate is used as the vehicle for delivery. In addition, glucose may be added to crystalloid cardioplegic solutions. Although isolated heart studies have demonstrated the deleterious effects of adding glucose to cardioplegic solutions, especially if insulin is included, these studies did not provide for washout of the undesirable end products of anaerobic metabolism and correction of the resulting acidosis, which impairs myocardial function.[171,172] Such corrections occur to some degree in the clinical setting because of the variable degree of noncoronary collateral blood flow and repeated infusions of cardioplegic solution. When these factors are taken into account, the addition of glucose and insulin has been shown to have beneficial effects.[173,174] Adding small amounts of glucose to cardioplegic solutions does not appear to be harmful clinically.

WARM CARDIOPLEGIC INDUCTION

The concept of pretreatment of energy-depleted hearts with normothermic blood cardioplegia to replenish high-energy phosphate levels prior to ischemic arrest has been used experimentally and clinically with favorable results.[12,13] This technique has not come into wide clinical use, but it may be an important adjunct in the treatment of selected patients.

GLUTAMATE

L-Glutamate is an amino acid extracted by the heart during anaerobic conditions and utilized to produce additional energy stores. Deamination of glutamate produces α-ketoglutarate, a Krebs-cycle intermediate, which is then oxidized to succinate, producing one additional mole of ATP per mole of glutamate oxidized. Glutamate may also increase energy production by its role in the molate–asparate shuttle under anaerobic and aerobic conditions. The addition of glutamate to cardioplegic solutions has been shown to have beneficial effects during the reperfusion period.[175,176] Robertson and associates have shown that glutamate enrichment of blood cardioplegia had no beneficial effects in the normal heart subjected to prolonged ischemia; however, when the same technique was used in energy-depleted hearts, metabolic and functional recovery was improved.[177,178] The best results were obtained when glutamate enrichment was combined with warm cardioplegic induction. Ribose, creatine phosphate, and erythro-9 (2-hydroxy-3-nonyl) adenine hydrochloride (EHNA) have also been used experimentally with beneficial results, but these agents have not yet been used clinically.[179–181]

METHODS TO REDUCE REPERFUSION INJURY

SECONDARY CARDIOPLEGIA

The concept of administering an infusion of normothermic blood cardioplegic solution for 5 minutes prior to release of the aortic clamp was introduced in 1979 by Lazar and Buckberg.[11] The theoretical advantages of this technique include the following: (1) the reparative processes are optimized by normothermic conditions, (2) energy utilization by electromechanical work is avoided, and (3) the limited ability to utilize oxygen is reduced for the cellular repair process, which has been shown to improve metabolic and functional results following global myocardial ischemia.[11,44]

OXYGEN FREE-RADICAL SCAVENGERS

Free radicals are atoms, group of atoms, or molecules with an unpaired electron in their outer shell. The role of oxygen free radicals in cellular injury has only recently been appreciated, and their role in the pathophysiology of reperfusion injury is currently under investigation. Normally, most oxygen undergoes tetravalent reduction to water and generates ATP; however, 1% to 2% undergoes univalent reduction and produces hydrogen peroxide, superoxide, and hydroxyl radicals, which are highly reactive and potent oxidation/reduction agents. Cellular mechanisms to prevent free-radical damage include reduction of the superoxide radical to hydrogen peroxide by superoxide dismutase, and reduction of hydrogen peroxide to hydroxyl radicals and then to water by catalases and peroxidases. Such oxygen free-radicals may cause a cascade of cytotoxic radical species production, resulting in damage to cell membranes, lysosomes, and mitochondria. This process may be the mechanism for the increase in myocardial injury seen on reperfusion (reoxygenation) of the heart following myocardial ischemia. It has been shown in experimental studies that superoxide dismutase plus catalase improves myocardial protection during global ischemia, as evidenced by better preservation of left ventricular function when compared with no enzyme treatment using both standard cardioplegia and oxygenated perfluorocarbon cardioplegia.[32,35,36] Stewart and associates found smilar preservation of left ventricular function using superoxide dismutase plus mannitol.[33,34] Casale found no effect on the time of administration of the free-radical scavengers during ischemia, suggesting that most of the injury produced by oxygen free radicals occurs during the early reperfusion period.[36] Chambers and associates, using a canine model, have demonstrated a reduction in infarct size following reversible coronary artery occlusion when superoxide dismutase was given.[182] The significance of this free-radical mechanism for creating reperfusion injury and ways to modify it by specific scavengers await further experimental and clinical trials.

COENZYME Q 10

Coenzyme Q 10 is a naturally occurring component of mitochondria that transports electrons between flavoproteins and cytochromes during oxidative phosphorylation. This coenzyme is known to be a potent antioxidant against lipid peroxidation in the myocardial mitochondrial membrane *in vitro*, and therefore it has a membrane-stabilizing effect.[183,184] Its ability to protect the myocardium may be related to blocking the effects of oxygen free radicals on the cell membrane. This protective action may also be related to its ability to avoid calcium overloading of the mitochondria.[185] Mori and Mohri, in an experimental study in which they added coenzyme Q 10 to a potassium cardioplegic solution, found improved myocardial levels of ATP and creatine phosphate as well as improved myocardial oxygen utilization and accelerated recovery of myocardial metabolism following ischemia.[186] Tanaka and associates, in a randomized prospective trial, pretreated patients undergoing valve replacement with oral coenzyme Q 10 and found a reduced incidence of low cardiac output syndrome following operation.[187] Further experimental and clinical trials will be needed before coenzyme Q 10 can be accepted into clinical use in the Unied States.

Khuri and associates have reported on a modified measurement of intramyocardial pH.[188] This technique allows serial assessments of myocardial integrity. It has already been applied to the study of reperfusion acidosis and offers, potentially, an on-line detection system for identifying early myocardial ischemia.

CONCLUSION

A review of recent developments in myocardial protection and currently accepted clinical techniques has been presented. The discussion in this chapter has concentrated on current topics of controversy and new investigations in this field. Although some investigators would argue that very little important new information is available in myocadial protection; we disagree. It is our impression that the field is not "dead" and that further progress requires imagination, ingenuity, and careful scientific analysis. It is our hope that this review will be useful to the practicing cardiac surgeon and will stimulate a review of his own current techniques for myocardial protection.

REFERENCES

1. Bigelow WG, Lindsay WK, Greenwood WF: Hypothermia: Its possible role in cardiac surgery: An investigation of factors governing survival in dogs at low body temperatures. Ann Surg 132:849, 1950

2. Bigelow WG, Mustard WT, Evans JG: Some physiologic concepts of hypothermia and their application to cardiac surgery. J Thorac Cadiovasc Surg 28:463, 1954

3. Lewis FJ, Taufic M: Closure of atrial septal defects with the aid of hypothermia: Experimental accomplishments and the report of one successful case. Surgery 33:52, 1953

4. Nizaz SA, Lewis FJ: Tolerance of adult rats to profound hypothermia and simultaneous cardiac standstill. Surgery 36:25, 1954

5. Melrose DG, Dreyer B, Nental HH et al: Elective cardiac arrest. Lancet 2:21–22, 1955

6. Bretschneider JH: Uberlebenszeit and Wiederbelebunszeit des Herzens be: Normo-und Hypothermie. Verh Dtsch Ges Herz Kreislaufforsch 30:11, 1964

7. Cross FS, Jones RD, Berne RM: Localized cardiac hypothermia as an adjunct to elective cardiac arrest. Surg Forum 8:355, 1957

8. Shumway NE, Lower RR, Stofer RC: Selective hypothermia of the heart in anoxic cardiac arrest. Surg Gynecol Obstet 104:750, 1959

9. Gay WA, Ebert PA: Functional, metabolic and morphologic effects of potassium-induced cardioplegia. Surgery 74:284, 1973

10. Follette DM, Mulder DG, Maloney JV, Jr et al: Advantages of blood cardioplegia over continuous coronary perfusion or intermittent ischemia: Experimental and clinical study. J Thorac Cardiovasc Surg 76:604–619, 1978

11. Lazar H, Manganara A, Foglia R et al: Reversal of ischemic damage with secondary blood cardioplegia. J Thorac Cardiovasc Surg 78:688–697, 1979

12. Rosenkranz ER, Okamoto F, Buckberg G et al: Benefits of normothermic induction of blood cardioplegia in energy-depleted hearts with maintenance or arrest by multidose cold blood cardioplegia. J Thorac Cardiovasc Surg 84:667–677, 1982

13. Rosenkranz ER, Buckberg GD, Laks H et al: Warm induction of cardioplegia with glutamate-enriched blood in coronary patients with cardiogenic shock who are dependent on inotropic drugs and intra-aortic balloon support: Initial experience and operative strategy. J Thorac Cardiovasc Surg 86:507–518, 1983

14. Levitsky S, Feinberg H: Biochemical changes of ischemia. Ann Thorac Surg 20:21–29, 1975

15. Reibel DK, Rovetto JJ: Myocardial ATP synthesis and mechanical function following oxygen deficiency. Am J Physiol 234:620–624, 1978

16. Rudiger L, Kloner RA, Zierler M et al: Time course of ischemic alterations during normothermic and hyperthermic arrest and its reflection by on-line monitoring of tissue pH. J Thorac Cardiovasc Surg 86:418–434, 1983

17. Williamson JR, Schaffer SW, Ford C, Safer B: Contribution of tissue acidosis to ischemia and infarction. Circulation (Suppl 1)53:3–14, 1976

18. Brachfeld N: Ischemic myocardial metabolism and cell necrosis. Bull NY Acad Med 50:261, 1974

19. Leaf A: Cell swelling: A factor in ischemic tissue injury. Circulation 48:455, 1973

20. Jennings RB, Ganote CE: Structural changes in myocardium during acute ischemia. Circ Res (Suppl 3)34(35):156–172, 1974

21. Katz AM, Tada M: The "Stone Heart" and other challenges to the biochemist. Am J Cardiol 39:1073, 1977

22. Campeau L, Crochet D, Lesperance J et al: Postoperative changes in aortocoronary saphenous vein grafts revisited: Angiographic studies at two weeks and at one year in two series of consecutive patients. Circulation 52:369, 1975

23. Rona G, Chappel GI, Balazs T, Gaudry R: An infarct-like myocardial lesion and other toxic manifestations produced by Isoproterenol in the rat. Arch Pathol Lab Med 67:443, 1959

24. Ridolfi RL, Hutchins GM: The relationship between coronary lesions and myocardial infarcts: Ulceration of atherosclerotic plaques precipitating coronary thrombosis. Am Heart J 93:468, 1977

25. Whalen DA, Jr, Hamilton DG, Ganote CE, Jennings RB: Effect of a transient period of ischemia on myocardial cells. I. Effect on cell volume regulation. Am J Pathol 74:381, 1974

26. Kloner RA, Ganote CE, Whalen DA, Jr, Jennings RB: Effect of a transient period of ischemia on myocardial cells. II. Fine structure during the first few minutes of reflow. Am J Pathol 74:399, 1974

27. Bulkley BH, Hutchins GM: Myocardial consequences of coronary artery bypass graft surgery: The paradox of necrosis in areas of revascularization. Circulation 56(6):906–913, 1977

28. Jennings RB, Ganote CE: Mitochondrial structure and function in acute myocardial injury. Circ Res (Suppl I)38:1–80, 1976

29. Nayler WG, Ferrari R, Williams A: Protective effect of pretreatment with Verapamil, Nifedipine, and Propranolol on mitochondrial function in the ischemic and reperfused myocardium. Am J Cardiol 46:242–248, 1980

30. Peng CF, Kane JJ, Murphy ML, Straub KD: Abnormal mitochondrial oxidative phosphorylation of ischemic myocardium reversed by CA 2^+-chelating agents. J Mol Cell Cardiol 9:897–908, 1977

31. Feinberg H, Rosenbaum DS, Levitsky S et al: Platelet deposition after surgically induced global myocardial ischemia: An etiologic factor for reperfusion injury. J Thorac Cardiovasc Surg 84:815, 1982

32. Shlafer M, Kane FS, Kirsch MM: Superoxide dismutase plus catalase enhances the efficacy of hypothermic cardioplegia to protect the globally ischemic, reperfused heart. J Thorac Cardiovasc Surg 83:830–839, 1982

33. Stewart JR, Blackwell WH, Crute SL et al: Prevention of myocardial ischemia/reperfusion injury with oxygen free-radical scavengers. Surg Forum 33:317–320, 1982

34. Stewart JR, Blackwell WH, Crute SL et al: Inhibition of surgically induced ischemia/reperfusion injury by oxygen free-radical scavengers. J Thorac Cardiovasc Surg 86:262–272, 1983

35. Casale AS, Bulkley GB, Bulkley BH et al: Oxygen free-radical scavengers protect the arrested, globally ischemic heart upon reperfusion. Surgical Forum 34:313–316, 1983

36. Casale AS, Hornetter PJ, Gott VL, Gardner TH: Oxygenated perfluorocarbon cardioplegia prevents oxygen free-radical reperfusion injury. Surgical Forum 35:282–285, 1984

37. Stewart JR, Blackwell WH, Crute SL et al: Prevention of free-radical induced myocardial reperfusion injury with allopurinol. J Thorac Cardiovasc Surg 90:68, 1985

38. Iyengar SR, Ranch S, Charrette EJ et al: Anoxic cardiac arrest: An experimental and clinical study on its effects. Part I. J Thorac Cardiovasc Surg 66:722–730, 1973

39. Sink JD, Pellom GI, Currie WD et al: Response of hypertrophied myocardium to ischemia. J Thorac Cardiovasc Surg 81:805–872, 1981

40. Jones RN, Currie WD, Olson CD et al: Recovery of metabolic function in hypertrophied cancine hearts following global ischemia (abstr). Circulation (Suppl III)62:30, 1980

41. Jones RN, Peton RB, Savina RC et al: Transmural gradient in high energy phosphate content in patients with coronary artery disease. Ann Thorac Surg 32:546–553, 1981

42. Dawson JT, Hall RJ, Hallman GL, Cooley DA: Mortality in patients undergoing coronary artery bypass surgery after myocardial infarction Am J Cardiol 33:483–486, 1974

43. Feinstein MB: Effects of experimental congestive heart failure, Ouabain, and asphyxia on the high energy phosphate and creatine content of the guinea pig heart. Circ Res 10:333–346, 1962

44. Rosenkranz ER, Buckberg GD: Myocardial protection during surgical coronary reperfusion. J Am Coll Cardiol 1:235–246, 1983

45. Hottenrott CE, Buckberg GD: Studies of the effects of ventricular fibrillation on the adequacy of regional myocardial flow. II. Effects at ventricular distension. J Thorac Cardiovasc Surg 68:626–633, 1974

46. Hottenrott CE, Towers B, Kirkzi JH et al: The hazard of ventricular fibrillation in hypertrophied ventricles during cardiopulmonary bypass. J Thorac Cardiovasc Surg 66:742–753, 1973

47. Olinger GN, Boncheck LI: Ventricular venting during coronary revascularization: Assessment or benefit by intraoperative ventricular function curves. Ann Thorac Surg 26:525, 1978

48. Kanter KR, Schaff HV, Gott VL, Gardner TJ: Reduced oxygen consumption with effective left ventricular venting during postischemic reperfusion. Circulation (Suppl I)66:50, 1982

49. Okies JE, Phillips SJ, Crenshaw R, Starr A: "No-vent" technique of coronary artery bypass. Ann Thorac Surg 19:191, 1975

50. Breyer RH, Meredity JW, Mills SA et al: Is a left ventricular vent necessary for coronary artery bypass operation performed with cardioplegic arrest? J Thorac Cardiovasc Surg 6:338–349, 1983

51. Salerno TA, Charrette EJP: Elimination of venting in coronary artery surgery. Ann Thorac Surg 27:340, 1979

52. Zwart JJH, Brainard JZ, DeWall RA: Ventricular fibrillation without left ventricular venting: Observations in humans. Ann Thorac Surg 20:481, 1975

53. Roberts AJ, Faro RS, Williams LA et al: Relative efficacy of left ventricular venting and venous drainage techniques commonly used during coronary artery bypass graft surgery. Ann Thorac Surg 36:444–452, 1983

54. Lucas SK, Gardner TJ, Elmer EB et al: Comparison of the effects of left ventricular fibrillation. Circulation (Suppl I)62:42, 1980

55. Ogilby JD, Apstein CS: Preservation of myocadial compliance and reversal of contracture ("stone heart") during ischemic arrest by applied intermittent ventricular sketch. Am J Cardiol 46:397, 1980

56. Little AG, Lin CY, Wernly JA et al: Use of the pulmonary artery for left ventricular venting during cardiac operations. J Thorac Cardiovasc Surg 87:532–538, 1984

57. Arom KV, Ellestad C, Grover FL: Objective evaluation of the efficacy of various venous cannulas. J Thorac Cardiovasc Surg 81:464, 1981

58. Bennett EV, Fewel JG, Ybarra J et al: Comparison of flow differences among venous cannulas. J Thorac Cardiovasc Surg 81:464, 1981

59. Bennett EV, Fewel JG, Grover FL et al: Myocardial preservation: Effect of venous drainage. Ann Thorac Surg 36:132–142, 1983

60. Techervenkov CJ, Wynands JE, Symes JF et al: Persistent atrial activity during cardioplegic arrest: A possible factor in the etiology of postoperative supraventricular tachyarrhythmias. Ann Thorac Surg 36:437–443, 1983

61. Novick RJ, Stefaniszyn JH, Morin JE et al: Atrial electrical activity and its suppression during cardioplegia arrest in pigs. J Thorac Cardiovasc Surg 86:235–241, 1983

62. Novick RJ, Stefaniszyn JH, Malcolm ID et al: Differential electrical activity of the atria during cardioplegic arrest in pigs. Ann Thorac Surg 37:154–158, 1984

63. Vanden Dungen JJ, Karliczek GF, Brenken U et al: Clinical study of blood trauma during perfusion with membrane and bubble oxygenators. J Thorac Cardiovasc Surg 83:108–116, 1982

64. Peterson KA, Dewanjee MK, Kaye MP: Fate of Indium 111 labeled platelet during cardiopulmonary bypass performed with membrane and bubble oxygenators. J Thorac Cardiovasc Surg 84:39–43, 1982

65. Tabak C, Eugene J, Stemmer EA: Erythrocyte survival following extracorporeal circulation: A question of membrane versus bubble oxygenators. J Thorac Cardiovasc Surg 81:30–33, 1981

66. Trumbull HR, Howe J, Mohl K et al: A comparison of the effects of membrane and bubble oxygenators on platelet counts and platelet size in elective cardiac operations. Ann Thorac Surg 30:52–57, 1980

67. Edmunds LH, Ellison N, Colman RW et al: Platelet function during cardiac operations: Comparison of membrane and bubble oxygenators. J Thorac Cardiovasc Surg 83:805–812, 1982

68. Hessel EA, Johnson DD, Ivey T et al: Membrane versus bubble oxygenators for cardiac operations: A prospective randomized study. J Thorac Cardiovasc Surg 80:111–112, 1980

69. Boers M, Vanden Dungen JJ, Karliczek GF et al: Two membrane oxygenators and a bubble: A clinical comparison. Ann Thorac Surg 35:455–462, 1983

70. Hearse DJ, Erol C, Robinson LA et al: Particle-induced coronary vasoconstriction during cardioplegic infusion. Characterization and possible mechanisms. J Thorac Cardiovasc Surg 89(3):428, 1985

71. Ellis RJ, Wisnewski A, Potts R et al: Reduction of flow rate and arterial pressure at moderate hypothermia does not result in cerebral dysfunction. J Thorac Cardiovasc Surg 79:173–180, 1980

72. Hickey RF, Hoar PE: Whole-body oxygen consumption during low-flow hypothermic cardiopulmonary bypass. J Thorac Cardiovasc Surg 86:903–906, 1983

73. Watkins WD, Peterson MJB, King DL et al: Thromboxane and prostacyclin changes during cardiopulmonary bypass with and without pulsatile flow. J Thorac Cardiovasc Surg 84(250):256, 1982

74. Silverman NA, Levitsky S, Kohler J et al: Prevention of reperfusion injury following cardioplegic arrest by pulsatile flow. Ann Thorac Surg 35:493–499, 1983

75. Edmunds LH: Pulseless cardiopulmonary bypass. J Thorac Cardiovasc Surg 84:800–804, 1982

76. Hickey PR, Buckley MJ, Philbin DM: Pulsatile and non-pulsatile cardiopulmonary bypass: Review of a counterproductive controversy. Ann Thorac Surg 36:720–737, 1984

77. Philbin DM, Hickey PR, Buckley MJ: Should we pulse? J Thorac Cardiovasc Surg 84:805–806, 1982

78. Christlieb IY, Clark RE: Adequacy of the perfusate. Its influence on successful myocardial protection. J Thorac Cardiovasc Surg 84:689, 1982

79. Rosenblum HM, Haasler GB, Spotnitz WD et al: Effects of simulated clinical cardiopulmonary bypass and cardioplegia on mass of the canine left ventricle. Ann Thorac Surg 39(2):139, 1985

80. Neptune WB, Weller R, Bailey CP: Experimental lung transplantation. J Thorac Cardiovasc Surg 26:275–289, 1953

81. Neptune WB, Cookson BA, Bailey CP et al: Complete homologous heart transplantation. Arch Surg 66:174–178, 1953

82. Sealy WC, Brown IW, Jr, Young WG, Jr et al: Hypothermia, low-flow extracorporeal circulation and controlled cardiac arrest for open heart surgery. Surg Gynecol Obstet 104:441, 1957

83. Buckberg GD, Brazier JR, Nelson RL et al: Studies of the effects of hypothermia on regional myocardial blood flow and metabolism during cardiopulmonary bypass. I. The adequately perfused, beating, fibrillating, and arrested heart. J Thorac Cardiovasc Surg 73:87, 1977

84. Buckberg GD: A proposed "solution" to the cardioplegic controversy. J Thorac Cardiovasc Surg 77:803–815, 1979

85. Grover FL, Fewel JG, Ghidoni JJ, Trinkle JK: Does lower systemic temperature enhance cardioplegic myocardial protection. J Thorac Cardiovasc Surg 81:11–20, 1981

86. Laschinger JC, Catinella FB, Cunningham JN et al: Myocardial cooling: Beneficial effects of topical hypothermia. J Thorac Cardiovasc Surg 84:807–814, 1982

87. Landymore RW, Tice D, Trehan N et al: Importance of typical hypothermia to ensure uniform myocardial cooling during coronary artery bypass. J Thorac Cardiovasc Surg 82:832–836, 1981

88. Nelson RL, Goldstein SM, McConnell DH et al: Studies of the effects of hypothermia on regional myocardial blood flow and metabolism during cardiopulmonary bypass: V. Profound topical hypothermia during ischemia in arrested hearts. Surgery 73:201, 1977

89. Bonchek LI, Olinger GN: An improved method of topical cardiac hypothermia. J Thorac Cardiovasc Surg 82:878–882, 1981

90. Rosenfeldt FL, Arnold M: Topical cardiac cooling by recirculation: Comparison of a closed system using a cooling pad with an open system using a topical spray. Ann Thorac Surg 34:138–145, 1982

91. Schachner A, Schimert G, Lajos TS et al: Selective intracavitary and coronary profound hypothermic cardioplegia for myocardial preservation: A new technique. Ann Thorac Surg 23:154, 1977

92. Force TL, Reabe DS, Coffin LH et al: Coronary ostial stenosis following aortic valve replacement without continuous coronary perfusion. J Thorac Cardiovasc Surg 80:537–641, 1980

93. Hilton CJ, Teubl W, Acker M et al: Inadequate cardioplegic protection with obstructed coronary arteries. Ann Thorac Surg 28:323, 1979

94. Tyers GFO, Williams EH, Hughes HC et al: Effect of perfusate temperature on myocardial protection from ischemia. J Thorac Cardiovasc Surg 73:766–771, 1977

95. Digerness SB, Vanini V, Wideman FE: Oxygen delivery to the ischemic myocardium. Circulation (Suppl 3)62:324, 1980

96. Balderman SC, Binette JP, Chan AWK et al: The optimal temperature for preservation of the myocardium during global ischemia. Ann Thorac Surg 35:605, 1983

97. Tyers GFO, Williams EH, Hughes HC, Jr et al: Optimal myocardial hypothermia at 10–15°C. Surgical Forum 26:233, 1976

98. Shragge BW, Digerness SB, Blackstone EH: Complete recovery of myocardial function following cold exposure. Circulation (Suppl 2)58:97, 1978

99. Kao RL, Conti VR, Williams EH: Effect of temperature during potassium arrest on myocardial metabolism and function. J Thorac Cardiovasc Surg 84:243–249, 1982

100. Magovern GJ, Jr, Flaherty JT, Gott VL et al: Optimal myocardial protection with fluosol. Ann Thorac Surg 34:249–257, 1982

101. Rosenfeldt FL: The relationship between myocardial temperature and recovery after experimental cardiac arrest. J Thorac Cardiovasc Surg 84:656–666, 1982

102. Magovern GJ, Jr, Flaherty JT, Gott VL et al: Failure of blood cardioplegia to protect myocardium at lower temperatures. Circulation (Suppl 1)66:60–67, 1982

103. Chiu RCJ, Blundell PJ, Scott HJ, Cain S: The importance of monitoring intramyocardial temperature during hypothermic myocardial protection. Ann Thorac Surg 28:317–322, 1979

104. Daggett WM, Jacocks MA, Coleman WS et al: Myocardial temperatures mapping: Improved intraoperative myocardial presevation. J Thorac Cardiovasc Surg 82:883–888, 1981

105. Becker H, Vinten–Johansen J, Buckberg GD et al: Critical importance of ensuring cardioplegic delivery with coronary stenosis. J Thorac Cardiovasc Surg 81:507, 1981

106. Vandersalm JJ, O'Kike ON, Cutler BS et al: Improved myocardial preservation by improved distribution of cardioplegic solutions. J Thorac Cardiovasc Surg 83:767–771, 1982

107. Roberts AJ, Faro RS, Watson WD et al: Coronary artery bypass graft surgery: Relative efficacy of initial proximal versus distal anastomoses. Ann Thorac Surg 38:15–20, 1984

108. Weisel RD, Hoy FB, Baird RJ et al: Comparison of alternative cardioplegic techniques. J Thorac Cardiovasc Surg 86:97–107, 1983

109. Weisel RD, Hoy FB, Baird RJ et al: Improved myocardial protection during a prolonged cross-clamp period. Ann Thorac Surg 36:664–674, 1983

110. Lillihei CW, DeWall RA, Gott VL et al: The direct vision correction of calcific aortic stenosis by means of a pump-oxygenator and retrograde coronary sinus perfusion. Chest 30:123, 1956

111. Williams GD, Burnett HF, Derrick BL et al: Retrograde venous cardiac perfusion for myocardial revascularization: An experimental evaluation. Ann Thorac Surg 22:322, 1976

112. Menasche P, Kural S, Fauchet M et al: Retrograde coronary sinus perfusion: A safe alternative for ensuring cardioplegic delivery in aortic valve surgery. Ann Thorac Surg 34:647, 1982

113. Gundry SR, Kirsch MM: A comparison of retrograde cardioplegia versus antegrade cardioplegia in the presence of coronary artery obstruction. Circulation (Suppl II)66:152, 1984

114. Gundry SR, Kirsch MM: A comparison of retrograde cardioplegia versus antegrade cardioplegia in the presence of coronary artery obstruction. Ann Thorac Surg 38:124–127, 1984

115. Fabiani JN, Relland J, Carpentier AF: Myocardial protection via the coronary sinus in cardiac surgery. Comparative evaluation of two techniques. In Mohl W, Wolner E, Glogar D (eds): The Coronary Sinus, p 305. Darmstadt, Steinkopff Verlag, 1984

116. Mohl W, Roberts AJ: Coronary sinus retroperfusion and pressure-controlled intermittent coronary sinus occlusion (PICSO) for myocardial protection. Surg Clin North Am 65(3):477, 1985

117. Molina JE, Gani KS, Voss DM: Pressurized rapid cardioplegia versus administration of exogenous substrate and topical hypothermia. Ann Thorac Surg 33:434–444, 1982

118. Johnson RE, Dorsey LM, Moye SJ et al: Cardioplegic

infusion: The safe limits of pressure and temperature. J Thorac Cardiovasc Surg 83:813–823, 1982

119. Engleman RM, Rousou JH, Lemeshow S: High-volume crystalloid cardioplegia: An improved method of myocardial preservation. J Thorac Cardiovasc Surg 86:87–96, 1983

120. Ebert PA; Editorial: Aspects of myocardial protection. Ann Thorac Surg 26:495–496, 1978

121. McGoon DC: The ongoing quest for ideal myocardial protection: A catalog of the recent English literature. J Thorac Cardiovasc Surg 89:639–653, 1985

122. Nwaneri NJ, Levitsky S, Silverman NA, Feinberg H: Induction of cardioplegia with blood and crystalloid potassium solutions during prolonger aortic cross-clamping. Surgery 94:836–841, 1983

123. Takamoto S, Levine FH, LaRaia PJ et al: Comparison of single-dose and multiple-dose crystalloid and blood potassium cardioplegia during prolonged hypothermic aortic occlusion. J Thorac Cardiovasc Surg 79:19–28, 1980

124. Feindel CM, Tait GA, Wilson GJ et al: Multidose blood versus crystalloid cardioplegia: Comparison by quantitative assessment of irreversible myocardial injury. J Thorac Cardiovasc Surg 87:585–595, 1984

125. Catinella FP, Cunningham JN, Spencer FC: Myocardial protection during prolonged aortic cross-clamping: Comparison of blood and crystalloid cardioplegia. J Thorac Cadiovasc Surg 88:411–423, 1984

126. Robertson JM, Buckberg DG, Vinten–Johansen J, Leaf JO: Comparison of distribution beyond coronary stenoses of blood and asanguineous cardioplegic solutions. J Thorac Cardiovasc Surg 86:80–86, 1983

127. Shapira N, Kirsh M, Jochim K, Behrendt DM: Comparison of the effect of blood cardioplegia to crystalloid cardioplegia on myocardial contractility in man. J Thorac Cardiovasc Surg 80:647–655, 1980

128. Roberts AJ, Moran JM, Sanders JH et al: Clinical evaluation of the relative effectiveness of multidose crystalloid and cold blood potassium cardioplegia in coronary artery bypass graft surgery: A nonrandomized matched-pair analysis. Ann Thorac Surg 33:421–433, 1982

129. Barner HB, Kaiser GC, Godd JE et al: Clinical experience with cold blood as the vehicle for hypothermia potassium cardioplegia. Ann Thorac Surg 29:224–227, 1980

130. Iverson LIH, Young JN, Ennix CL et al: Myocardial protection: A comparison of cold blood and cold crystalloid cardioplegia. J Thorac Cardiovasc Surg 87:509–516, 1984

131. Cunningham JN, Adams PX, Knopp EA et al: Protection of ATP, ultra-structure, and ventricular function after aortic cross-clamping and reperfusion: Clinical use of blood potassium cardioplegia. J Thorac Cardiovasc Surg 78:708–720, 1979

132. Singh AK, Farrugia R, Teplitz C et al: Electrolyte versus blood cardioplegia: Randomized clinical and myocardial ultrastructural study. Ann Thorac Surg 33:218–231i, 1982

133. Chen YF, Lin YT: Comparison of blood cardioplegia to electrolyte cardioplegia on the effectiveness of preservation of right atrial myocardium: Mitochondrial morphometric study. Ann Thorac Surg 39:434–438, 1985

134. Codd JE, Barner HB, Pennington DG et al: Intraoperative myocardial protection: A comparison of blood and asanguineous cardioplegia. Ann Thorac Surg 39:125–133, 1985

135. Bodenhamer RM, DeBoer LWV, Geffin GA et al: Enhanced myocardial protection during ischemic arrest: Oxygenation of a crystalloid cardioplegic solution. J Thorac Cardiovasc Surg 85:769–780, 1983

136. Kanter KR, Jaffin JH, Ehrlichman RJ et al: Superiority of perfluorocarbon cardioplegia over blood or crystalloid cardioplegia. Circulation (Suppl 2)64:75–80, 1981

137. Rousou JH, Dobbs WA, Engleman RM: Fluosol cardioplegia: A method of optimizing aerobic metabolism during arrest. Circulation (Suppl 2)66:55–59, 1982

138. Hicks GL, Arnold W, DeWall RA: Fluorocarbon cardioplegia and myocardial protection. Ann Thorac Surg 35:500–503, 1983

139. Gardner TJ, Flaherty JT, Kanter KR, Magovern GJ, Jr: Improved myocardial protection with perfluorocarbon cardioplegia. Prog Clin Biol Res 122:405–417, 1983

140. Flaherty JT, Jaffin JH, Magovern GJ, Jr et al: Maintenance of aerobic metabolism during global ischemia with perfluorocarbon cardioplegia improves myocardial preservation.

141. Novick RJ, Stefaniszny HJ, Michel RP et al: Protection of the hypertrophied pig myocardium: A comparison of crystalloid, blood, and Fluosol-DA cardioplegia during prolonged aortic clamping. J Thorac Cardiovasc Surg 89:547–566, 1985

142. Vander Woude JC, Christlieb Y, Sicard GA, Clark RE: Imidazole-buffered cardioplegic solution. Improved myocardial preservation during global ischemia. J Thorac Cardiovasc Surg 90:225, 1985

143. Follette DM, Fey K, Mulder DM et al: Prolonged safe aortic cross-clamping by combining membrane stabilization, multidose cardioplegia, and physiologic reperfusion. J Thorac Cardiovasc Surg 74:682, 1977

144. Wildenthal K, Mierzwaik DS, Mitchell JI: Acute effects of increased serum osmolality of left ventricular performance. Am J Physiol 216:898, 1969

145. Tyers GFO, Todd GJ, Niebauer IM et al: The mechanism

of myocardial damage following potassium citrate (Melrose) cardioplegia. Surgery 78:45, 1975

146. Fey K, Follette D, Bugyi H et al: Effects of membrane stabilization on the safety of hypothermic arrest after aortic cross-clamping. Circulation (Suppl 2)56:771, 1977

147. Levinsky L, Schimert G, Lajos TZ et al: The use of steroids as a potentiator of hypothermic myocardial preservation in man. J Surg Res 26:629–651, 1979

148. Hearse DJ, Stewart DA, Braimbridge MV: Metabolic and myocardial protection during elective cardiac arrest. Circ Res 36:481, 1975

149. Ellis RJ, Mavroudis C, Gardner C et al: Relationship between atrioventricular arrhythmias and the concentration of K^+ ion in cardioplegic solution. J Thorac Cardiovasc Surg 80:517–526, 1980

150. Rousou JH, Engleman RM, Dobbs WA et al: The optimal potassium concentration in cardioplegic solutions. Ann Thorac Surg 32:75–79, 1981

151. Jellinek M, Standeven JW, Menz LJ et al: Cold blood potassium cardioplegia: Effects of increasing concentrations of potassium. J Thorac Cardiovasc Surg 82:26–37, 1981

152. Rich TL, Brady AJ: Potassium contracture and utilization of high-energy phosphates in rabbit heart. Am J Physiol 226:105, 1974

153. Engelman RM, Avvil J, O'Donoghue MJ, Levitsky S: Significance of multidose cardioplegia and hypothermia in myocardial preservation during ischemic arrest. J Thorac Cardiovasc Surg 75:555, 1978

154. Hearse DJ, Stewart DA, Braimbridge MV: Myocardial protection during ischemic cardiac arrest: Importance of magnesium in cardioplegic infusates. J Thorac Cardiovasc Surg 75:877, 1978

155. Frank JS, Langer GA, Nudd LM, Seraydarian K: The myocardial cell surface, its histochemistry, and the effect of sialic acid and calcium removal on its structure and cellular ionic exchange. Circ Res 41:702, 1977

156. Yates JC, Dhalla NS: Structural and functional changes associated with failure and recovery of hearts after perfusion with Ca^{2+} free medium. J Mol Cell Cardiol 7:91, 1975

157. Vouche PR, Helias J, Grandin CM: Myocardial protection through cold cardioplegia using diltiazem, a calcium channel blocker. Ann Thorac Surg 30:342–348, 1980

158. Standeven JW, Jellinke M, Menz LJ et al: Cold blood potassium diltiazem cardioplegia. J Thorac Cardiovasc Surg 87:201–212, 1984

159. Clark RE, Christlieb IY, Fergusen TB et al: The first American clinical trial of nifedipine in cardioplegia. J Thorac Cardiovasc Surg 82:848–859, 1981

160. Clark RE, Magovern GJ, Christlieb IY et al: Nifedipine cardioplegia experience: Results of a 3 year cooperative clinical study. Ann Thorac Surg 36:654–663, 1983

161. Guyton RA, Dorsey LM, Colgan TI et al: Calcium-channel blockade as an adjunct to heterogenous delivery of cardioplegia. Ann Thorac Surg 35:626–632, 1983

162. Clark RE, Christlieb IY, Henry PD et al: Nifedipine: A myocardial protective agent. Am J Cardiol 44:825, 1979

163. Nayler WG: Protection of the myocardium against postischemic reperfusion damage: The combined effect of hypothermia and nifedipine. J Thorac Cardiovasc Surg 84:897–965, 1982

164. Lupinetti FM, Hammon JW, Huddleston CB et al: Global ischemia in the immature canine ventricle: Enhanced protective effect of Verapamil and potassium. J Thorac Cardiovasc Surg 87:213–219, 1984

165. Robb–Nicholsen C, Currie WD, Wechsler AS: Effects of Verapamil on myocardial tolerance to ischemic arrest. Circulation (Suppl 2)58:1–119, 1978

166. Fumio Y, Manning AS, Braimbridge MV et al: Cardioplegia and slow-channel blockers: Studies with Verapamil. J Thorac Cardiovasc Surg 86:252–261, 1983

167. Hicks GL, Jr, Salley RK, DeWeese JA: Calcium channel blockers: An intraoperative and postoperative trial in women. Ann Thorac Surg 37:319–323, 1984

168. Balderman SC, Chan AK, Gage AA: Verapamil cardioplegia: Improved myocardial preservation during global ischemia. J Thorac Cardiovasc Surg 88:57–66, 1984

169. Flameng W, Borgers M, Vander Vusse GJ: Cardioprotective effects of Lidoflazine in extensive aorta-coronary bypass grafting. J Thorac Cardiovasc Surg 85:758–768, 1983

170. Kales RA, Dorsey LM, Kaplan JA: Pretreatment with Lidoflazine, a calcium channel blocker: Useful adjunct to heterogenous cold potassium cardioplegia. J Thorac Cardiovasc Surg 85:278–286, 1983

171. Rovetto MJ, Whitmer JT, Neely JR: Comparison of the effects of anoxia and whole heart ischemia of the carbohydrate utilization in isolated working rat hearts. Circ Res 32:699, 1973

172. Hearse DJ, Stewart DA, Braimbridge MV: Myocardial protection during ischemic cardiac arrest: Possible deleterious effects of glucose and mannitol in coronary infusates. J Thorac Cardiovasc Surg 76:16, 1978

173. Hewitt RL, Lolley DM, Adrouny GA et al: Protective effect of glycogen and glucose on the anoxic arrested heart. Surgery 75:1, 1974

174. Austen WG, Greenberg JJ, Piccinini JC: Myocardial

function and contractile force affected by glucose loading of the heart during anoxia. Surgery 67:839, 1965

175. Lazar HL, Buckberg GD, Manganero AJ et al: Reversal of ischemic damage with amino acid substrate enhancement during reperfusion. Surgery 88:702–710, 1980

176. Lazar HL, Buckberg GD, Manganaro AM, Becker H: Myocardial energy replenishment and reversal of ischemic damage by substrate enhancement of secondary blood cardioplegia with amino acids during reperfusion. J Thorac Cardiovasc Surg 80:350–359, 1980

177. Robertson JM, Vinten–Johansen J, Buckberg GD et al: Safety of prolonged aortic clamping with blood cardioplegia. I. Glutamate enrichment in normal hearts. J Thorac Cardiovasc Surg 88:395–401, 1984

178. Rosenkranz ER, Okamoto F, Buckberg GD et al: Safety of prolonged aortic clamping with blood cardioplegia. II. Glutamate enrichment in energy-depleted hearts. J Thorac Cardiovasc Surg 88:402–410, 1984

179. Pasque MK, Sprag TL, Pellam GL et al: Ribose-enhanced myocardial recovery following ischemia in the isolated working rat heart. J Thorac Cardiovasc Surg 83:390–398, 1982

180. Robinson LA, Braimbridge MV, Hearse DJ: Creatine phosphate: An additive myocardial protective and antiarrhythmic agent in cardioplegia. J Thorac Cardiovasc Surg 87:190–200, 1984

181. Humphrey SM, Seeley RN: Improved functional recovery of ischemic myocardium by suppression of adenosine catabolism. J Thorac Cardiovasc Surg 84:16–22, 1982

182. Chambers DE, Parks DA, Patterson G et al: Role of oxygen derived radicals in myocardial ischemia. Fed Proc 47:1093, 1983

183. Mellors A, Tappel AL: The inhibition of mitochondrial peroxidation by ubiquinone and ubiquinol. J Biol Chem 241:4353, 1966

184. Takeshige K, Takayanagi R, Minakami S: Reduced coenzyme Q_{10} as an antioxidant of lipid peroxidation in bovine heart mitochondria. In Yamamura Y, Folkers K, Ito Y (eds): Biomedical and Clinical Aspects of Coenzyme Q, Vol 2, p 3. Amsterdam, Elsevier Biomedical Press, 1980

185. Nayler WG: The use of coenzyme Q_{10} to protect ischemic heart muscle. In Yamamura Y, Foklers K, Ito Y (eds): Biomedical and Clinical Aspects of Coenzyme Q, Vol 2, p 409. Amsterdam, Elsevier, 1980

186. Mori F, Mohri H: Effects of coenzyme Q_{10} added to a potassium cardioplegic solution for myocardial protection during ischemic cardiac arrest. Ann Thorac Surg 39:30–36, 1985

187. Tanaka J, Tominaga R, Yoshitoshi M et al: Coenzyme Q_{10}: The prophylactic effect on low cardiac output following cardiac valve replacement. Ann Thorac Surg 33:145–151, 1982

188. Khuri SF, Marston WA, Josa M et al: Observations on 100 patients with continuous intraoperative monitoring of intramyocardial pH. The adverse effects of ventricular fibrillation and reperfusion. J Thorac Cardiovasc Surg 89:170, 1985

PEDIATRIC CARDIAC SURGERY

Thomas L. Spray

Since its beginnings more than 40 years ago, surgery for congenital heart disease has progressed to the point that virtually all forms of congenital heart disease can be managed surgically with some degree of success. The prodigious operative risks of early repairs are now being significantly reduced, and more and more children are presented with the prospect of a normal life. These advances have been related not only to improvement in the surgical techniques but to improvements in postoperative care and intraoperative perfusion and monitoring. As many surgical techniques have evolved, the opportunity to examine the long-term results of successful congenital heart operations has altered approaches that were initially believed to give excellent results.

Although a comprehensive evaluation of the state of the art of congenital heart disease is beyond the scope of this chapter, several areas of surgery for congenital heart disease have undergone significant changes in attitude or emphasis over the past 5 years. These areas will be covered in this chapter.

COARCTATION OF THE AORTA

MORPHOLOGY

Classic coarctation of the aorta is an infolding of aortic media in the portion of the circumference of the aorta that is opposite or just proximal to the ductus arteriosus. Often associated with this infolding is a localized ridge of intimal hyper-

trophy resembling ductal tissue, which progressively narrows the lumen.[1] The intimal hypertrophy may be a progressive change related to hemodynamic forces that decrease the lateral pressure on the aortic wall distal to a site of narrowing. Narrowing then progresses until a critical size at which the resistance to flow allows for no further drop in pressure beyond the narrowing.[2] In some patients with coarctation, a more diffuse narrowing of the aortic isthmus between the subclavian artery and the coarctation is found and has been termed *tubular hypoplasia of the aortic arch*. Occasionally, this narrowing may be severe enough to cause a pressure gradient across the site without an associated intimal shelf. Rudolph's theory of hemodynamic molding suggests that the type of coarctation seen is related to flow patterns through the ductus and aortic arch complex in fetal life (Fig. 17–1).[3,4] In normal fetal life, the flow across the aortic isthmus is approximately 60% of that across the ductus arteriosus (Fig. 17–1A). This fact has been used to explain the smaller diameter of the aortic isthmus compared with that of the descending aorta in normal humans. The infolding of the aortic media then may result from the angle at which the ductus meets the aorta; the tendency for intimal proliferation and therefore exacerbation of the coarctation will be exaggerated when ductal flow is large. This situation occurs when associated defects such as a ventricular septal defect are present (Fig. 17–1B). Even further hypoplasia of the aortic isthmus occurs when lesions of left ventricular outflow obstruction are associated with the increased ductal blood flow (hy-

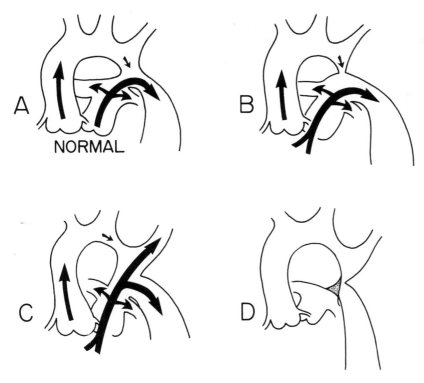

FIG. 17–1. (A) Normal fetal flow patterns with the majority of flow across the ductus arteriosus and relatively little flow across the aortic isthmus (small arrow). **(B)** The association of a ventricular septal defect results in increased ductal flow at the expense of aortic isthmus flow. Here isthmic flow may be only 25% to 30% of the amount of ductal flow. **(C)** Direction of ductal flow toward the left subclavian artery, resulting in hypoplasia between the carotid and subclavian vessels (small arrow). **(D)** Obliteration of ductal tissue involving the aortic wall, resulting in significant aortic coarctation.

poplastic left ventricular complex). Although a few cases of coarctation in association with lesions that decrease ductal blood flow have been reported, the extreme rarity of these defects suggests that diminished ductal blood flow allows for an enlargement of the isthmus and descending aorta from a relative increase in blood flow through these areas.[5–7]

Occasionally, narrowing of the aorta in the juxtaductal position appears to be delayed until the onset of ductal closure. Recent studies have suggested that ductal tissue may be present around the circumference of the aorta at the site of ductal insertion and, therefore, that the ductus and descending aorta are a common channel.[8,9] The obliteration of the ductus arteriosus then may cause narrowing in the portion of the aorta that is made up of ductal tissue (Fig. 17–1D).

Coarctation or hypoplasia between the origin of the left subclavian and common carotid arteries is explained by reorientation of the intimal shelf such that increased ductal flow is channeled to the subclavian artery in addition to the descending aorta, resulting in an area of low flow between the carotid and subclavian vessels (Fig. 17–1C).

Consideration of the possible causes of the various anatomical types of coarctation of the aorta has become important to determine the optimal surgical management to reduce the long-term recurrence rate.

CLINICAL PRESENTATION

Neonates with coarctation of the aorta often are admitted in critical condition and congestive heart failure. Associated cardiac anomalies are present in approximately 85% of cases in the neonatal period and include bicuspid aortic valve, ventricular septal defect, and mitral valve anomalies.[10] A chest film often shows marked cardiomegaly and congestion with increased pulmonary vascularity. The electrocardiogram may show right ventricular hypertrophy in the neonate. Echocardiography can often determine the site of coarctation and rule out associated defects whereas angiocardiography may still be necessary in some cases to delineate the anatomy. While the preliminary investigations are performed, the patient is treated medically with the institution of prostaglandin E_1 at 0.1 μ/kg/minute in neonates less than 10 days of age to maintain ductal patency and to improve peripheral perfusion. Digitalis and diuretics, or in more severe cases, mechanical ventilation and inotropic support, may be necessary. After the patient is clinically stablized, operation is undertaken. In older children who present with coarctation, symptoms are often notably absent and the diagnosis is made by routine physical examination, which reveals cardiac murmur or a discrepancy in blood pressure between the upper and lower extremities. When coarctation presents in childhood, associated cardiac anomalies occur much less frequently.[10] Surgical treatment is usually recommended at between 3 and 5 years of age to allow for regression of left ventricular hypertrophy and maximal resolution of hypertension.

SURGICAL TREATMENT

The classic repair for coarctation of the aorta involves resection of the coarctation segment with end-to-end anastomosis (Fig. 17–2A).[11,12] The anterior suture line used to complete the repair is generally performed with an interrupted technique to allow for some future growth. Although early results have been quite good, concerns about recoarctation at the repair site and the persistence of gradients and hypertension as the child grows have resulted in several modifications of the technique. One initial approach was a patch aortoplasty across the coarctation segment using a portion of Dacron graft or Gore-Tex material (Fig. 17–2C).[13–15] Although results are also excellent with this technique and it allows the advantages of not requiring complete dissection of the proximal and distal aorta or sacrificing of collateral vessels, long-term follow-up has suggested that aneurysm formation opposite the site of the patch may be a relatively frequent long-term complication requiring reoperation.[16] The aneurysm formation appears to be related to differences in compliance between the native aorta and the patch material, resulting in distortion of hemodynamic forces across the repair site. Problems with the patch aortoplasty and end-to-end anastomoses on long-term follow-up have led to the widespread utilization of subclavian-flap angioplasty, initially popularized by Waldhausen and associates (Fig. 17–2B).[17] This technique involves ligation of the left subclavian artery at the origin of the vertebral artery with or without compromise of the vertebral vessel. The coarctation area is then incised longitudinally, and the coarctation shelf and intimal proliferation are excised as much as possible. The flap of open subclavian artery is then brought down beyond the coarctation site and the anastomosis is completed. The width of the opened subclavian artery determines the maximal circumferential widening of the coarctation site. Because there is no circumferential suture line, there is evidence to suggest that the area of repair may grow with time.[18] In addition, to maximize the possible growth potential at the site of the anastomosis, some authors have recommended the use of monofilament absorbable suture for completion of the anastomosis. Preliminary studies suggest that growth will be acceptable at this anastomosis, although long-term data are not yet available.[19] The use of the Waldhausen subclavian-flap aortoplasty has resulted in extremely low operative mortality rates for coarctation repair in infants. In several series, the operative mortality ranges from 0% to 3%.[20,21,22] Even at a very

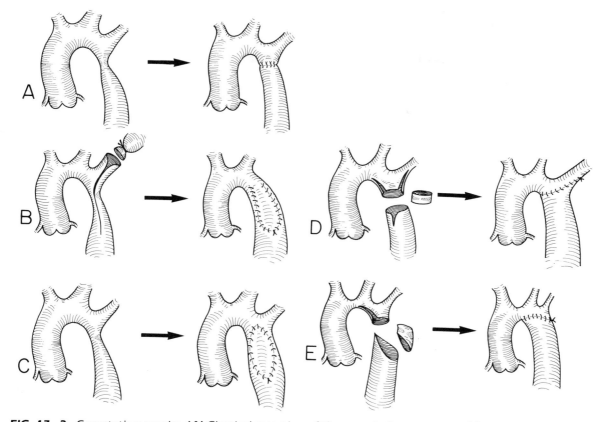

FIG. 17–2. Coarctation repairs. **(A)** Classical resection of the coarctation segment with end-to-end anastomosis using interrupted sutures. **(B)** Subclavian flap aortoplasty, turning down the flap of the left subclavian artery to patch across the coarctation site. **(C)** Patch graft aortoplasty using a portion of prosthetic material to enlarge the area of coarctation. **(D)** Modification of resection with end-to-end anastomosis. Excision of coarctation site and enlargement of the proximal aorta under the arch and onto the left subclavian artery. **(E)** Extensive enlargement of the undersurface of the aortic arch in severe tubular hypoplasia of the aortic arch. The lack of prosthetic material allows for potentially greater future growth.

young age and very small size, operative risk is below 10%, the mortality being associated with coexisting congenital anomalies[18,22] Hospital mortality for repair of coarctation in older children or adults likewise has approached zero, with a current operative mortality of approximately 1%.[21,23]

INCIDENCE OF RECOARCTATION

In most series of coarctation repair, a small but significant incidence of restenosis at the coarctation repair site has been reported.[21,23,24] It is unclear whether these "recoarctations" are merely inadequate relief of the initial obstruction, lack of sufficient anastomotic growth, or proliferation of tissue causing narrowing of the previously adequate lumen. Clearly, the incidence of recoarctation is related to the age at which the initial repair was performed. The incidence of recoarctation after end-to-end anastomosis approaches 50% when the operation is performed in neonates and decreases to approximately 15% at 6 months and less than 5% after infancy.[21] The incidence of stenosis appears to be less in some series and has been reported to be as low as 10% in end-to-end anastomoses using modified techniques.[25] The subclavian-flap repair has apparently lowered the incidence of persistent or recurrent coarctation in neonates and infants to 0% to 6%, although Cobanoglu and associates suggest that recurrent coarctation is excessive when subclavian-flap angioplasty is performed in patients less than 8 weeks of age.[25] Recoarctation in this situation appears to result from progressive constriction of the posterior aorta, which contains the intimal shelf, possibly related to involution of the ductal material in the aortic wall.

Concerns about recoarctation in the small infant with coarctation repair and the relative disadvantage of sacrifice of the left subclavian artery have prompted the use of a modified end-to-end anastomosis in small infants with favorable anatomy. In this technique, the coarctation area and presumably the ductal tissue are completely excised, and the aorta is mobilized freely and enlarged proximally or distally to create a widely patent anastomosis (Fig. 17–2D and E). Monofilament absorbable or nonabsorbable sutures have been used in these techniques. Early results suggest excellent relief of obstruction using variations of this technique, however, long-term results are not currently available.[26]

SUMMARY

Although coarctation of the aorta can now be repaired even in extremely small neonates with excellent results and hospital mortality is approaching 0% in the absence of associated defects, concern persists about the possibilities of late recoarctation or residual stenosis. Although the subclavian-flap repair has gained in popularity and is currently the most widely used technique in infants, the possibility of abnormal ductal tissue retained in the aortic wall and therefore a higher incidence of recoarctation in very small neonates have prompted reevaluation of this technique. In situations of favorable anatomy, modified end-to-end anastomoses may provide optimal results even in very small infants. Superior results may now be possible by individualizing the technique of operation to the anatomical type of coarctation and the magnitude and location of associated tubular hypoplasia of the aortic arch. Optimal surgical therapy may also vary with age and associated cardiovascular abnormalities.

TRANSPOSITION OF THE GREAT VESSELS

MORPHOLOGY

Complete transposition of the great vessels is present when the aorta rises entirely, or in large part, from the right ventricle and the pulmonary artery arises from the left ventricle. Systemic oxygenation is maintained by a shunt at the level of the atrial septum, the ventricular septum, or the pulmonary artery. Associated abnormalities include ventricular septal defect, patent ductus arteriosus, or subpulmonic left ventricular outflow tract obstruction. Initial approaches to palliative surgery for transposition included the Blalock–Hanlon operation, in which a large portion of atrial septum is excised to allow for mixing of pulmonary and systemic blood.[27] Balloon atrial septostomy to create the atrial septal defect was pioneered by Rashkind in 1966 and is effective palliation in the neonatal period.[28] Surgical attempts to correct transposition of the great vessels were directed at the arterial or atrial levels. In 1954 Albert proposed redirection of the atrial septum so that caval return was directed to the left ventricle and pulmonary venous return to the right ventricle.[29] In 1959 Senning performed the first operation of this type by using the walls of the atria as baffles to redirect pulmonary and systemic venous blood flow.[30] To provide larger atrial chambers, Mustard created similar baffles with homologous or prosthetic material.[31] Problems with baffle obstruction and arrhythmias following the Mustard repair resulted in a resurgence in popularity of the Senning operation with a modification by Quaeguebuer and Brom in 1977.[32] Refinements in the Senning operation have now resulted in large series of patients with simple transposition of the great vessels not associated with ventricular septal defect (VSD) or left ventricular outflow tract obstruction with operative mortalities of 0% to 5%.[33,34] The Mustard procedure has also resulted in low operative mortality, although concern over baffle obstruction and arrhythmias persists.[35,36]

The disappointing results of atrial switch operations for transposition associated with other anomalies, including left ventricular outflow tract obstruction and large ventricular septal defect, stimulated interest in surgery to correct the anomaly at the arterial level. In 1975 Jatene reported successful arterial switch in children with transposition of the great vessels and associated ventricular septal defect.[37] Attempts, however, to apply the arterial switch operation to neonates with intact ventricular septum were initially frustrated by the inability of the left ventricle to handle the systemic load when the switch operation was done after the first few weeks of life. Yacoub attributed this to alteration in left ventricular function as the pulmonary vascular resistance dropped, and he proposed pulmonary artery banding as a first procedure with resulting preparation of the ventricle for increased systemic work. With the use of this technique, improvements in survival following the repair were

reported.[38] As an alternate approach, several groups performed the operation in the first few weeks of life when the left ventricle was adequately prepared to handle the workload of the systemic circulation. Currently, an increasing number of centers are gaining experience with arterial switch operations in the first few days and weeks of life with markedly improving early results (Fig. 17–3).[39–41]

At the present time, the early results of atrial repairs of transposition of the great vessels in patients with intact ventricular septum appear to be somewhat more favorable than the early results with the arterial switch operation. Pulmonary banding as a preliminary to later arterial switch operation in patients with intact septum appears to carry a higher mortality than that of infants of the same age on whom an atrial switch operation is performed.[38] Therefore, the current interest in arterial switch operations in the neonatal age range is of great importance. The long-term follow-up of arterial switch operations performed in infancy appears to show good growth of the aortic and coronary anastomoses, although problems with pulmonary stenosis at the suture line and some aortic valve insufficiency raise questions about the long-term durability of the procedure.[41] Nevertheless, left ventricular function appears to remain adequate, and therefore there is optimism about the possibility of better long-term functional results in older children and adults who have had a more anatomical repair during infancy. The problems of supraventricular arrhythmias seen with the atrial repairs have not yet been seen following the arterial repair, suggesting that these abnormal rhythms are indeed a postoperative complication rather than part of the preexisting congenital defect.[42] Nevertheless, the majority of children and young adults who have had atrial switch operations such as the Senning procedure in infancy continue to do well. Although there are definable alterations in right ventricular geometry and function, these appear to be associated with

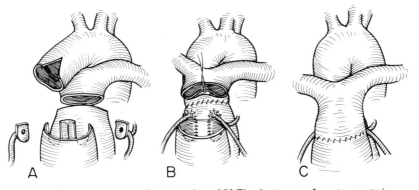

FIG. 17–3. Arterial switch operation. **(A)** The buttons of aorta containing the coronary artery ostia are excised and the great vessels mobilized. **(B)** The coronary arteries are reimplanted into appropriate sites of the adjacent pulmonary artery wall, and the aorta is enlarged and connected to the proximal pulmonary artery. The defects in the anterior aorta are closed with patches of pericardium. **(C)** The completed procedure results in an anterior pulmonary vessel sewn to the proximal aorta and a posterior vessel containing the neocoronary ostia and the ascending aorta. The aorta now contains what was once a pulmonary valve.

physiological abnormalities in only a relatively small proportion of patients.[43]

TETRALOGY OF FALLOT

Tetralogy of Fallot is characterized by right ventricular infundibular hypoplasia with anterior and leftward displacement of the infundibular septum and its parietal extension. It is associated with pulmonary stenosis or atresia and a mal-alignment type of ventricular septal defect that is located primarily beneath the aorta but occasionally may be located beneath both the aorta and pulmonary artery. The aorta overrides onto the right ventricle.

Clinically, children with tetralogy of Fallot defect present in the first several months of life with progressively increasing cyanosis due to the associated pulmonary stenosis and infundibular

hypertrophy. The excellent results of surgical treatment for tetralogy of Fallot have permitted some authors to recommend complete primary repair in infancy rather than the more traditional creation of a palliative systemic-to-pulmonary-artery shunt followed by complete repair in childhood.[44] The complications of systemic-to-pulmonary-artery shunts, with distortion of pulmonary artery anatomy and possible problems with ventricular failure or bacterial endocarditis, has lead to the desire to perform complete repair at the earliest age consistent with good results. Kirklin and associates have performed elaborate studies evaluating the effect of age and prior shunt on mortality after repair of tetralogy of Fallot. The incremental risk factor of small size appears to be present up until approximately 3 months of age, and by 6 months of age, the risk of total correction appears to be equivalent to or less than the risk of combined operations in which a shunt procedure is followed by later repair in cases with uncomplicated anatomy.[46] This type of risk analysis is based on predictions of the residual right ventricular outflow tract obstruction following repair with or without a transannular patch.

Although operative mortality is low in tetralogy of Fallot, there does appear to be an incremental decrease in long-term survival with increases in pulmonary valvar insufficiency and residual right ventricular outflow tract obstruction.[47-49] Kirklin has shown that the ratio of right ventricular pressure (PRV) to left ventricular pressure (PLV) in the immediate postoperative period can be predictive of the need for transannular patching.[46] PRV/PLV of 0.7 or less is generally associated with a good postoperative result. If infundibular resection alone is associated with a PRV/PLV of less than 0.85, a significant proportion of patients will have a progressive drop in the pressure ratio to 0.7 by the day after surgery.[46] Thus, in these patients, transannular patching may not be necessary, and therefore the magnitude of pulmonary insufficiency should be decreased. Equations developed to predict the postoperative PRV/PLV ratio have resulted in the realization that transannular patching is not required in a significant proportion of patients with tetralogy of Fallot, and they have been used to select patients for whom two-staged repair may be preferable to early complete repair.[50]

Concern about the magnitude of pulmonary insufficiency and resulting right ventricular dysfunction later in life after successful repair of tetralogy of Fallot has led to attempts to repair the defect with minimal or no right ventriculotomy.[51,52] The surgical approach is through the right atrium, with patch closure of the ventricular septal defect through the tricuspid valve and resection of infundibular obstructing muscle either from the right atrium or across the pulmonary valve, or both.[53-56] This approach may be augmented in selected cases by minimal right ventriculotomy or extension of a pulmonary arteriotomy minimally across the annulus if annulus enlargement is required. These approaches have resulted in lower incidences of pulmonary insufficiency, right bundle-branch block, and right ventricular dysfunction following surgery with quite acceptable early mortality.[56]

When shunts are required for palliation in infancy prior to a later-staged complete repair, the "classic" Blalock–Taussig shunt or the "Great Ormond Street shunt" using a 4- or 5-mm portion of Gore-Tex prosthesis from the subclavian vessel to the pulmonary artery may be used. The advantages using the prosthetic graft are the ability to create a shunt of sufficient length without tenting or kinking of the pulmonary artery and maintenance of subclavian artery flow. Excellent patency rates, even in small neonates, have been obtained with this technique.[57-59] Although the Blalock–Taussig anastomosis is still the shunt of choice when it can be created on the side of the innominate artery, when this is not feasible, the Gore-Tex shunt is the next most desirable alternative. The problems of distortion of pulmonary artery anatomy from the Waterston–Cooley anastomosis or the difficulty in later closure of Potts shunts have made their use generally undesirable at present.

CONDUITS, HOMOGRAFTS, AND VALVES

Many corrective procedures for congenital heart disease require the placement of prosthetic material as conduits or valves between chambers of the heart. Although prosthetic grafts and valves have been used extensively in adults, the materials used present specific problems in children. In many conduit repairs (including repair of truncus arteriosus in which a valved conduit is used to connect the right ventricle to the pulmonary arteries, or the Fontan operation), the use of bioprosthetic-valve–containing Dacron conduits has been associated with a high incidence of prosthetic-valve dysfunction with calcification and degeneration of the tissue valve and with formation of a fibrous peel in the conduit, which can dissect from the wall of the conduit and obstruct flow.[60-62] Because more patients are surviving repairs with this type of conduit material, a significantly higher incidence of conduit dysfunction has been encountered.[61] Therefore, the current trend has been to perform repairs with valveless conduits or conduits made of homologous material.

Current modifications of the Fontan operation, which connects the right atrium to the right ventricle or directly to the pulmonary artery, use portions of right atrium and homologous pericardium without valves for maintenance of a patulous connection (Bjork modification) (Fig. 17–4).[63,64] In some instances, the pulmonary artery, with or without its valve, can be transposed to the right atrium for direct anastomosis (Kreutzer procedure).[65] In all cases, use of prosthetic material is to be avoided whenever possible. In certain truncus repairs, especially in very small infants, the current valve-containing conduits or homografts are too large for implantation. Experience has been gained with the use of nonvalved conduits in these children with quite acceptable results.[66,67] Therefore, it is possible that nonvalved Gore-Tex or homologous pericardial conduits may be used increasingly for right ventricular outflow tract reconstruction, even in complex situations such as truncus arteriosus. The associated pulmonary insufficiency appears to be well tolerated in the absence of pulmonary obstruction. In the future, greater availability of small-sized homograft valve conduits may eliminate the need to accept the insufficiency inherent in valveless conduits.

In conduits containing bioprosthetic valves that are currently available, actuarial-projected

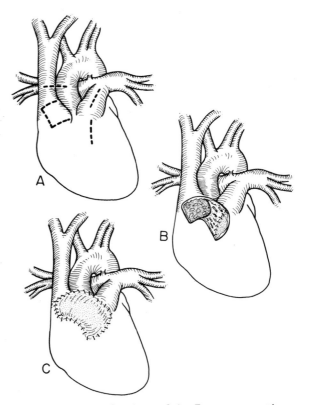

FIG. 17–4. Modifications of the Fontan operation. **(A)** Sites of incision for connection of the right atrium **(rectangular dashed line)** to the main pulmonary artery or right ventricular outflow tract. **(B)** Use of a flap of atrial appendage to fashion the posterior portion of the conduit, in this case, to the right ventricular outflow tract (Bjork modification). **(C)** Completion of the connection using a portion of autologous pericardium for the anterior aspect of the conduit.

reoperation rates for conduit obstruction have ranged from 4% to 10% per patient-year.[68-70] These disturbing results have led to an increased interest in the use of homograft valves for conduit reconstructions of the right ventricular outflow tract in children (Fig. 17–5). Large series from Fontan and the ''Great Ormond Street''

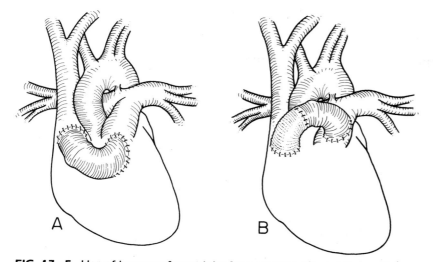

FIG. 17–5. Use of homograft conduits for reconstruction of the outflow tract in children. **(A)** Homograft valve-containing aorta connecting the right atrium to the right ventricular outflow tract. **(B)** Homograft valve-containing aorta elongated by a portion of crimped Dacron conduit extending from the right atrium to the main pulmonary artery directly. These modifications may be used in patients with pulmonary atresia with adequate-sized pulmonary arteries or certain cases of tricuspid atresia with ventricular septal defect.

group have demonstrated that homograft conduit survival at 9 years is projected to be 75% to 80%[71,72] Although the aortic wall calcifies with time, the leaflet tissue appears to remain resistant to the calcification process.[73,74] The dramatic increase in the development of organ donor programs for cardiac transplantation and multiple-organ procurement has permitted the opportunity to harvest greater numbers of homograft valves for use as conduits for right or left ventricular outflow tract reconstruction in children.

The disappointing results with the use of bioprosthetic valve-containing conduits in children have also been reflected in the problems of mechanical and bioprosthetic valve replacement in infants and children. Mechanical valves have been associated with high incidences of thromboembolism or thrombosis with or without chronic anticoagulation therapy.[68,75,76] In addition, anticoagulation therapy has been associated with significant complications of its own.[68]

The bioprosthetic heart valves were initially believed to be a marked improvement over mechanical prostheses, because chronic anticoagulation was not required. However, the rapid calcification of these valves in children, and therefore the need for frequent reoperation with its attendant operative risks, has resulted in the abandonment of tissue prosthetics in children except in isolated instances in the right side of the heart.[77–79] The calcification process and tissue destruction of the bioprosthetics appear to be somewhat less rapid in the tricuspid and pulmonic positions than in the left side of the

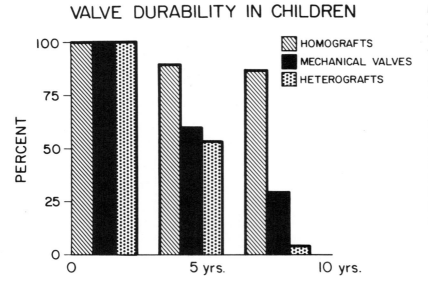

VALVE DURABILITY IN CHILDREN

HOMOGRAFTS
MECHANICAL VALVES
HETEROGRAFTS

FIG. 17–6. Estimated valve durability in children for various types of prosthetic valves. At 5 years, the homograft valves retain the greatest durability, which is maintained at approximately 10 years. Significant problems with mechanical valves occur primarily because of thromboembolism and thrombosis. The heterograft valves perform most poorly at 10 years following implantation because of calcification and degeneration.

heart.[80] Therefore, currently, mechanical prostheses are recommended for valve replacement in the left side of the heart and mechanical or biologic prostheses for tricuspid or pulmonic valve replacement.

In the future, the availability of aortic homografts may permit the use of unstented ("freehand") preserved aortic homograft-valve replacement for the aortic-valve position in greater numbers. Certainly data suggest that the long-term results with this type of material would be superior to either mechanical or heterograft bioprosthetic valves (Fig. 17–6). Unfortunately, attempts to mount antibiotic-treated homografts on stents for placement in the mitral or tricuspid position have been associated with high rates of structural failure, precluding their use in this position.[81]

HYPOPLASTIC LEFT-SIDED HEART SYNDROME

The hypoplastic left-sided heart syndrome, which consists of severe hypoplasia of the left ventricle with aortic or mitral atresia, atrial septal defect, and frequently coarctation of the aorta, has been particularly resistant to surgical approaches. The majority of infants with this syndrome are of normal birth weight and have few other associated abnormalities. Death usually occurs in the first few weeks of life because of progressive congestive heart failure. Palliative approaches to the therapy of these children have been developed by Norwood and others.[82,83] The Norwood procedure creates a single-ventricle physiology (morphologically a right ventricle). Blood exits the heart through a neoaorta created from the pulmonary artery and a large patch of material that is used to enlarge the ascending aorta and arch beyond any area of coarctation. The proximal ascending aorta then becomes functionally a common coronary artery. Pulmonary blood flow is maintained by a systemic-to-pulmonary shunt (Fig. 17–7). Modifications of the Norwood-type procedure include (1) use of a homograft connecting the pulmonary artery to the descending aorta, (2) shunts of Gore-Tex from the right ventricle or pulmonary artery to the distal pulmonary vessel or direct controlled 3-mm aortopulmonary connection, or (3) plica-

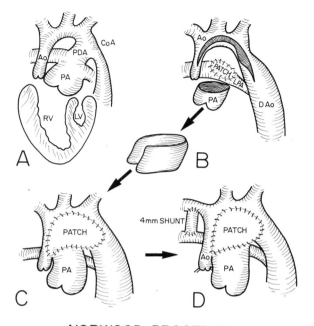

NORWOOD PROCEDURE

FIG. 17–7. Diagrammatic representation of the steps in the Norwood procedure for hypoplastic left-sided heart syndrome. **(A)** General anatomy of hypoplastic left ventricle, large pulmonary artery, and ductus arteriosus with associated coarctation of the aorta and extremely small, hypoplastic ascending aorta containing the coronary arteries. **(B)** Detachment of the proximal pulmonary artery from the confluence of the pulmonary vessels and closure of the defect with a patch of Gore-Tex or pericardium. A large incision is made in the underside of the aorta beyond any coarctation site. **(C)** A patch of Gore-Tex or pericardial material is also used to then connect the proximal pulmonary artery to the underside of the aortic arch. **(D)** Finally, a 4-mm Gore-Tex shunt is connected from the innominate artery to the right pulmonary artery to establish pulmonary blood flow.

tion of the right and left pulmonary artery orifices to maintain pulmonary blood flow while the main pulmonary artery is connected to the ascending aorta (Sade modification) (Fig. 17–8).[*,†,84–86]

At the present time, the survival rate for the initial palliative procedure in a few series approaches 50%.[‡,§] However, there appears to be significant interim mortality prior to the second stage of the repair, which consists of a Fontan-type operation connecting the right atrium directly to the pulmonary circuit and closure of the atrial septal defect and palliative systemic-to-pulmonary shunt (see Fig. 17–8). Only a few children have survived to successful completion of the second stage of the repair, and therefore long-term prognosis and functional results are unknown at this time, although pulmonary resistance in survivors of the first stage appears to return to normal.[88] However, the dismal results without surgical palliation and the progressively decreasing mortality from the first stage of repair in several centers suggests that some optimism is warranted.

The extremely poor prognosis in children with hypoplastic left ventricular syndrome and the initial high mortality with the other palliative procedures have encouraged Dr. Leonard Bailey to consider cross-species transplantation for some children with this problem. The initial transplantation of a baboon heart to an infant with hypoplastic left heart syndrome was successful until rejection intervened, possibly caused by blood transfusion incompatibility.[‖] Although this procedure can be considered only experimental at the present time, modifications of immunosuppression regimens and further re-

---

* Sade RM: Personal communication, 1985
† Jonas RA: Personal communication, 1985
‡ Jonas RA: Personal communication, 1985
§ Norwood WI: Personal communication, 1985
‖ Bailey L: Personal communication, 1985

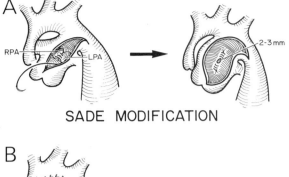

SADE MODIFICATION

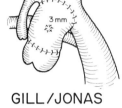

GILL/JONAS

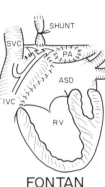

FONTAN

FIG. 17–8. Modifications of the Norwood procedure. **(A)** The Sade modification plicates the right **(RPA)** and left **(LPA)** pulmonary arteries, leaving a 2-mm to 3-mm opening into the main pulmonary vessel. **(B)** The Jonas modification uses a portion of prosthetic conduit or aortic homograft to connect the proximal pulmonary artery and arch of the aorta, and then a 3-mm opening is made between this homograft vessel and the confluence of the pulmonary arteries. **(C)** The final repair, which is completed at a later date for all of the initial palliative procedures, involves a Fontan operation connecting the inferior **(IVC)** and superior **(SVC)** vena cava directly by way of the atrial appendage **(ASD)** to the confluent pulmonary arteries **(PA) (open arrows).** A patch is placed in the atrium to baffle pulmonary venous blood into the right ventricle **(RV)**, and the Gore-Tex shunt is ligated.

search on interspecies transplantation may result in more enthusiasm for this approach. The extreme scarcity of donors for allogeneic heart transplantation in the neonatal age range makes it less likely as an initial treatment for these infants, despite the fact that it is a much more desirable alternative.

If palliative procedures, such as the Norwood procedure, can result in a low enough early and late mortality, they may prove to be satisfactory compromises to be followed by cardiac transplantation in later years.

CARDIOVASCULAR ASSIST DEVICES IN INFANTS AND CHILDREN

Although there has been much interest in assist devices for the circulation of adults, there have also been several recent advances in use of extracorporeal assist devices for support of neonates, infants, and children who have undergone cardiac procedures. Intra-aortic balloon pumping has been used in small series of patients in varying ages, sizes, and weights.[89,90] Commercially available small balloon catheters can now be obtained, and in situations of primary left ventricular dysfunction, they may result in some improvement. Nevertheless, the total experience is small and severe right ventricular dysfunction, which is the more common lesion in children, does not appear to be particularly responsive to intra-aortic balloon pumping.

Right ventricular assist devices, or pulmonary artery balloon counterpulsation, may offer greater cardiac support in infants with congenital heart disease, who often have primarily right ventricular dysfunction, but use of these modalities often presupposes a competent pulmonary valve—a situation that may be uncommon in children after repair of right ventricular lesions.[91,92]

Other forms of circulatory assist include intermittent compression of either the extremities or the abdomen for optimal systemic venous blood return to the pulmonary circuit in patients immediately following Fontan operations. Use of these devices has resulted in less ascites and pulmonary effusions and in improved left-sided hemodynamics immediately following operation.[93,98]

More complete circulatory assistance has been popularized by Bartlett with the use of prolonged

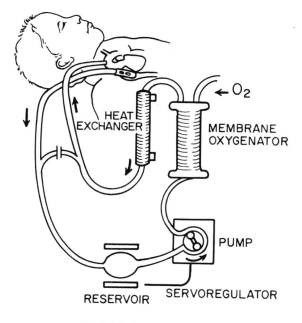

ECMO CIRCUIT

FIG. 17–9. *Diagrammatic representation of the extracorporeal membrane oxygenation (ECMO) circuit for neonates. Arterial cannulation is placed in the internal carotid artery and is positioned at the aortic arch; the venous cannulation through the internal jugular vein is positioned in the right atrium. Blood passes first through a reservoir and servoregulated pump, then through a membrane oxygenator and heat exchanger, and finally back into the arterial system, bypassing the lungs.*

extracorporeal membrane oxygenation (ECMO) for infants and children with reversible pulmonary insults, including meconium-aspiration syndrome and persistent fetal circulation.[95,96] In addition, the technology has been extended for use in patients with congenital diaphragmatic hernia and for right ventricular assistance following some cardiac procedures, such as cardiac transplantation with coexisting pulmonary hypertension, or right ventricular failure following tetralogy of Fallot repair.[97,98] In some patients with total anomalous pulmonary venous return, ECMO has maintained good perfusion up to and following surgery while the pulmonary vascular resistance drops. Using membrane oxygenators and a closed system with integral heat exchangers and reservoirs, infants can be maintained on extracorporeal oxygenation for several weeks (Fig. 17–9). As the number of survivors of this type of therapy increases, the indications for ECMO will probably be extended.

SUMMARY

Although cardiac surgery for reconstruction of congenital heart disease has reached a high level of sophistication, with markedly improving results in even the most complex anatomies, considerable room for improvement still exists. Most operations for congenital cardiac anomalies can result in a return to more normal physiology, but anatomical abnormalities remain. Often, cardiac structures are absent or extremely hypoplastic. Bioprosthetic materials and surgically created connections between chambers may become obstructive or alter physiologic flow in the developing child. The peculiar problems of size and the differences in pediatric cardiovascular physiology make reoperation much more common in the pediatric population. In addition, the relatively short postoperative experience with most major cardiovascular repairs means that the long-term functional results remain obscure. The greatest activity in pediatric cardiac surgery at the present time involves refinements and modifications of current techniques to allow for the most "normal" physiological and anatomical repair with the minimal possible use of prosthetics. With these modifications, an ever greater number of infants and children are reaching adulthood with adequate functional capabilities.

REFERENCES

1. Pellegrino A, Deverall PB, Anderson RH, et al: Aortic coarctation in the first three months of life. An anatomo-pathological study with respect to treatment. J Thorac Cardiovasc Surg 89:121, 1985
2. Rodbard S: Vascular modifications induced by flow. Am Heart J 51:926, 1956
3. Rudolph AM, Heymann MA, Spitzner U: Haemodynamic considerations in the development of narrowing of the aorta. Am J Cardiol 30:514, 1972
4. Weldon CS: Congenital obstruction to left ventricular outflow. In Ravitch M, Welch JK, Benson DC et al (eds): Pediatric Surgery, 3rd ed, vol 1, pp 633–649. Chicago, Year Book Medical Publishers, 1978
5. Nagao GI, Daoud GI, McAdams AJ et al: Cardiovascular anomalies associated with tetralogy of Fallot. Am J Cardiol 20:206, 1967
6. Becker AE, Becker MJ, Edwards JE: Anomalies associated with coarctation of the aorta: Particular reference to infancy. Circulation 41:1067, 1970
7. Bullaboy CA, Derkac WM, Johnson DH, Jennings RB, Jr: Tetralogy of Fallot and coarctation of the aorta: Successful repair in an infant. Ann Thorac Surg 38:400, 1984
8. Brom AG: Narrowing of the aortic isthmus and enlargement of the mind. J Thorac Cardiovasc Surg 50:166, 1965
9. Ho SY, Anderson RH: Coarctation, tubular hypoplasia and the ductus arteriosus. Histological study of 35 specimens. Br Heart J 41:268, 1979
10. Shinebourne EA, Elseed AM: Relation between fetal flow patterns, coarctation of the aorta and pulmonary blood flow. Br Heart J 36:498, 1974
11. Gross RE, Hufnagel CA: Coarctation of the aorta. Experimental studies regarding its surgical correction. N Engl J Med 233:287, 1945
12. Gross RE: Surgical correction for coarctation of the aorta. Surgery 18:673, 1945
13. Vosschulte K: Isthmusplastik Zur Behandlung der Aortenisthmusstenose. Thoraxchirurgie 4:443–450, 1957
14. Reul GJ, Kabbani SS, Sandiford FM et al: Repair of coarctation of the thoracic aorta by patch graft aortoplasty. J Thorac Cardiovasc Surg 68:696–704, 1974
15. Sade RM, Crawford FA, Hohn AR et al: Growth of the aorta after prosthetic patch aortoplasty for coarctation in infants. Ann Thorac Surg 38:21, 1984
16. Bergdahl L, Ljundqvist A: Long-term results after repair of coarctation of the aorta by patch grafting. J Thorac Cardiovasc Surg 80:177–181, 1980
17. Waldhausen JA, Nahrwold DL: Repair of coarctation of the aorta with a subclavian flap. J Thorac Cardiovasc Surg 51:532, 1966
18. Moulton AL, Brenner JI, Roberts G et al: Subclavian flap repair of coarctation of the aorta in neonates. Realization of growth potential. J Thorac Cardiovasc Surg 87:220, 1984
19. Myers JL, Waldhausen JA, Pae WE, Jr, et al: Vascular anastomosis in growing vessels: The use of absorbable sutures. Ann Thorac Surg 34:529, 1982
20. Penkoske PA, Williams WG, Olley PM et al: Subclavian arterioplasty. Repair of coarctation of the aorta in the first year of life. J Thorac Cardiovasc Surg 87:894, 1984
21. Kirklin JW, Barratt–Boyes BG: Coarctation of the aorta and aortic arch interruptions. In Kirklin JW, Barratt–Boyes BG: Cardiac Surgery, pp 1035–1080. New York, John Wiley & Sons, 1985
22. Hammon JW, Jr, Graham TP, Jr, Boucek RJ, Jr, et al: Repair of coarctation of the aorta in infants: Improved results with prostaglandin E$_1$ infusion and subclavian flap angioplasty. J Am Coll Cardiol 1:663, 1983
23. Pennington DG, Liberthson RR, Jacobs M et al: Critical review of experience with surgical repair of coarctation of the aorta. J Thorac Cardiovasc Surg 77:217–229, 1979
24. Beekman RH, Rocchini AP, Behrendt DM, Rosenthal A: Re-operation for coarctation of the aorta. Am J Cardiol 48:1108, 1981
25. Cobanoglu A, Teply JF, Grunkemeier GL et al: Coarctation of the aorta in patients younger than three months. A critique of the subclavian flap operation . J Thorac Cardiovasc Surg 89:128–135, 1985
26. Brown JW, Fiore AC, King H: Isthmus flap aortoplasty: An alternative to subclavian flap aortoplasty for long-segment coarctation of the aorta in infants. Ann Thorac Surg 40:274–279, 1985
27. Blalock A, Hanlon, CR: The surgical treatment of complete transposition of the aorta and pulmonary artery. Surg Gynecol Obstet 90:1, 1950
28. Rashkind WJ, Miller WW: Creation of an atrial septal

defect without thoracotomy: A palliative approach JAMA 196:991, 1966

29. Albert HM: Surgical correction of transposition of the great vessels. Surg Forum 5:74, 1954

30. Senning A: Surgical correction of transposition of the great vessels. Surgery 45:966, 1959

31. Mustard WT: Successful two-stage correction of transposition of the great vessels. Surgery 55:469, 1964

32. Quaegebeur JM, Rohmer J, Brom AG: Revival of the Senning operation in the treatment of transposition of the great arteries. Preliminary report on recent experience. Thorax 32:517, 1977

33. Pacifico AD: Concordant transposition: Senning operation. In Stark J, de Leval M (eds): Surgery for Congenital Heart Defects, pp 345–361. New York, Grune & Stratton, 1983

34. Marx GR, Hongen TJ, Norwood WI et al: Transposition of the great arteries with intact ventricular septum: Results of Mustard and Senning operations in 123 consecutive patients. J Am Coll Cardiol 1:476, 1983

35. Stark J, Silove ED, Taylor JF, Graham GR: Obstruction to systemic venous return following the Mustard operation for transposition of the great arteries. J Thorac Cardiovasc Surg 68:742, 1974

36. El-Said G, Rosenberg HS, Mullins CE et al: Dysrhythmias after Mustard's operation for transposition of the great arteries. Am J Cardiol 30:526, 1972

37. Jatene AD, Fontes VF, Paulista PP et al: Anatomic correction of transposition of the great vessels. J Thorac Cardiovasc Surg 72:364, 1976

38. Yacoub MH, Radley–Smith R, Maclaurin R: Two-stage operation for anatomical correction of transposition of the great arteries with intact ventricular spectum. Lancet 1:1275, 1977

39. Radley–Smith R, Yacoub MH: One stage anatomic correction of simple complete transposition of the great arteries in neonates. Br Heart J 51:685, 1984

40. Idriss FS, Albanic MN, DeLeon SY et al: Transposition of the great arteries with intact ventricular septum: Arterial switches in the first month of life (abstr). J Am Coll Cardiol 5:477, 1985.

41. Castaneda AR, Norwood WI, Jonas RA et al: Transposition of the great arteries and intact ventricular septum: Anatomical repair in the neonate. Ann Thorac Surg 28:438, 1984

42. Arensman FW, Bostock J, Radley–Smith R, Yacoub MH: Cardiac rhythm and conduction before and after anatomic correction of transposition of the great arteries. Am J Cardiol 52:836, 1983

43. Park SC, Neches WH, Mathews et al: Hemodynamic function after the Mustard operation for transposition of the great arteries. Am J Cardiol 51:1514, 1983

44. Castaneda AR, Freed MD, Williams RG, Norwood WI: Repair of tetralogy of Fallot in infancy. J Thorac Cardiovasc Surg 74:372, 1977

45. Kirklin JW, Westaby S, Chenoweth D et al: Complement and the damaging effects of cardiopulmonary bypass. J Thorac Cardiovasc Surg 86:845, 1983

46. Kirklin JW, Barratt–Boyes BG: Ventricular septal defect and pulmonary stenosis or atresia. In Kirklin JW, Barratt–Boyes BG: Cardiac Surgery pp 699–819. New York, John Wiley & Sons, 1985

47. Zhao, HX, Miller, DC, Reitz, BA, Shumway, NE: Surgical repair of tetralogy of Fallot. J Thorac Cardiovasc Surg 89:204, 1985.

48. Goldman BS, Mustard WT, Trusler GS: Total correction of tetralogy of Fallot. Br Heart J 30:563, 1968

49. Kirklin JW, Wallace RB, McGoon DC, DuShane JW: Early and late results after intracardiac repair of tetralogy of Fallot: 5-year review of 337 patients. Ann Surg 162:578, 1965

50. Blackstone EH, Kirklin JW, Bertranou EG et al: Preoperative prediction from cineangiograms of postrepair right ventricular pressure in tetralogy of Fallot. J Thorac Cardiovasc Surg 78:542, 1979

51. Graham TP, Cordell D, Atwood GF et al: Right ventricular volume characteristics before and after palliative and reparative operation in tetralogy of Fallot. Circulation 54:417–423, 1976

52. Bove EL, Byrum CJ, Thomas FD et al: The influence of pulmonary insufficiency on ventricular function following repair of tetraology of Fallot. Evaluation using radionuclide ventriculography. J Thorac Cardiovasc Surg 85:691–696, 1983

53. Hudspeth AS, Cordell AR, Johnston FR: Transatrial approach to total correction of tetraology of Fallot. Circulation 27:796–800, 1963

54. Edmunds LH, Saxena NC, Friedman S et al: Transatrial resection of the obstructed right ventricular infundibulum. Circulation 54:117–122, 1976

55. Binet JP, Patane L, Nottin R: Correction of tetralogy of Fallot by combined transatrial and pulmonary approach. Mod Probl Paediatr 22:152–156, 1963

56. Kawashima Y, Matsuda H, Hirose H, et al: Ninety consecutive operations for tetralogy of Fallot with or without minimal right ventriculotomy. J Thorac Cardiovasc Surg 90:856–863, 1985

57. Arciniegas E, Farooki ZQ, Hakimi M et al: Classic shunting operations for congenital cyanotic heart defects. J Thorac Cardiovasc Surg 84:88, 1982

58. de Leval MR, McKay R, Jones M et al: Modified Blalock–Taussig shunt. Use of subclavian artery orifice as flow regulator in prosthetic systemic-pulmonary artery shunts. J Thorac Cardiovasc Surg 81:112, 1981

59. Kay PH, Capuani A, Franks R, Lincoln C: Experience with the modified Blalock–Taussig operation using polytetrafluoroethylene (Impra) grafts. Br Heart J 49:359, 1983

60. Ben–Shachar G, Nicoloff DM, Edwards JE: Separation of neointima from Dacron graft causing obstruction: Case following Fontan procedure for tricuspid atresia. J Thorac Cardiovasc Surg 82:268–271, 1981

61. Agarwal KC, Edwards WD, Feldt RH et al: Clinicopathologic correlates of obstructed right-sided, porcine-valved, extracardiac conduits. J Thorac Cardiovasc Surg 81:591–601, 1981

62. Laks H, Williams WG, Hellenbrand WE et al: Results of right atrial to right ventricular and right atrial to pulmonary artery conduits for complex congenital heart disease. Ann Surg 192:382–389, 1980

63. Bjork VO, Olin CL, Bjarke BB, Thoren CA: Right atrial–right ventricular anastomosis for correction of tricuspid atresia. J Thorac Cardiovasc Surg 77:452–458, 1979

64. Doty DB, Marvin WJ, Laver RM: Modified Fontan procedure: Methods to achieve direct anastomosis of right atrium to pulmonary artery. J Thorac Cardiovasc Surg 81:470, 1981

65. Kreutzer G, Galindez E, Bono H et al: An operation for the correction of tricuspid atresia. J Thorac Cardiovasc Surg 66:613, 1973

66. Spicer RL, Behrendt D, Crowley DC et al: Repair of truncus arteriosus in neonates with the use of a valveless conduit. Circulation (Suppl I) 70:I–26, 1984

67. Ebert PA, Turley K, Stanger P et al: Surgical treatment of truncus arteriosus in the first six months of life. Ann Surg 200:451, 1984

68. Shore DF, de Leval MR, Stark J: Valve replacement in children: Biologic versus mechanical valves. In Cohn LH, Gallucci V (eds): Cardiac Bioprostheses, Chap 22, pp 239–247. New York, Yorke Medical Books, 1982

69. Williams DB, Danielson GK, McGoon DC et al: Porcine heterograft valve replacement in children. J Thorac Cardiovasc Surg 84:446–450, 1982

70. Miller DC, Stinson EB, Oyer PE et al: The durability of porcine xenograft valves and conduits in children. Circulation (Suppl I) 66:172–185, 1982

71. Fontan F, Choussat A, Deville C et al: Aortic valve homografts in the surgical treatment of complex cardiac malformations. J Thorac Cardiovasc Surg 87:649, 1984

72. di Carlo D, Stark J, Revignas A, de Leval MR: Conduits containing antibiotic-preserved homografts in the treatment of complex congenital heart defects. In Cohn LH, Gallucci V: Cardiac Bioprostheses, Chap 25, pp 259–265. New York, Yorke Medical Books, 1982

73. Saravalli OA, Sommerville J, Jefferson KE: Calcification of aortic homografts used for reconstruction of the right ventricular outflow tract. J Thorac Cardiovasc Surg 80:909–920, 1980

74. Moore CH, Martelli V, Ross DN: Reconstruction of right ventricular outflow tract with a valved conduit in 75 cases of congenital heart disease. J Thorac Cardiovasc Surg 71:11–19, 1976

75. Klint R, Hernandez A, Weldon C et al: Replacement of cardiac valves in children. J Pediatr 80:980–987, 1972

76. Sade RM, Ballenger JF, Hohn AR et al: Cardiac valve replacement in children: Comparison of tissue with mechanical prostheses. J Thorac Cardiovasc Surg 78:123–127, 1979

77. Wada J, Yokoyama M, Hashimoto A et al: Long-term followup of artificial valves in patients under 15 years old. Ann Thorac Surg 29:519–521, 1980

78. Silver MM, Pollock J, Silver MD et al: Calcification in porcine heterograft valves in children. Am J Cardiol 45:685–689, 1980

79. Geha AS, Laks H, Stansel HC, Jr, et al: Late failure of porcine valve heterografts in children. J Thorac Cardiovasc Surg 78:351–364, 1979

80. Dunn JM: Porcine valve durability in children. Ann Thorac Surg 32:357–368, 1981

81. Christie GW, Gavin JB, Barratt–Boyes BG: Graft detachment, a cause of incompetence in stent-mounted aortic valve allografts. J Thorac Cardiovasc Surg 90:901–907, 1985

82. Norwood WI, Lang P, Castaneda AR, Campbell DN: Experience with operations for hypoplastic left heart syndrome. J Thorac Cardiovasc Surg 82:511, 1981

83. Doty DB, Marvin WJ, Jr, Schicken RM, Lauer RM: Hypoplastic left heart syndrome: Successful palliation with a new operation. J Thorac Cardiovasc Surg 80:148, 1980

84. Behrendt DM, Rocchini A: An operation for the hypoplastic left heart syndrome: Preliminary report. Ann Thorac Surg 32:284, 1981

85. Mohri H, Horiuchi T, Haneda K et al: Surgical treatment of hypoplastic left heart syndrome. J Thorac Cardiovasc Surg 78:223, 1979

86. Norwood WI, Kirklin JK, Sanders SP: Hypoplastic left heart syndrome. Experience with palliative surgery. Am J Cardiol 45:87, 1980

87. Norwood WI, Lang P, Hansen D: Physiologic repair of aortic atresia–hypoplastic left heart syndrome. N Engl J Med 308:23, 1983

88. Lang P, Norwood WI: Hemodynamic assessment after

palliative surgery for hypoplastic left heart syndrome. Circulation 68:104, 1983

89. Pollock JC, Charlton MC, Williams WG et al: Intraaortic balloon pumping in children. Ann Thorac Surg 29:522–528, 1980

90. Veasy LG, Blalock RC, Orth JL, Boucek MM: Intra-aortic balloon pumping in infants and children. Circulation 68:1095–1100, 1983

91. Miller DC, Moreno–Cabral RJ, Stinson EB et al: Pulmonary artery balloon counterpulsation for acute right ventricular failure. J Thorac Cardiovasc Surg 80:760–763, 1980

92. Parr GVS, Pierce WS, Rosenberg G, Waldhausen JA: Right ventricular failure after repair of left ventricular aneurysm. J Thorac Cardiovasc Surg 80:79–84, 1980

93. Hecks HA, Doty DB: Assisted circulation by phasic external lower body compression. Circulation (Suppl II) 64:118–122, 1981

94. Laks H, Milliken JC, Perloff JK et al: Experience with the Fontan procedure. J Thorac Cardiovasc Surg 88:939–951, 1984

95. Bartlett RH, Gazzaniga AB: Extracorporeal circulation for cardiopulmonary failure. Current Probl in Surg 15:5, 1978

96. Bartlett RH, Andrews AF, Toomasian JM et al: Extracorporeal membrane oxygenation (ECMO) for newborn respiratory failure: 45 cases. Surgery 92:425–433, 1982

97. Hardesty RL, Griffith BP, Debski RF et al: Extracorporeal membrane oxygenation: Successful treatment of persistent fetal circulation following repair of congenital diaphragmatic hernia. J Thorac Cardiovasc Surg 81:556–563, 1981

98. Soeter JR, Mamiya RT, Sprague AY, McNamara JJ: Prolonged extracorporeal oxygenation for cardiorespiratory failure after tetralogy correction. J Thorac Cardiovasc Surg 66:214–218, 1973

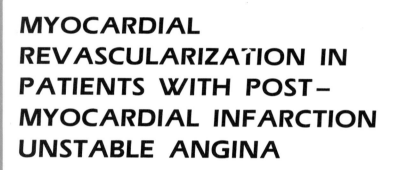

18

MYOCARDIAL REVASCULARIZATION IN PATIENTS WITH POST-MYOCARDIAL INFARCTION UNSTABLE ANGINA

John R. McCormick
Ahmad Rajaii Khorasani
Harold L. Lazar
Arthur J. Roberts

The term *unstable angina,* in a general sense, defines a clinical syndrome experienced by a very heterogeneous group of patients. A characteristic grouping of subsets is that employed in the coronary artery surgery study (CASS).[1] We tend to look to this study for information about the surgical management of coronary artery disease because of its large patient population and extensive clinical and angiographic data. Patients in CASS were characterized as having unstable angina if their chest pain fell into one or more of the following patterns: new onset, rest angina, acute coronary insufficiency, or changing pattern. Other authors have identified three subgroups of patients with unstable angina: progressive anginal pain of recent onset; anginal pain, at rest, of a sufficient intensity to warrant coronary care unit admission and to exclude an acute myocardial infarction; and pain after recovery from an acute myocardial infarction over a period starting immediately after or up until 3 months from the initial event.[2,3] Patients in the second subgroup in the three-group classification system are similar to patients with acute coronary insufficiency as defined in the CASS study. The patients in the first subgroup are similar to the other patients with unstable angina in CASS. There is no counterpart in CASS to the group of post–myocardial infarction unstable angina patients.

Many patients in this very heterogeneous population are not at a particularly high risk for acute myocardial infarction or death. To emphasize this point, CASS is again useful. For example, many patients enrolled in CASS, characterized as experiencing unstable angina, did not have angina during their admission for cardiac catheterization. Furthermore, many individuals who eventually underwent coronary artery bypass graft (CABG) surgery were discharged from the hospital and readmitted for elective operation.

The foregoing illustrations serve to highlight the difficulty of formulating a general plan of clinical management for patients with "unstable angina." Such arguments provide a rationale for limiting the scope of this chapter to a precisely definable subset of unstable angina patients. Thus, the focus in this chapter will be those patients with unstable angina during the early (<30-day) recovery period after an acute myocardial infarction. Our personal experience and that of our surgical colleagues leads us to believe that the post–myocardial infarction unstable angina patient is being seen with increasing frequency.[4] In addition, we and others feel that these patients represent the subset of unstable angina patients that are at the highest risk for recurrent myocardial infarction or death, and require the most aggressive medical and surgical management.[5-7]

PATHOPHYSIOLOGY

The mechanisms responsible for the clinical syndrome of unstable angina are not completely understood. Coronary spasm, thrombosis, increased coronary artery tone, circulating platelet aggregates, and prostaglandins may all be responsible for the clinical instability of patients experiencing unstable angina.[8-19] One study showed that post–myocardial infarction unstable angina patients have more extensive coronary artery disease than patients who do not experience unstable angina after an acute myocardial infarction.[20] Consideration of the above as possible causes of unstable angina forms the basis for the initial pharmacologic management of these patients. This management has been detailed in Chapter 23 and will not be reviewed in this chapter.

PROGNOSIS FOR POST–MYOCARDIAL INFARCTION UNSTABLE ANGINA WITHOUT MYOCARDIAL REVASCULARIZATION

It is important to know the frequency of occurrence of unstable angina after acute myocardial infarction, as well as the natural history of the disease in those patients who have not had myocardial revascularization. The particular circumstances of the acute myocardial infarction to be evaluated may include the following: (1) whether the infarction is transmural or subendocardial, (2) the status of underlying left ventricular function accompanying the acute event, and (3) whether the ischemia producing the unstable angina occurs at the site of the acute myocardial infarction or at a distance (*i.e.,* in the area of another coronary artery).[21]

Twelve percent of all patients experiencing an acute myocardial infarction can be expected to develop unstable angina within 7 days, and 25% within a 12-month interval.[22] The mortality of post–myocardial infarction unstable angina patients with medical treatment is not well known. An estimate from the information that is available indicates that the likelihood of death is within the range of 25% to 56% at a average interval of 6 months.[21-23]

Nontransmural myocardial infarction has been shown to have an increased likelihood of sudden death, death from all cardiac causes, and angina pectoris or recurring infarction when compared with transmural myocardial infarction.[7,14,24,25] Other authors have shown that patients who have infarct extension are at a higher risk for early and late mortality if the infarct extension is a nontransmural (non–Q wave) as opposed to a transmural (Q wave) associated infarction.[25,26] Patients with repetitive rest angina with marked anterior ST-segment elevation and mild increases in serum creatine kinase (CK)-MB enzymes may progress rapidly to massive myocardial infarction.[7] One investigation showed that early recurring myocardial infarction frequently occurred after subendocardial infarction and was associated with an increased mortality.[6] In another important study, Schuster and Bulkley showed that angina after recent myocardial infarction was associated with a 56% mortality at a 6-month interval.[21] The above data indicate that patients with unstable angina after myocardial infarction are at particularly high risk for mortality or other cardiac events and that the risk may be even higher if the myocardial infarction was subendocardial. Conventional medical therapy has not been particularly effective in the treatment of this subgroup of patients.

MANAGEMENT OF PATIENTS WITH POSTINFARCTION UNSTABLE ANGINA

The appearance of angina in the early post–myocardial infarction period, especially when it is associated with ST–T wave changes on the electrocardiogram (ECG) signifies a potentially serious complication of myocardial infarction.[6] Most such patients should be closely monitored in the coronary care unit (CCU). Careful observation of the duration and frequency of chest pain, the serial ECG changes, patterns of change in serial samples of serum CK-MB and invasive hemodynamic monitoring when necessary permit the identification of recurrent myocardial infarction with reasonable accuracy. However, the sensitivity and specificity of the diagnosis for anterior myocardial infarction is superior to that achieved in inferior wall infarction.[6] In addition, serial studies with radionuclide ventriculography have shown that in the presence of initial subendocardial myocardial infarction, recurrent infarction is usually not associated with the development of new Q waves. Furthermore, repeat radionuclide ventriculograms are helpful in documenting the site or extent of recurrent myocardial infarctions and subsequent changes in regional and global left ventricular function.[6] Several studies have shown that high-risk subsets of patients with post–myocardial infarction angina can be identified.[21] The modified exercise-tolerance test is an example of a reasonably predictive test that is used in patients whose condition is stable enough to undergo such physical stress.[27] The development of angina at a low exercise load, ST-segment depression, and inadequate blood pressure response are characteristic of a high-risk group for subsequent cardiac events or death. In patients who are too sick to undergo stress testing, persistent ST-segment alterations, rest pain, and ventricular tachycardia have been identified as factors associated with a poor prognosis.[28] It has been suggested that since the advent of aggressive medical therapy for patients with acute myocardial infarction, the extent of myocardium infarcted has been reduced, compared with earlier periods when more conventional medical therapy was instituted. Consequently, following this reasoning, a greater portion of the myocardium that is at risk for subsequent myocardial infarction will probably remain viable. This is a major explanation for the increasing incidence of post–myocardial infarction angina in the CABG surgery population.

Medical therapy includes adequate sedation, oxygenation, and psychological reassurance. For persistent myocardial ischemia, morphine and intravenous nitroglycerin are important forms of therapy.[29,30] In addition, beta blockers and calcium channel blockers are warranted when clinically indicated.[31,32] Some investigators would argue that intravenous heparin therapy and/or platelet antagonists may also play a beneficial role in the treatment of unstable post–myocardial infarction angina. If the measures described previously are unsuccessful in controlling recurring myocardial ischemia, the intra-aortic balloon pump (IABP) should be inserted, when possible, using the percutaneous insertion technique.[33–36] In our experience, an inability to insert the balloon pump is relatively uncommon. However, in certain cases, the peripheral arterial circulation may not allow the insertion of the balloon pump and emergency catheterization and urgent myocardial revascularization must be considered. Prompt relief of chest pain is seen in approximately 98% of patients with unstable angina, 82% of patients with postinfarction angina, and 88% of patients with slowly evolving myocardial infarction.[37]

The timing of cardiac catheterization and consideration for myocardial revascularization remain controversial. In patients who become clinically stable with medical treatment that does not include IABP, catheterization and revascularization may proceed more slowly. In patients who have refractory myocardial ischemia despite IABP, cardiac catheterization should be undertaken at an early time and myocardial revascularization should follow within a few days of the delineation of cardiac anatomy. At the present time, myocardial revascularization may be achieved by either percutaneous transluminal coronary angioplasty or CABG. The choice of the particular form of myocardial revascularization depends on the particular cardiac anatomy and the relative availability and expertise of the cardiac angiography and cardiac surgery teams.

In our experience, however, the majority of patients with post–myocardial infarction unstable angina tend to have diffuse coronary artery disease. Consequently, more often than not CABG surgery is indicated for these patients. The surgical approach to unstable patients with post–myocardial infarction angina is not unlike that used for any patient having elective CABG surgery. The factors that are associated with an increased operative mortality in the subgroup of patients with postinfarction angina include advanced age coupled with significant depression in left ventricular function (ejection fraction [EF] < 30%) and the clinical syndromes of cardiogenic shock or recurrent ventricular tachycardia — fibrillation. In the operating room, particular attention is given to myocardial protection and an expeditious operation. Because it is quicker to use the saphenous vein of the leg as a bypass conduit than to dissect the internal mammary artery from the chest wall, unstable patients, for the most part, receive saphenous vein bypass grafts. However, if the patient is stable hemodynamically at the time of surgery, we feel that either single or bilateral internal mammary artery implants should be included in the surgical revascularization plan.

RESULTS OF SURGICAL TREATMENT

We are aware of 15 reports, including our own, that relate specifically to CABG surgery in patients with postinfarction angina receiving operations within approximately 60 days of the initial myocardial infarction[4,5,38–50] (Table 18–1). The timing of such operations is determined chiefly by the severity of clinical symptomatology and the particular selection preferences existing at a given institution. Approximately 1300 patients are represented in the combined clinical experience illustrated in Table 18-1. The sample size in each report varies from 17 to 280 patients. The

use of IABP preoperatively ranged from near 0% to 100%. Mean EF preoperatively fluctuated between 34% and 55%, and mean preoperative left ventricular end-diastolic pressure (LVEDP) varied from 18 mm Hg to 25 mm Hg. The operative mortality for postinfarction angina ranged from 0% to 31% with a mean value of nearly 7%. Perioperative myocardial infarction rate varied from 1% to 15% with a mean of 6%. Late death rates were approximately 2% per year, but in the reported experience, the follow-up period was limited to 1 to 3 years. In terms of early postoperative changes in left ventricular function, Roberts and colleagues reported that patients with preoperative subendocardial myocardial infarction show an increase in EF postoperatively, which is similar to that observed in patients without any recent preoperative myocardial infarction.[45] However, patients with preoperative transmural myocardial infarction showed an early decrease in EF and no later increase in EF postoperatively. Despite these postoperative changes in left ventricular function, there does not appear to be a difference in operative mortality between groups of patients with preoperative subendocardial or transmural myocardial infarction when the subgroup with cardiogenic shock is excluded.

In our clinical experience, we have observed that operative mortality in patients with post–myocardial infarction angina can be divided temporally into two groups; those patients operated on less than 30 days after myocardial infarction and those operated on more than 30 days after the acute event (Table 18–2). However, in patients operated on less than 30 days after myocardial infarction, there appear to be two somewhat distinct clinical subgroups. These groups can be differentiated by the presence or absence of certain high-risk factors. Those patients with high-risk factors might be expected to have an operative mortality between 10% and 20% whereas those patients without such factors have a 3% to 5% projected mortality. Those patients

TABLE 18–1
POST–MYOCARDIAL INFARCTION ANGINA: PATIENTS RECEIVING CABG SURGERY WITHIN 60 DAYS

Report	No. of Cases	Duration Post–MI (Days)	IABP Usage (%)	LV Function EF	LV Function Mean EDP	Operative Mortality (%)	Perioperative MI (%)	Late Death (%)	Follow-up (Months)
1. Dawson (1974) Texas Heart Institute	145	0–60	—	—	—	14.5	—	—	—
	76	0–30				31			
2. Bardet (1977) Ambroise Hospital (Paris)	17	2–15	100	42	18	5.8	5.8	0	18
3. Levine (1978) MGH (Boston)	80	0–30	72	—	—	8.8	2.5	1.4	32
4. Brundage (1980) University of San Francisco	22	0–30	5	50	20	9	14	9	33
5. Jones (1981) Emory University	116	1–30	3.4	55	18	0	5	4.4	18
6. Fudge (1982) Methodist Hospital (Memphis)	280	0–60	2.5	50	—	1	—	3.5	39
	60	0–30							
7. Roberts (1983) Northwestern (Chicago)	20	2–28	56	47	18	0	15	0	12
8. Nunley (1983) University of Oregon	80	1–14	2.5	48	—	5	2.5	—	33
9. Molina (1983) University of Minnesota	38	0–14	32	34	25	10.5	—	5.2	36
10. Williams (1983) University of Washington	103	0–30	7	50	16	1.9	1	1	15
11. Baumgartner (1984) Johns Hopkins	34	1–30	41	52	—	9	15	3.5	14
12. Hochberg (1984) Beth Israel (New Jersey)	174	1–48	25	41	—	16	—	4	24
13. Rankin (1984) Duke University	52	0–30	21	45	—	3.8	3.8	8	24
14. Breyer (1985) Baystate Hospital (Massachusetts)	75	0–30	39	53	18	8	—	0	13
15. McCormick (1986) Boston University	50	1–30	100	50	21	4	4	2	13

TABLE 18–2
OPERATIVE MORTALITY IN PATIENTS WITH POST–MYOCARDIAL INFARCTION ANGINA

Post–MI Angina CABG Surgery (Days)	Risk	Operative Mortality (%)
<30	High risk	10–20
<30	Low risk	5
≥30	Low risk	5

operated on more than 30 days after acute infarction are in a low-risk group, with mortality approximating the mortality found among elective CABG surgery groups (2%).

Factors that define "high risk" in patients undergoing early surgery after myocardial infarction are shown in Table 18–3. They include cardiogenic shock, reinfarction during clinical observation, and the combination of depressed EF (<30%) coupled with age greater than 70 years. We have found the following clinical findings, which are not associated with independent predictive value, related to early surgical outcome (Table 18-3). They include the need for IABP, the level of preoperative EF alone, and the time from initial acute myocardial infarction to CABG surgery.

OPERATIVE MORTALITY

A number of authors have published reports about the operative mortality of the surgical treatment of post–myocardial infarction unstable angina pectoris. In part, the large variability in reported series relates to patient selection within the spectrum of patients with post–myocardial infarction angina. Baumgartner and colleagues, at Johns Hopkins Hospital showed an operative mortality of 9% in a study containing 34 patients.[47] Levine and associates, at the Massachusetts General Hospital, published their report on a series of 80 patients with an operative mortality of 8.8%.[40] Jones and associates from the Emory University group reported no deaths in 116 patients.[42] Williams and colleagues, from the University of Washington, had 1.9% operative mortality in a group of 103 patients.[5] Breyer and associates, in a recent publication from Baystate Medical Center, had an operative mortality of 8% with 75 operative patients.[4] Hochberg and coworkers, from the Beth Israel Hospital in Newark, New Jersey, had 27 deaths in 147 patients, with an operative mortality of 18%.[48] Molina and colleagues, in a smaller series, had a 10.5% operative mortality in 30 patients.[46] Conversely, Rahimtoola, reporting on the overall approach to several subgroups of patients with unstable preinfarction angina in the *New England Journal of Medicine,* reported a 1.8% mortality.[3]

Thus, there seems to be little doubt that coronary artery bypass grafting can be accomplished in post–infarction angina patients with a reasonable operative mortality. Indeed, nearly one half of the reported series state that the operative mortality for this subgroup is no different than it would be for coronary artery bypass grafting in a

TABLE 18–3
POST–MYOCARDIAL INFARCTION ANGINA: FACTORS RELATED TO OUTCOME OF CABG SURGERY

High-Risk Factors	Factors Not Independently Predictive of Outcome
Operation < 30 days (relative)	Need for IABP
Cardiogenic shock	Level of EF alone
Reinfarction and depressed EF (<30%)	Length of time from MI to
Age > 70 years and operation <30 days	surgery

population of patients with stable angina. Nevertheless, about half of the investigators also show an increased operative mortality in the 8% to 10% range, which is higher than would be expected in surgery for chronic stable angina.

ROLE OF PERCUTANEOUS TRANSLUMINAL CORONARY ANGIOPLASTY (PTCA) IN POSTINFARCTION ANGINA

In recent years some patients with unstable anginal syndrome have been treated by thrombolysis and/or PTCA.[51,52] The initial approach to such patients with postinfarction angina is medical stabilization. If these patients cannot be relieved of chest pain, early cardiac catheterization is indicated. If the coronary artery obstructions are amenable to thrombolysis (within a few hours of infarction) or PTCA, these measures may be attempted. If the coronary anatomy is unfavorable for such therapeutic catheterization laboratory techniques or if such attempts fail, CABG surgery should be used for patients with postinfarction angina.[4,53] Regardless of the treatment modality employed, the long-term results are better with "complete" revascularization. The appearance of the contrast ventriculogram has also been reported as an important indicator of subsequent myocardial viability and, consequently, as a factor in the choice of therapeutic modality.[53] At the present time, there are no prospective, randomized studies comparing the available means for myocardial revascularization. Until further information about the early and late consequences of such treatment plans is available, it appears that PTCA will be increasingly performed for anatomically suitable patients. However, our experience suggests that the majority of refractory postinfarction angina patients have diffuse, multivessel coronary disease, and, therefore, CABG surgery will remain the most common initial treatment modality for these patients.

CONCLUSION

Patients with postinfarction unstable angina are at a high risk for infarct extension, serious ventricular arrhythmia, and death. Consequently, an aggressive management policy is necessary to minimize life-threatening sequelae and to maximize left ventricular function. Initial management requires careful observation in the CCU. Intensive medical therapy, including IABP when necessary, should be used to attain medical stabilization. Early delineation of the coronary artery anatomy and the level of ventricular function should be obtained by cardiac catheterization. Serial assessment of left ventricular function by radionuclide ventriculography may be helpful, especially when contrast ventriculography is deemed risky because of the clinical circumstances. The appropriate choice of therapy for refractory cases and the optimal timing for such therapeutic interventions remains uncertain. Our bias favors very early and aggressive intervention. If PTCA is technically possible, such a procedure is indicated, because the initial experience has been promising and PTCA is relatively less invasive as well as inexpensive compared with CABG surgery. If PTCA is unsuccessful, urgent CABG surgery is necessary. If PTCA is not possible, early CABG surgery should be employed. The operative mortality for patients with postinfarction angina is relatively high compared with that of patients who have elective CABG surgery, and certain subgroups with this disease complex are among the most difficult management problems in CABG surgery. In this patient group, medical management alone is associated with a poor prognosis, even with recent advances in medical therapy. There are relatively few reports of long-term survival (>3 years) after PTCA and/or CABG surgery for postinfarction angina. Consequently, the clinical impact of these treatment modalities remains to be clarified. Our bias is that long-term survival in this relatively high-risk group of patients is less than that observed for patients with chronic stable angina following myocardial infarction.

REFERENCES

1. McCormick JR, Schick EC, McCabe CH et al: Determinants of operative mortality and long-term survival in patients with unstable angina. The CASS experience. J Thorac Cardiovasc Surg 89:683–688, 1985
2. Rahimtoola SH: Coronary bypass surgery for unstable angina. Circulation 69:842–848, 1984
3. Rahimtoola SH, Nunley D, Grunkemeier G et al: Ten year survival after coronary bypass surgery for unstable angina. N Engl J Med 308:676–681, 1983
4. Breyer RH, Engleman RM, Rousou JA, Lemeshaw S: Post infarction angina: An expanding subset of patients undergoing coronary artery bypass. J Thorac Cardiovasc Surg 90:532–540, 1985
5. Williams DB, Ivey TD, Bailey WW et al: Post infarction angina: Results of early revascularization. J Am Coll Cardiol 2:859–864, 1985
6. Marmor A, Sobel B, Roberts R: Factors presaging early recurrent myocardial infarction (extension). Am J Cardiol 49:603–610, 1981
7. Madigian NP, Rutherford BO, Frye RL: The clinical course, early prognosis and coronary anatomy of subendocardial infarction. Am J Med 60:634, 1976
8. Rahimtoola SH: Unstable angina: Current status. Modern concept of cardiovascular disease. JAMA 54:19–23, 1985
9. Maseri A, L'Abbate, Baroldi G et al: Coronary vasospasm as a possible cause of myocardial infarction: A conclusion derived from the study of "Preinfarction" angina. N Engl J Med 299:1271–1277, 1978
10. Maseri A, Severi S, Denes M et al: Variant angina. One aspect of the continuous spectrum of vasospastic myocardial ischemia: Pathogenic mechanisms, estimated incidence and clinical and coronary arteriographic findings in 138 patients. Am J Cardiol 42:1010–1035, 1978
11. Dunn RE, Kelly OT, Sadick N, Wren R: Multi-vessel coronary artery spasm. Circulation 60:451–455, 1979
12. Mautner R, Kanade A, Phillips J: Coronary artery spasm in patients with unstable angina pectoris. South Med J 71(6):729–732, 1978
13. Robertson RM, Robertson D, Friesinger GC: Platelet aggregate in peripheral and coronary sinus blood in patients with spontaneous coronary artery spasm. Lancet 2:829, 1980
14. Mehta J, Mehta P, Pepine CJ: Platelet aggregation in aortic and coronary venous blood in patients with and without coronary disease: III. Role of tachycardia, stress and propanolol. Circulation 58:881, 1978
15. Mehta P, Mehta J, Pepine CJ: Platelet aggregation across the myocardial vascular bed in man: Normal versus diseased coronary arteries. Thromb Res 14:623, 1979
16. Telford A, Wilson C: Trial of heparin versus atenolol in prevention of myocardial infarction in intermediate coronary syndrome. Lancet 1:1225–1228, 1981
17. Folts JD, Crowell EB Jr, Rowe CG: Platelet aggregation in partially obstructed vessels and its elimination with aspirin. Circulation 54:365–370, 1976
18. Lewis HD Jr, Davis JW, Archibald GD et al: Protective effects of aspirin against acute myocardial infarction and death in men with unstable angina: Results of a Veterans Administration cooperative study. N Engl J Med 309:396–403, 1983
19. Stone PH, Muller JE: Nifedipine therapy for recurrent ischemic pain following myocardial infarction. Clin Cardiol, 5:223–230, 1982
20. Schuster EH, Bulkley BH: Ischemia at a distance after acute myocardial infarction. A case of early post infarction angina. Circulation 62:509–515, 1980
21. Schuster EH, Bulkley BH: Early post infarction angina. Ischemia at a distance and ischemia in the infarct zone. New Engl J Med 305:1101–1105, 1981
22. Moss AJ, DeCamilla J, David H et al: The early posthospital phase of myocardial infarction: Prognostic stratification. Circulation 54:58, 1976
23. McQuay NW, Edwards JE, Burchell HB: Type of death in acute myocardial infarction. Arch Intern Med 96:1–10, 1955
24. Hutter AM Jr, Desanctis RW, Flynn T et al: Nontransmural myocardial infarction. A comparison of hospital and late clinical course of patients with that of matched patients with transmural anterior and transmural inferior myocardial infarction. Am J Cardiol 48:595–602, 1981
25. Piffare R, Spinazzola A, Wemickas R et al: Emergency aortocoronary bypass for acute MI. Arch Surg 103:535–538, 1971
26. Maisel AS, Ahnve S, Gilpin E et al: Prognosis after extension of myocardial infarction: The role of Q-wave or non–Q-wave infarction. Circulation 71:211–217, 1985
27. Starling MR, Crowford MH, Kennedy GT, O'Rourke RA: Exercise testing early after myocardial infarction: Predictive value for subsequent unstable angina and death. Am J Cardiol 46(6):909–914, 1980
28. Johnson SM, Mauritson DR, Winniford MD et al: Continuous electrocardiographic monitoring in patients with unstable angina pectoris: Identification of high-risk subgroups with severe coronary disease, variant angina and/or impaired early prognosis. Am Heart J 103(1):4–12, 1982

29. Roubin GS, Harris PJ, Eckhardt I et al: Intravenous nitroglycerine in refractory unstable angina pectoris. Aust NZ J Med 12(6):598–602, 1982

30. Hakki AH, Spielman SR, Segal BL: Intravenous nitroglycerine for rest angina. Potential pathophysiologic mechanisms of action. Arch Intern Med 142(10)1806–1809, 1982

31. Mehta J, Conti CR: Verapamil therapy for unstable angina pectoris: Review of double blind placebo-controlled randomized clinical traits. Am J Cardiol 50(4):919–922, 1982

32. Stone PH, Muller JE: Nifedipine therapy for recurrent ischemic pain following myocardial infarction. Clin Cardiol 5:223–230, 1982

33. Williams DO, Korr KS, Gewirtz H, Most AS: The effect of intra-aortic balloon counterpulsation on regional myocardial blood flow and oxygen consumption in the presence of coronary artery stenosis in patients with unstable angina. J Am Coll Cardiol 2:859–864, 1983

34. Gold HK, Leinbach RC, Buckley MJ et al: Refractory angina pectoris follow-up after intra-aortic balloon pumping and surgery. Circulation (Suppl 3) 54(6):41–46, 1976

35. Aroesty JM, Weintraub RM, Paulin S, O'Grady GP: Medically refractory unstable angina pectoris. II. Hemodynamic and angiographic effects of intra-aortic balloon counterpulsation. Am J Cardiol 43:883–887, 1979

36. Weintraub RM, Aroesty JM, Paulin S et al: Medically refractory unstable angina pectoris: Long-term follow-up of patients undergoing IABP counterpulsation. Am J Cardiol 43(5):877–882, 1979

37. Michels R, Kint PP, Hagemeijer F et al: Intra aortic balloon pumping in coronary artery disease. Herz 4(5):397–409, 1979

38. Dawson JT, Hall RJ, Hallman GL, Cooley DA: Mortality in patients undergoing coronary artery bypass surgery after myocardial infarction. Am J Cardiol 33:483–486, 1979

39. Bardet J, Rigaud M, Kahn JC et al: Treatment of post-myocardial infarction angina by intra-aortic balloon pumping and emergency revascularization. J Thorac Cardiovasc Surg 74:299–306, 1977

40. Levine FH, Gold HK, Leinbach RC et al: Safe early revascularization for continuing ischemia after acute myocardial infarction. Circulation (Suppl I) 60:1–9, 1979

41. Brundage BH, Ullyot DJ, Winokur S et al: The role of aortic balloon pumping in post infarction angina: A different perspective. Circulation (Suppl I) 62:1–123, 1980

42. Jones EL, Waites TF, Craver JM et al: Coronary bypass for relief of persistent pain following acute myocardial infarction. Ann Thorac Surg 32:33–43, 1981

43. Fudge TL, Harrington OB, Crosby VG et al: Coronary artery bypass after recent myocardial infarction. Arch Surg 117:1418–1420, 1982

44. Roberts AJ, Sanders JH Jr, Moran JH et al: The efficiency of medical stabilization prior to myocardial revascularization in early refractory postinfarction angina. Ann Surg 197:91–97, 1983

45. Nunley DL, Grunkemeier GL, Teply JF et al: Coronary bypass operation following acute complicated myocardial infarction. J Thorac Cardiovasc Surg 85:485–491, 1983

46. Molina JE, Dorsey JS, Emanuel DA, Reyes J: Coronary bypass operation for early postinfarction angina. Surg Gynecol Obstet 157:455–460, 1983

47. Baumgartner WA, Borkon AM, Zibulewsky J et al: Operative intervention for postinfarction angina. Ann Thorac Surg 38:265–267, 1984

48. Hochberg MS, Parsonnet V, Gielchinsky I et al: Timing of coronary revascularization after acute myocardial infarction. Early and late results in patients revascularized within seven weeks. J Thorac Cardiovasc Surg 88:914–921, 1984

49. Rankin JS, Newton, JR Jr, Califf RM et al: Clinical characteristics and current management of medically refractory unstable angina. Ann Surg 200:457–465, 1984

50. McCormick JR, Khorasani AR, Lazar HL et al: Current therapy for post infarction angina pectoris. Manuscript in preparation.

51. Meyer J, Erbel R, Schmitz HJ et al: Transluminal angioplasty—unstable angina fresh infarct. Z Kardiol (Suppl 2) 73:167–176, 1984

52. Faxon DP, Detre KM, McCabe CH et al: Role of percutaneous transluminal coronary angioplasty in the treatment of unstable angina. Report from the National Heart, Lung, and Blood Institute. Percutaneous transluminal coronary angioplasty and coronary artery surgery study registries. Am J Cardiol 53(12):131C–135C, 1984

53. Phillips SJ, Zeff RH, Skinner JR et al: Reperfusion protocol and results in 738 patients with evolving myocardial infarction. Ann Thorac Surg 41:119–125, 1986

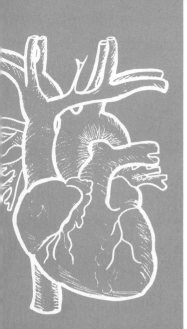

19

SURGERY IN EVOLVING ACUTE MYOCARDIAL INFARCTION

Steven J. Phillips

Emergency surgical reperfusion during an evolving myocardial infarction is an intervention that is directed toward the primary mechanical obstructive process affecting a coronary artery.[1-11] Reperfusion is not appropriate for all patients with myocardial infarction, but timely reperfusion in selected patients can inhibit infarct evolution and can reduce or reverse myocardial injury.[12-18] This review describes a 10-year experience with emergency reperfusion in patients with acute evolving myocardial infarction and emphasizes surgical reperfusion. Analysis of our patients has allowed us to recommend clinical criteria to select patients who should undergo emergency coronary angiography, which can predict those patients who would benefit from emergency reperfusion.

METHODS

Our treatment plan for acute evolving myocardial infarction parallels that used for acute trauma. An all-encompassing educational program aimed toward public, paramedical, and medical personnel has evolved over the past 10 years. This program urges rapid transport of patients with evolving myocardial infarction to a hospital equipped for reperfusion. Readily available transport includes land, rotary-wing, or fixed-wing vehicles. Trained paramedical personnel accompany the patient and are in radiotelephone contact with the hospital. A physical environment has been created wherein the emergency room, cardiac catheterization laboratories, and operating rooms are adjacent to each other. Cardiac catheterization and reperfusion modalities are available 24 hours a day, 7 days a week. Patients with evolving myocardial infarction have immediate catheterization priority over patients scheduled for elective procedures. One of our three cardiac operating rooms is available 24 hours a day for emergency cardiac surgery. Patients who are scheduled for elective catheterization or surgery are aware of a potential delay or cancellation if an emergency occurs. Our operating room contains all the appropriate equipment needed for cardiac surgery, including a mini-laboratory. Instruments and drapes are prepackaged and positioned, unopened, in the operating room. This system eliminates most of the delays associated with operating room preparation and patient transport. Patients are transported directly from the cardiac catheterization laboratory to the operating room, which can be readied within 15 minutes from the time of request. An intra-aortic balloon pump and percutaneous cardiopulmonary bypass are available for use in the emergency room or cardiac catheterization laboratory if necessary.[19]

The cardiologist functions as the triage physician. A patient who exhibits signs and symptoms of an evolving myocardial infarction or post–myocardial infarction angina undergoes cardiac catheterization. Once catheterization is performed, then the patient is triaged to standard coronary care or reperfusion (Fig. 19–1). The choice for reperfusion depends on the catheteri-

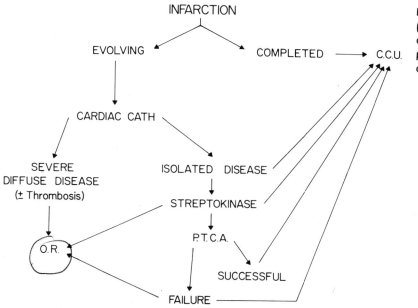

INFARCTION

EVOLVING   COMPLETED ———→ C.C.U.

CARDIAC CATH

SEVERE
DIFFUSE DISEASE   ISOLATED DISEASE
(± Thrombosis)

STREPTOKINASE

O.R.   P.T.C.A.

SUCCESSFUL

FAILURE

FIG. 19–1. Triage protocol. (**O.R.,** operating room; **C.C.U.,** coronary care unit; **P.T.C.A.,** percutaneous transluminal coronary angioplasty)

zation findings, which indicate whether or not the myocardial region affected shows potential for recovery.

CORONARY CARE UNIT THERAPY

Conventional coronary care unit therapy is applied to patients whose endocardial architecture on ventriculography shows no potential for recovery. The criteria for choosing these patients will be described below. In addition, patients who are unconscious or have noncardiac contraindications for reperfusion (malignancy, and so forth) are usually treated by conventional therapy.

REPERFUSION TECHNIQUES

The method of reperfusion depends on the catheterization findings. Until 1979 all patients with evolving myocardial infarction were treated by surgical reperfusion. Since 1979 patients with

angiographically proven single-vessel disease are usually managed with intracoronary streptokinase and/or angioplasty. Patients with evolving myocardial infarction who have multiple-vessel disease undergo emergency coronary revascularization because it is believed that multiple angioplastic dilatations in the evolving infarction are inappropriate.

The surgical techniques utilized have been described previously and are similar to those used for elective surgery.[4,6,7,11,20,21] In past years, the bypasses have been limited to the use of the saphenous vein. However, more recently, the internal mammary artery has been used. The internal mammary artery is prepared on bypass. In general, the proximal anastomoses to the aorta are carried out first, followed by sequential distal anastomosis. Thrombectomy of the affected artery is usually attempted (Fig. 19–2). The heart is arrested utilizing cold potassium cardioplegia with an attempt to maintain the myocardial temperature at approximately 5°C to 10°C.[21]

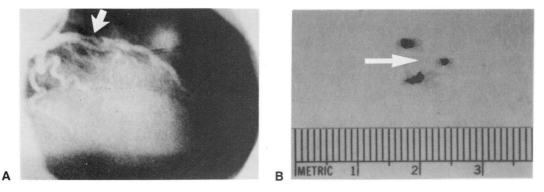

FIG. 19–2. (A) Right anterior oblique view of left anterior descending coronary artery with a filling defect **(arrow)**. **(B)** Large arrow indicates clot removed from the artery at surgery.

PATIENT PROFILE

From June 1975 until January 1985, 863 patients had emergency cardiac catheterization during the evolving phase of myocardial infarction. There were 699 males whose ages ranged from 39 to 85 years with an average of 59.8 years, and 164 females whose ages ranged from 36 to 81 years with an average of 62.3 years. Chest pain was the major indicator of evolution. As long as clinical evidence of evolution persisted, time from the onset of chest pain, the hemodynamic state, and the electrocardiographic presence of Q waves were not considered contraindications for catheterization. Cardiac catheterization with multiple views was performed by way of the groin, utilizing systemic heparinization. Coronary anatomy was defined by direct injection of dye into the coronary arteries and ventricular function by direct ventriculography. Fifty percent, or 432 patients, had primarily single-vessel disease. Thirty percent, or 259 patients, had double-vessel disease, and 172, or 20 percent of the total patient group, had triple-vessel disease. The location of the evolving infarct on patients with single-vessel disease was equal in anterior and inferior location. Those with multiple-vessel dis-

ease showed a slight predominance for anterior over inferior.

Of the 863 patients studied, 717 were treated by reperfusion, and 146 patients were treated by conventional coronary care unit therapy. Three hundred ninety-one patients had emergency surgical reperfusion. Two hundred thirty-seven patients were reperfused surgically as the treatment of choice. The remaining 154 patients who were operated on included 76 patients who received streptokinase in an unsuccessful attempt to reperfuse them in the catheterization laboratory, and 78 patients with catastrophic coronary artery closure who were reperfused during elective percutaneous transluminal coronary angioplasty (PTCA). Not included were hemodynamically stable patients whose elective angioplasty failed and who eventually had surgery.

RESULTS

MORTALITY

There were 22 deaths (5.4%) among the 391 patients who were reperfused surgically. Further analysis revealed that the 237 patients who, by first choice, were reperfused surgically contained 9 deaths (3.9%). Among 76 patients in whom reperfusion in the catheterization laboratory failed and who crossed over to surgical reperfusion, there were 9 deaths (12%). Among 78 patients who had catastrophic hemodynamic instability during elective coronary angioplasty, there were 4 deaths (5%). Fourteen deaths (4.2%) occurred in the 326 patients reperfused in the catheterization laboratory. The group of 146 patients who were studied but not reperfused contained 25 deaths (17%) (Table 19–1).

Overall, patients who had unstable hemodynamics and who could not be reperfused had an 85% mortality compared with similar patients who were reperfused (11% mortality). Patients who had stable hemodynamics but were not reperfused had a 6.8% mortality, compared with a 1.8% mortality in those patients who were reperfused. Thus the group of 717 patients who were reperfused by any technique contained 36 deaths (4.9%), as compared with the 25 deaths (17%) in the 146 patients who were not reperfused.

FACTORS INFLUENCING WALL MOTION RECOVERY

Endocardial Anatomy. All patients exhibited wall motion abnormalities in the area of absent or reduced flow. Restudy of the patients who demonstrated a predominantly smooth and finely trabeculated endocardium (normal) in the area of ischemia revealed improved function of that wall after reperfusion (Fig. 19–3). The majority of these patients also demonstrated some flow to the infarct area either by way of collaterals or antegrade through a stenotic vessel. Those patients whose nonmoving endocardial surface appeared irregular with a loss of normal trabeculation or contained filling defects (endocardial

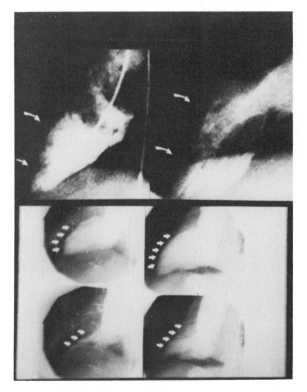

FIG. 19-3. (Top Frames) Systole pre-reperfusion **(right)** and postreperfusion **(left)** with streptokinase into the left anterior descending coronary artery. **(Bottom Frames)** Presystole **(right)** and postsystole **(left)** and diastole of surgical reperfusion of the left anterior descending coronary artery. Reperfusion allowed recovery of regional wall motion. (**Arrows** indicate a ''normal''-appearing endocardial surface.)

TABLE 19–1
MORTALITY RATES IN 832 PATIENTS

Reperfused	No. of Patients	Mortality
Not reperfused	146	25 (17%)
Totally reperfused	717	36 (4.9%)
PTCA/SK	326	14 (4.2%)
Surgical (failed catheterization laboratory)	76	9 (12%)
Failed PTCA	78	4 (5%)
Primary surgical	237	9 (3.9%)

PTCA, percutaneous transluminal coronary angioplasty; SK, streptokinase

edema or clot) did not generally demonstrate improvement in wall motion (Fig. 19–4). The majority of these patients exhibited no flow to the region of ischemia either by collaterals or through the myocardial infarction artery.

Time. No correlation with time and regional myocardial salvage could be made in patients who exhibited blood flow either by way of collaterals or antegrade to a myocardial infarction wall that showed "normal" endocardial architecture on the pre-reperfusion ventriculogram. Time to reperfusion in these patients averaged 8 hours, with a range from 1 to 36 hours. If no flow to the myocardial infarction wall was present, the cutoff time for wall motion improvement was 4 hours or less. In this group of patients, angiographic abnormalities (mottled, fuzzy surface) predominated after 4 hours from the onset of symptoms, and less than 10% of these patients exhibited wall motion improvement (Fig. 19–4).

Choice of Reperfusion Technique. Prior to 1979 all patients with evolving myocardial infarction were reperfused surgically. These patients included those with single- and multiple-vessel disease and the above-mentioned mortality of patients primarily treated surgically was 3.9%. After 1979 streptokinase and angioplasty became available in our hospital, and reperfusion in the catheterization laboratory was initially attempted in 549 of the 863 patients. Reperfusion was achieved in 326 (60%) of these patients (4.2% mortality), most of whom had single-vessel disease. Reperfusion in the catheterization laboratory was unsuccessful in the residual 222 patients, who had predominantly multiple-vessel disease. Seventy-six of patients with evolving myocardial infarction had emergency surgical reperfusion (11% mortality) because their endocardial anatomy indicated good potential for recovery. Seventy-eight additional patients had emergency surgery following failed coronary angioplasty. Thus, 391 patients (35%) were reperfused surgically. The remaining 146 (20%) patients, who were not reperfused, were treated conventionally (17% mortality). Our review demonstrates that patients with multiple-vessel disease had a high incidence of failed reperfusion in the catheterization laboratory. We recommend

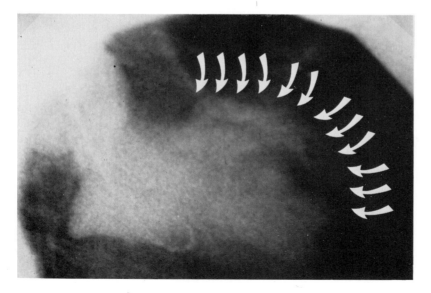

FIG. 19-4. Note the abnormal endocardial surface with associated filling defects **(arrows),** which may represent clot formation and/or endocardial edema.

TABLE 19–2
TECHNIQUES AND RESULTS OF REPERFUSION

No. of Patients	No. of Vessels	Catheterization Laboratory/Deaths	Operating Room/Deaths
48	Single	40/1 (2.5%)	8/0
117	Multiple	16* (5/0)	101/3 (3%)
			11/3† (36%)

* Eleven of sixteen patients (69%) with multiple-vessel disease could not be completely reperfused with multiple-vessel dilatations in the catheterization laboratory.
† These 11 "surgically delayed" patients were reperfused in the operating room, with 3 deaths.

that patients with evolving myocardial infarction and multiple-vessel disease have immediate surgery and that techniques for reperfusion in the catheterization laboratory be reserved for patients with predominantly single-vessel disease (Table 19–2).

Patients receiving streptokinase prior to surgery had a higher incidence of postoperative bleeding than those who did not receive streptokinase. This was not a contraindication to surgery; however, these patients required an average of 8.5 units of blood compared with the 1.5 units required for those who had elective surgery.[22] Hemodynamic studies in a subgroup of patients showed general improvement, with the most improvement occurring in patients who had unstable hemodynamics (Table 19–3). Long-term follow-up is summarized in Table 19–4.

DISCUSSION

The treatment protocol is based on the philosophy of using our facilities as a "cardiac trauma center." Transport to the hospital utilizes monitored land or air vehicles with high-level paramedical and medical support. Transport vehicles have the ability to communicate with the hospital, to monitor cardiac rhythm and hemodynamics, to defibrillate, to utilize drugs, and, if needed, to transport the patient with an intraaortic balloon pump in place. The cardiologist functions as the triage physician and determines the therapeutic regimen to be utilized on the basis of the findings at cardiac catheterization. Reperfusion is a therapy, and the technique for reperfusion is determined by catheterization findings. As with any therapy, successful reperfusion depends on appropriate patient selection.

TABLE 19–3
HEMODYNAMIC DATA: PRE- VERSUS POSTREPERFUSION (10 DAYS) IN 165 PATIENTS

	Pre-reperfusion	Post-reperfusion	% Change	P
EF (%)	40 ± 9	51 ± 11	+22	0.05
LVEDP (mm Hg)	22 ± 8	13 ± 4	−41	0.01
SV (cc)	71 ± 19	93 ± 15	+24	0.05
ESV (cc)	141 ± 41	97 ± 17	−31	0.05
EDV (cc)	212 ± 63	186 ± 71	−12	0.1

EF, ejection fraction; LVEDP, left ventricular end diastolic pressure; SV, stroke volume; ESV, end systolic volume; EDV, end diastolic volume

TABLE 19–4
MORBIDITY IN 404 PATIENTS FOLLOWED 1–9
YEARS POSTREPERFUSION (MEAN 3.5 YEARS)

Measure	Morbidity
Treadmill	76%—normal (308 patients)
	10%—abnormal (42 patients)
Chest pain	7% (26 patients)
Disabled	7% (28 patients)

The experiences of our group, Berg, and others, suggest that rapid and complete myocardial reperfusion in appropriately selected patients is associated with the lowest morbidity and mortality for evolving myocardial infarction.[3–18,22–28] Those patients described above, in whom reperfusion was attempted but failed, revert to the statistical category of morbidity and mortality equivalent to that of standard myocardial infarction therapy.[29]

Our data indicate that the most effective method for reperfusing patients with multiple-vessel disease is surgical. Most mortalities occurred in patients with multiple-vessel disease whose definitive therapy was attempted in the catheterization laboratory (multiple vessel dilatations) but failed (Table 19–2).

Pre-reperfusion angiography can often predict whether the regional wall motion abnormality associated with the evolving myocardial infarction will improve. We have noted that if the nonmoving endocardial surface in the area of hypoperfusion has a normal appearance (smooth and finely trabeculated), as opposed to mottled and fuzzy, which indicates endocardial edema and/or clot formation, then recovery can be expected.[30,31] This favorable appearance is usually associated with collateral or antegrade blood flow.

In general, the elapse of time could not be used to predict a beneficial outcome with reperfusion. Those patients who were 4 hours or more from the onset of symptoms and had no residual or collateral blood flow to the area of myocardial infarction generally demonstrated unfavorable endocardial anatomy and had a poor result with reperfusion. When a favorable-appearing endocardial surface was associated with residual or collateral blood flow to that area, then the length of time from the onset of symptoms to reperfusion could not be correlated with myocardial salvage. Thus, the decision of whether to reperfuse should not be based on time, but rather on endocardial anatomy and its potential for recovery.

In summary, a "cardiac trauma center" should manage evolving myocardial infarction. The cardiologist is the triage physician. Triage to conventional therapy or reperfusion should be based on clinical findings. If clinical symptoms of evolution persist, most specifically pain, emergency cardiac catheterization should be performed, and time from the onset of chest pain should not influence this decision. The findings at catheterization should then be used to predict the potential for myocardial salvage as well as to indicate the best reperfusion technique.

Single-vessel disease usually can be managed successfully in the catheterization laboratory; multiple-vessel disease should be treated with immediate surgery. Reperfusion therapy is not beneficial to those patients whose endocardial architecture in the myocardial infarction area has deteriorated to a mottled, irregular appearance. The protocol described previously (Fig. 19-1) combined with the criteria to predict regional wall salvage appears to be superior to conventional therapy for evolving myocardial infarction.

REFERENCES

1. Pifarré R, Spinazzola A, Nemickas R et al: Emergency aortocoronary bypass for acute myocardial infarction. Arch Surg 103:525–528, 1971
2. Keon J, Bedard P, Shankar KR et al: Experience with emergency aortocoronary bypass grafts in the presence

of acute myocardial infarction. Circulation 48(3):151–155, 1973

3. Berg R, Jr, Kendall RW, Duvosin GE et al: Acute myocardial infarction, a surgical emergency. J Thorac Cardiovasc Surg 70:432–437, 1975

4. Phillips SJ, Kongtahworn C, Zeff RH et al: Emergency coronary artery revascularization: A possible therapy for acute myocardial infarction. Circulation 60:241–246, 1979

5. DeWood MA, Spores J, Notske RN et al: Medical and surgical management of acute myocardial infarction. Am J Cardiol 44:1356–1364, 1979

6. Phillips SJ, Zeff RH, Kongtahworn C et al: Surgery for evolving myocardial infarction. JAMA 248(11):1325–1328, 1982

7. Phillips SJ, Kongtahworn C, Skinner JR, Zeff RH: Emergency coronary artery reperfusion: A choice therapy for evolving myocardial infarction. J Thorac Cardiovasc Surg 86(5):679–688, 1983

8. Zeff RH, Phillips SJ: The case for early direct myocardial reperfusion. Int. J Cardiol 4:99–103, 1983

9. Selinger SL, Berg R, Leonard J et al: Surgical treatment of acute evolving anterior myocardial infarction. Circulation 64(2), 1981

10. Berg R, Selinger SL, Leonard JJ et al: Immediate coronary artery bypass for acute evolving myocardial infarction. J Thorac Cardiovasc Surg 81:493, 1981

11. Phillips SJ: Role of surgery in evolving acute infarction: Indications and special aspects of technique. In Surgery of Coronary Artery Disease. London, Chapman & Hall Limited (in press)

12. Markis JE, Malagold M, Parker JA et al: Myocardial salvage after intracoronary thrombolysis with streptokinase in acute myocardial infarction. Assessment by intracoronary thallium-201. N Engl J Med 305:77–78, 1981

13. Reduto LA, Freund GC, Gaeta JM et al: Coronary artery reperfusion in acute myocardial infarction: Beneficial effects of intracoronary streptokinase on left ventricular salvage and performance. Am Heart J 102:1168, 1981

14. Mathey DG, Rodewalk G, Rentrop P et al: Intracoronary streptokinase thrombolytic recanalization and subsequent surgical bypass of remaining atherosclerotic stenosis in acute myocardial infarction. Complementary combined approach effecting reduced infarct size, preventing reinfarction, and improving left ventricular function. Am Heart J 102:1194–1201, 1981

15. Markis JE, Malagold M, Parker A et al: Myocardial salvage after intracoronary thrombolysis with streptokinase in acute myocardial infarction. N Engl J Med 305:777, 1981

16. Maddahi J, Ganz W, Ninomiya K et al. Myocardial salvage by intracoronary thrombolysis in evolving acute myocardial infarction: Evaluation using intracoronary injection of thallium-201. Am Heart J 102:664, 1982

17. Ludbrook PA, Geltman EM, Tiefenbrunn AJ et al: Restoration of regional myocardial metabolism by coronary thrombolysis in patients. Circulation 68(III):325, 1983

18. Sobel BE, Geltman EM, Tiefenbrunn AJ et al: Improvement of regional myocardial metabolism after coronary thrombolysis induced with tissue-type plasminogen. Basic Res Cardiol 78:210, 1983

19. Phillips SJ: Percutaneous cardiopulmonary bypass and innovations in clinical counterpulsation. In Critical Care Clinics. Philadelphia, WB Saunders (in press)

20. Okies JE, Phillips SJ, Crenshaw R, Starr A: "No-vent" technique of coronary artery bypass. Ann Thorac Surg 70(4):696, 1975

21. Phillips SJ, Zeff RH, Kongtahworn C et al: Anoxic hypothermic cardioplegia compared to intermittent anoxic fibrillatory cardiac arrest: Clinical and metabolic experience with 1080 cases. Ann Surg (190)1:80–83, 1979

22. Skinner JR, Phillips SJ, Zeff RH, Kongtahworn C: Immediate coronary bypass following failed streptokinase infusion in evolving myocardial infarction. J Thorac Cardiovasc Surg 87(4):567–570, 1984

23. Mathey D, Kuck KH, Tilsner V et al: Nonsurgical coronary artery recanalization in patients with acute myocardial infarction. Circulation 63:489–497, 1981

24. Meyer J, Merx W, Schmitz H et al: Percutaneous transluminal coronary angioplasty immediately after intracoronary streptolysis of transmural myocardial infarction. Circulation 66:905, 1982

25. Krebber JH, Mathey D, Schofer J, Rodewald G: Indication for early aorto-coronary bypass surgery after successful intracoronary lysis. J. Thorac Cardiovasc Surg 31:50–53, 1983

26. Anderson JL, Marshall HW, Bray BE et al: A randomized trial of intracoronary streptokinase in the treatment of acute myocardial infarction. N Engl J Med 3308:1312, 1983

27. European Cooperative Study Group: Streptokinase in acute myocardial infarction. N Engl J Med 301:797, 1979

28. Mathey DG, Rodewald G, Rentrop P et al: Intracoronary streptokinase thrombolytic recanalization and subsequent surgical bypass of remaining atherosclerotic stenosis in acute myocardial infarction: Complementary combined approach effecting reduced infarct size, preventing reinfarction and improving left ventricular function. Am Heart J 1194–1201, 1981

29. Corday E, Corday SR: Advanced clinical management of acute myocardial infarction in the past twenty-five years. J Am Coll Cardiol 1:126–132, 1983

30. Haendchen RV, Corday E, Torres M et al: Increased end-diastolic wall thickness after reperfusion: A sign of irreversibly damaged myocardium. J Am Coll Cardiol 3(6):1444–1453, 1984

31. Weinreich DJ, Burke JF, Pauletto FJ: Left ventricular mural thrombi complicating acute myocardial infarction. Long-term follow-up with serial echocardiography. Ann Int Med 100:789, 1984

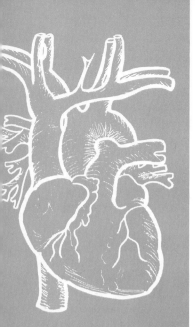

20

CARDIAC PACING:
PAST, PRESENT,
AND FUTURE

Paul A. Levine

The first fully implantable permanent pacemaker was placed in humans in 1958. This first device lasted approximately 3 hours, at which time it failed and had to be replaced.[1] Since that inauspicious beginning, major advances have occurred in biomedical engineering, in our understanding of pathophysiology, and in our ability to both diagnose and treat a multiplicity of rhythm disorders utilizing electrical stimulation techniques. Control of bradyarrhythmias remains a major objective of cardiac pacing. However, there is an increasing utilization of pacing techniques to control a number of tachyarrhythmias. Although some might argue that implantable devices capable of automatic cardioversion or defibrillation of life-threatening arrhythmias do not fall within the realm of cardiac pacing, they do fall within the broad spectrum of implantable electrical devices used to treat symptomatic cardiac rhythm disorders. This chapter will review the history of pacing with regard to technologic advances, clinical application of pacing technology for the control of bradycardias and tachycardias, and the future directions of this field.

TECHNOLOGICAL ADVANCES

In approximately one quarter of a century, pacing systems have progressed through several iterations, rendering them smaller, more durable, more versatile, and more reliable.[2,3] Advances in microelectronics and battery technology have resulted in a significant reduction in both their overall size and weight, while greatly increas-ing their functional life. The early fixed-rate, nonprogrammable, discrete-component devices powered by mercury – zinc oxide batteries had an expected longevity of only 2, possibly 3, years. Weighing 120 g to 150 g and having a thickness of 20 mm to 25 mm, complications such as erosion and local discomfort occurred because of size alone. The electronics were less than reliable, resulting in premature component failure. The implantation of the device required a major thoracotomy to fix the leads directly on the epicardial surface of the heart, resulting in significant disease and even death. As such, the indications for permanent pacing were extremely stringent, with these first units being recommended only to patients who could not survive without them. Thus the risk : benefit calculations still favored the patient.

Currently, pacemakers are powered by a variety of lithium salts, which can be hermetically sealed to protect them against the incursion of body fluids. Depending on the capacity of the battery and the reduced current drain secondary to improvements in circuit technology, present-generation pacemakers can be reasonably expected to function properly for 5 to 10 years following implantation.[4] Advances in electronics utilizing complementary metal oxide semiconductor (CMOS) and large-scale integration (LSI) technology have facilitated the development of more versatile and complex systems that allow for the noninvasive adjustment of multiple parameters, and dual-chamber and antitachycardia pacing. This has been achieved in a package that is considerably smaller than the older yet simpler units. Present-generation pacemakers weigh between 40 g and 80 g and vary from 6 mm to 15 mm in thickness (Fig. 20–1). Despite their increased complexity, these pacemakers are more reliable than earlier units because each integrated circuit, while doing the work equivalent to thousands of discrete components, has the statistical reliability of a single component.[5]

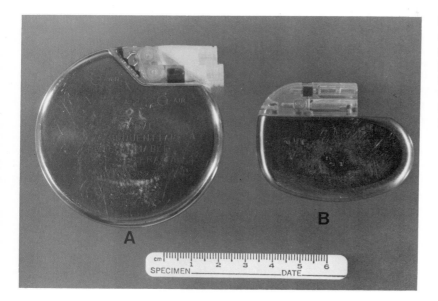

FIG. 20–1. Side-by-side comparison of **(A)** early generation and **(B)** present generation dual-chamber pacemakers from the same manufacturer. The two panels show different views of each pacemaker.

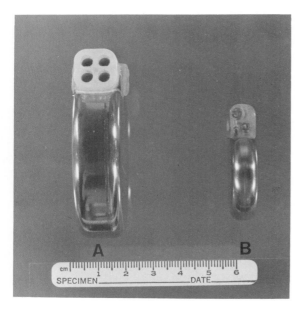

Previous problems associated with implantation, erosion, and patient acceptance have markedly decreased. Combining this with increases in our understanding of cardiac electrophysiology and hemodynamics and with the development of devices that can more closely restore the normal cardiac physiology, there has been an increase in the use of cardiac pacing as a major therapeutic modality.

The pulse generator, or pacemaker, is but one of three components of the pacing system. Although it is the most complex of the two man-made portions, it is totally ineffective without both the lead electrode and the heart itself. Changes in the lead, which is the insulated electrical conductor that connects the pulse generator to the electrode, have also been dramatic advances.[6,7] The first leads were simply single strands of wire covered by an insulating sheath. Repetitive contraction and relaxation of the heart as well as body motion led to a high incidence of conductor fracture, necessitating repeat operative intervention. This was a formidable procedure because it required a repeat thoracotomy. Initially, coiling of a single conductor followed by coiling of multiple conductor strands markedly enhanced the flexibility of the lead, reducing the incidence of fracture to its present level of less than 1% per year. Development of permanent leads that can be inserted transvenously enables the entire procedure to be performed under local anesthesia and avoids the need for thoracotomy.

Similar to the first pacemakers, the first transvenous leads were large and bulky, often requiring placement through an external or even internal jugular vein. There was also a 20% incidence of early lead dislodgement. The addition of Silastic, and more recently of polyurethane projections, just proximal to the electrode, facilitated passive fixation among the trabeculae in the right ventricle and, more recently, in the right atrial appendage. A variety of active fixation elements, including fixed or retractable screws, enable the use of endocardial leads in patients with large dilated right ventricles and/or atria without an atrial appendage. Improvements in insulation material have resulted in a reduction in the cross-sectional diameter of the leads, allowing two leads to be placed through veins that are too small to allow placement of a single early-generation lead.

Advances have also occurred in the electrode.[8-10] The electrode is the exposed metal that makes actual contact with the heart muscle, and it is connected to the pulse generator by way of the conductor coil within the lead. The first electrodes were large and thus required a larger amount of delivered energy to reach the critical threshold level. Capture threshold is a function of current density; by reducing the electrode surface area, one could achieve the critical current density with a smaller delivered energy level, thus reducing the drain on the battery and increasing pulse-generator longevity. Evaluation of a number of different electrode materials and configurations has led to a reduction in both polarization at the electrode–myocardial interface and in the fibrotic growth that usually surrounds the electrode. This combined reduction results in a lower chronic capture threshold, allowing for a further reduction in pacemaker output while still maintaining an adequate margin for consistent stimulation.

Much of the progress in cardiac pacing would not have been realized had it not been for major advances in battery, circuit, lead, and electrode technology.

PROGRAMMABILITY

With pacing systems presently capable of functioning properly for 5 and possibly 10 years and even longer without an intervening surgical procedure, the ability to program or to noninvasively adjust the functional parameters of the pacing system becomes extremely important.[11,14] The majority of pacemakers commercially available in 1985 have some degree of programmability. The North American Society of Pacing and Electrophysiology (NASPE) has officially stated that programmability is mandatory in modern pacemaker practice for patient safety as well as for reducing the need for secondary interventions.[15]

A pacemaker is a limited device. Based on design specifications and while it is functioning normally, it does exactly what the engineers designed it to do—no more, no less, despite any changes in the patient's clinical condition that may render the original parameters less than optimal. Programmability allows the physician to adjust one or more of the pacemaker's parameters to fit the pacemaker better to the patient, much as a physician might titrate the dose of a medication. Rate, output, sensitivity, pacing mode, and refractory period are only some of the aspects of the "dose" of pacing that may need to be altered to achieve optimal cardiac function within the limits imposed by the underlying disease process. Disease is an evolving process; hence, a nonprogrammable pacemaker, while initially appropriate and beneficial to a given patient, may become counterproductive as the disease evolves. The nuclear-powered pulse generators, with a predicted longevity of 50 years, are generally nonprogrammable and have not gained wide acceptance for this reason.

Prior to the availability of programmable pacemakers, a patient had to "live with" a less than optimal system, utilizing medication to compensate for any deficiencies in the pacing system, or he had to undergo another operative procedure. Only those patients who were markedly compromised by inappropriate parameters were subjected to replacement of their otherwise normally functioning pulse generator. Replacement of the pacemaker was no guarantee that the specifications of the new unit would remain appropriate for the patient. Changing the pacemaker was the

equivalent of clinical experimentation, and like any experiment, carried no guarantee of success. While multiparameter programmability will not solve all of the potential problems associated with pacing, it will solve (and has solved) many of them. It has facilitated the diagnostic evaluation of pacing-system malfunctions and has permitted the titration of pacing parameters to obtain optimum therapeutic benefit from a given pacing system for a specific patient. Some of the parameters that are currently capable of being programmed are detailed in Table 20–1.

The ability to program multiple parameters carries with it two potentially serious problems. The first is that the physician will program the pacemaker to settings that are inappropriate or unsafe for the patient. Thus it is imperative that the physician be knowledgeable about both the utility and limitation of these devices. The second problem is that a given set of parameters will be misinterpreted as a malfunction and the patient will be subjected to an unnecessary surgical procedure with replacement of a normally function-

TABLE 20–1
PROGRAMMABLE PARAMETERS IN IMPLANTED PACEMAKERS

Rate
    Demand or lower rate limit
    Maximum tracking rate
    Fallback rate
    Hysteresis escape rate
Output (on atrial or ventricular channel)
    Pulse amplitude
      Current
      Voltage
    Pulse duration
Sensitivity (on atrial or ventricular channel)
Refractory period (on atrial or ventricular channel)
Atrioventricular delay interval
Blanking period
Mode
Upper rate behavior
Lead polarity

ing device. Although all patients are given an identification card, many fail to carry it. In addition, a physician's records may not be immediately available, or changes in the pacemaker parameters instituted by one physician may not have been communicated to all the other individuals involved in the patient's care. Our patients are progressively more mobile, traveling for vacation as well as making permanent moves, and physicians who have no knowledge of the patients' prior history may become involved in their care. There must be a system by which the pacemaker can inform the physician about its programmed settings. A communication system termed "bidirectional telemetry and interrogation" allows the pacemaker not only to respond to a command from the programmer and to confirm the appropriate response to that command, but to also be "interrogated" about its programmed setting.[16] In some units, indices of battery and electrode function may also be assessed in this manner. This will help to clarify potential problems when a patient is seen in follow-up, particularly when he is seen by a physician other than the original monitoring or implanting physician. Is a given rate within specification or does it signify a device failure? Is the failure to sense a native signal caused by a pacemaker failure or was the pacemaker sensitivity merely set inappropriately, or is their an insulation defect on the lead? The ability to "question" the pacemaker about its programmed settings, to know exactly how the pacemaker is set when the patient is seen in follow-up and to identify a potential abnormality are essential to ensure safe and appropriate use of these sophisticated devices.

The increased longevity of the pacemakers being used today adds another wrinkle to the management of the pacemaker patient. How frequently and by what manner should patients receive follow-up care? When pacemakers were powered by mercury–zinc oxide batteries and expected to last only 2 and possibly 3 years, weekly transtelephonic follow-up beginning approximately 18 months after implantation was both safe and efficient, allowing one to obtain the maximum use of the pacemaker while maintaining patient safety. In this way, the frequency of operative interventions was reduced, thus helping to control overall medical costs. The recommended replacement time indicator of the early-generation pacemakers was a 10% reduction in the present or programmed rate, a relatively easy parameter to follow by transtelephonic monitoring techniques. In lithium-powered devices, which are capable of extensive programmability, a rate change remains only one of the recommended replacement time indicators.

If replacement does not occur for 10 years, weekly follow-up beginning at 2 years is excessive and unnecessary. Program mode, rate, output, and even the stimulation impedance on the electrode itself all affect the current drain and, hence, pulse-generator longevity. In addition, all lithium chemistries are not identical, so when should more frequent evaluation begin in a given patient? A number of systems now permit the direct measurement of the battery status and current drain out of the pacemaker by telemetry systems, making pacemaker follow-up analogous to the observation of a fuel gauge in an automobile. When a lithium–iodine battery is fully charged, it will have a low internal resistance. If this can be determined, only infrequent follow-up is required for assessment of battery status. Based on the rate of change of the battery resistance and the current drain, which might be assessed every 6 to 12 months initially, the follow-up schedule can be modified as the battery resistance rises, because this would indicate that the amount of available energy is falling and more frequent evaluations would then be appropriate. Waiting for the rate to change is analogous to watching the indicator lights in the automobile; when they flash, the car is already in trouble. When the rate change has already occurred, an emergency may be imminent. Following battery resistance and current drain of the pacemaker is equivalent to observing the fuel gauge of a car. As the fuel level decreases, a more diligent search for a service station is necessary to avoid running out of gasoline at an inopportune moment. As the resistance rises, more frequent evaluations of the pacing system become warranted so that a medical emergency may be avoided, and in this manner, the need for prophylactic replacement of the device may be eliminated.[17] Other factors, including the degree of pacemaker dependency, the track record of a given device, and the general medical status of the patient, all play a role in determining the frequency of the follow-up schedule.

Many of the same units that permit the noninvasive determination of battery status also permit the assessment of electrode function by measurement of the stimulation impedance. A normal impedance is determined by the conductor, the size of the electrode, and tissue reaction and polarization effects at the electrode–myocardial interface. Normal values range between 300 and 1000 ohms. A rise in the impedance signals a conductor fracture, whereas a fall in the impedance, when compared with the baseline measurement, heralds a defect in the insulation material. Both of these defects will interfere with the normal operation of the pacing system and may cause premature failure of the pulse generator itself. Neither of these problems, however, will be corrected by simple replacement of the pulse generator, and thus their preoperative identification is essential. Because pacemaker manufacturers have made quantum strides in the reliability and longevity of their devices, these units have become more complex, and the physicians' knowledge must become more sophisticated to ensure not only the proper function of

the device but also that its program settings remain appropriate for the patient.

PHYSIOLOGIC PACING

As the reliability, longevity, and ease of insertion of pacemakers has increased, so have the indications for pacing therapy. Whereas the early units were only implanted in a life-and-death situation associated with cardiac standstill, there is now a growing utilization of pacing in patients with marked sinus bradycardia, drug-induced bradyarrhythmias, the bradycardia–tachycardia syndrome, and intermittent second- and third-degree atrioventricular (AV) block. These conditions often do not manifest total asystole or syncope. In some cases, prophylactic pacing is employed after an acute myocardial infarction complicated by transient heart block. With the increased utilization of pacing, more patients are being identified in whom normally functioning ventricular pacing systems induce both adverse arrhythmias and hemodynamic states, all of which are generally classified under the diagnosis of "the pacemaker syndrome."[18,19] These include reentrant tachyarrhythmias from retrograde activation of the atrium and AV node, low cardiac output secondary to loss of appropriate AV asynchrony, development of overt congestive heart failure, and even syncope. All of these may accompany "normal" ventricular pacing. In this case, normal simply means that the device is functioning in the way that it is designed to function.

Returning to the original indications for pacing, chronic complete heart block and high-grade asystole, the increase in ventricular rate alone both prevents the patients' syncopal spells, improves cardiac output, and even increases longevity. Studies performed on patients with stable complete heart block demonstrated that the optimal rise in cardiac output at rest was achieved at a mean ventricular pace rate of 70 to 80 pulses per minute, although individual patients would vary from this, given one of the early indications for rate programmability. Because as pacemakers were implanted in patients with sick sinus syndrome or intermittent heart block, and in some cases prophylactically, ventricular pacing at 70 pulses per minute resulted in periods of pacing when pacing was not clearly required. This precipitated symptoms of weakness and fatigue that resulted from low cardiac output, edema and dyspnea from congestive heart failure, and occasionally even syncope, all due to the loss of appropriate AV synchrony. High pulmonary capil-

lary wedge and systemic venous pressures were seen with retrograde atrial activation or AV dissociation, with coincidental atrial and ventricular electrical activation leading to the contraction of the atrium against a closed value, which contributed to the patient's symptoms. Meanwhile, the ventricle itself was underfilled because of the loss of an appropriately timed atrial contraction leading to a fall in cardiac output that is characteristic of the Starling effect. It has become apparent that proper synchronization between atrial and ventricular contraction may be more important to the maintenance of cardiac output and low filling pressures at rest than rate alone is (Fig. 20-2). Similarly, the ability to increase the pacing rate

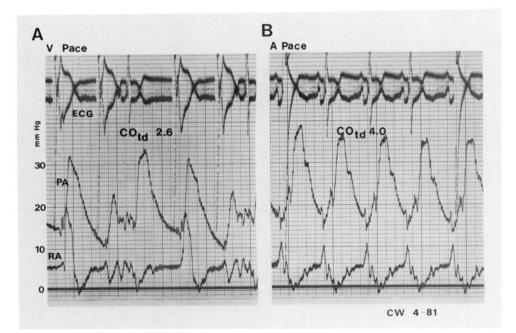

FIG. 20-2. (A) Marked variations are seen in pulmonary artery pressure and right atrial pressure during ventricular pacing, with a high arterial pressure and low filling pressure corresponding to the coincidental occurrence of a native P wave just before ventricular pacing. **(B)** Atrial pacing results in stable arterial and venous pressures that are higher and lower, respectively, than during ventricular pacing and yet with a higher cardiac output.

while maintaining AV synchrony may offer additional hemodynamic benefits over simply increasing the ventricular paced rate during periods of stress.

Thus, although a ventricular pacemaker will protect the patient from life-threatening bradycardias, it may induce the pacemaker syndrome and engender iatrogenic disease, which can be more limiting than the original problem for which the pacemaker was implanted. This has led to the development of pacemakers that allow for maintenance of AV synchronization and rate responsiveness, a concept generally termed *physiologic pacing*. As presently used by both the medical community and pacing industry, physiologic pacing refers specifically to dual-chamber pacemakers. I disagree with this limited use of the term and prefer to define physiologic pacing as a series of technological approximations that apply the available biomedical capabilities to restoration of the patient's rhythm as close to normal as is feasible within any limitations imposed by the patient's underlying disease process. Hence, in 1960, when only asynchronous fixed-rate ventricular pacing systems were available, this system was considered to be a physiologic pacemaker because it was certainly more physiologic than asystole. The demand ventricular pacemaker, by eliminating competition and reducing the incidence of pacemaker-induced ventricular fibrillation, was more physiologic than the asynchronous pacemaker. Present-generation physiologic pacemakers restore AV synchrony by pacing and/or sensing in both the atrium and ventricle and require two leads to accomplish this. Future physiologic pacemakers may require three or more leads, and they may utilize sensors to respond to metabolic or other biologic signals to guide not only the pacing rate but also energy output and AV interval to automatically maximize cardiac output. Hence, the "physiologic pacemaker" of 1985 may be viewed as a relatively primitive device and clearly not as

physiologic as the devices that are expected to be available 10 years from now.

The technology that is commercially available at this time enables the physician to choose a pacing system that will pace the ventricle, pace the atrium, or pace and sense in both chambers of the heart.[18,20-22] The optimal pacing system is not always a ventricular demand pacemaker. In patients who have sinus node dysfunction but intact AV nodal conduction, the ideal pacing system is a single-chamber atrial pacemaker that can improve cardiac output 20% to 40% over that of ventricular pacing at an identical rate. At the same time, atrial pacing may control many of the paroxysmal supraventricular tachyarrhythmias that appear to arise out of the bradycardia itself in the subgroup of patients with the bradycardia–tachycardia syndrome. Where there is sinus as well as AV-node disease, atrial pacing alone is unsafe because of the potential for AV block. If maintenance of atrial ventricular synchrony is deemed important in this setting, one needs to pace the atrium and then pace the ventricle in sequence, which is called *AV sequential pacing* (Fig. 20–3). When sinus node function is normal but AV conduction is impaired, one need only to synchronize the ventricular paced beat with the normal atrial activation, a form of pacing called *P-wave synchronous ventricular pacing* that provides rate responsiveness and allows the patient to obtain maximum hemodynamic benefits during exercise. Both P-wave synchronous and AV sequential pacing systems require two electrodes, one positioned in the atrium and one in the ventricle to detect or to stimulate the respective chamber. The present generation of dual-chamber pacemakers both pace and sense in each chamber, with coordination between the two controlled by a special logic circuit. This has been called the *fully automatic* or *AV universal pacemaker* and is designated DDD according to the Intersociety Commission on Heart Disease (ICHD) code.

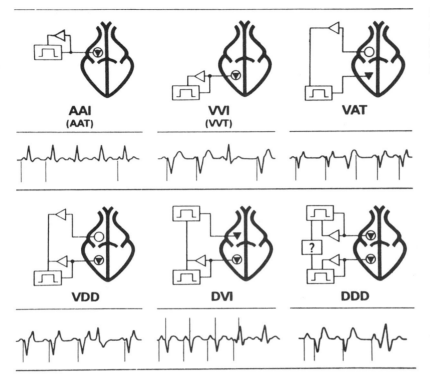

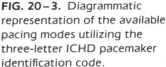

FIG. 20–3. Diagrammatic representation of the available pacing modes utilizing the three-letter ICHD pacemaker identification code.

ICHD CODE

As pacemakers become more complex and as they vary in their capabilities, it becomes imperative that the physician know generally what the pacing system is capable of doing. In 1980 the ICHD resources upgraded its former three-position code to a five-position code, which identifies the general function of presently available pacemakers.[23,24] This code simplistically describes the capability of the implanted device. The first position describes the chamber being paced: A means atrium, V means ventricle, and D means dual or double chamber. The second position describes the chamber that is being sensed: A, V, and D have the same meaning as in the first position. In this position, there can also be a zero, which can indicate the absence of sensing in either chamber. The third position describes the sensing modality: 0 signifies the absence of sensing, I signifies that the pacemaker is inhibited (*i.e.*, it recognizes a native complex and pacemaker timing is recycled), and T signifies that the pacemaker is triggered (*i.e.*, caused to discharge in response to a sensed native complex). The fourth and fifth positions are considered optional and may be separated from the first three letters of the code by a comma. The fourth position indicates the absence or presence of programmability, which is the ability to adjust one or more parameters of the pacemaker noninvasively after implantation. Zero indicates the absence of programmability. P indicates one- or two-parameter programmability, and M indicates three or more programmable functions and is called *multiparameter programmability*. C, in this position, indicates communicating or telemetric capability and implies multiparameter programmability. The fifth position relates to specific antitachycardia functions, such as the pacemaker emitting a burst of rapid stimuli (B), underdrive competition at a normal rate (N), or scanning of electrical diastole to interrupt the tachycardia (S). Suppression of the tachycardia by application of an exteral magnet or a radiofrequency transmitter is indicated by E, and, again, zero would indicate the absence of any antitachycardia function. This is the weakest section of the code, because E refers to how the device is activated, namely by some external control, but not what it does, and more than one letter is not allowed in the use of this code. Hence, while a device may be activated externally, when it does function, it may release a burst of rapid stimuli and we could not use both E and B in this position. Although not included in the present code, one might use a D in this fifth position to indicate automatic defibrillation. The code is detailed in Table 20–2.

IMPLANTABLE SENSORS

The ICHD code does not presently account for the multiplicity of physiologic sensors that are being evaluated.[25-28] At present they are being employed in single-chamber devices to provide rate responsiveness with exercise or other metabolic stresses. Among the systems presently under study are muscle noise, QT interval, respiratory rate, central venous oxygen saturation, and core temperature sensors. Others under study include *p*H, cardiac output, and minute ventilation-volume detectors. Eventually one or more of these systems may be incorporated into dual-chamber pacing systems, allowing automatic adjustment of both rate and AV delay to optimize cardiac output.

ANTITACHYCARDIA PACING

Until now pacemakers have been discussed primarily in relation to their use in the treatment of bradyarrhythmias. Major advances have occurred in both the basic science and clinical laboratories with respect to our understanding of cardiac rhythm disorders. Most paroxysmal tachycardias are sustained by a reentrant or circus-movement mechanism. This requires two functional pathways with the wave of depolarization proceeding down one and then up the other in a circular fashion, resulting in a sustained tachycardia. Maintenance of the tachycardia requires a critical balance between conduction and recovery times in these two pathways.

TABLE 20–2
INTERSOCIETY COMMISSION OF HEART DISEASE (ICHD) RESOURCES PACEMAKER IDENTIFICATION CODE

Position I Chamber Paced	Position II Chamber Sensed	Position III Mode of Sensing	Position IV Programmability	Position V Antitachycardia
A = atrial	A	O = no sensing	O = none	E = external
V = ventricle	V	I = inhibited	P = 1 or 2 parameters	N = normal rate
D = dual	D	T = triggered	M = 3 or more parameters	B = burst
	O = no sensing	D = both modes of sensing	C = communicating	S = scanning
S = single*	S			

* S is restricted for use by the manufacturer to indicate that the pacemaker can be used in either the atrium or ventricle but that it is a single-chamber device. Once the device is implanted, it becomes either an atrial or a ventricular pacemaker.

The tachycardia will stop if one pathway can be interrupted by any means. With paroxysmal supraventricular tachycardia, which is usually a reentrant mechanism either within the AV node or between the AV node and an accessory pathway (bypass track), increasing vagal tone, such as that achieved with carotid sinus massage or intravenous Tensilon, will both slow conduction and increase refractoriness in the AV node, upsetting this critical balance and terminating the tachycardia. Chronic pharmacologic therapy may have a similar effect. In the laboratory, both ventricular and supraventricular reentrant tachycardias can be reproducibly initiated by a variety of pacing techniques, including rapid pacing and single, double, and multiple extrastimuli. These tachyarrhythmias can often be terminated by properly timed pacing stimuli, which enter the reentrant pathway at a critical point, rendering it refractory to the circulating wave front, and thus interrupt and terminate the sustained tachycardia.

A variety of permanent pacing techniques have been utilized to control recurrent tachyarrhythmias. The simplest technique is the application of a magnet over a standard demand pacemaker; this converts it to a fixed rate unit, which will compete with the patient's intrinsic tachycardia. Chance occurrence of a properly timed paced beat will enter the reentrant pathway and terminate the fast, abnormal tachyarrhythmia. Some tachycardias will respond more rapidly to a burst of rapid stimuli. This may be achieved by holding an externally activated radiofrequency transmitter over an internally implanted receiving coil to initiate a burst of rapid stimuli, or it may be an automatic device that is fully implanted. The external systems require that the patient is hemodynamically stable and aware of the tachycardia, that he is sufficiently alert to activate the external control device, and that he has no associated bradyarrhythmias following termination of the tachycardia. Other pacemakers automatically recognize tachycardia and then initiate a brief burst of rapid stimuli, or they progressively scan the diastolic period with single or double premature stimuli until the tachycardia is terminated (Fig. 20-4). These units are gaining a wider degree of acceptance because they help to control many of the tachycardias otherwise resistant to pharmacologic therapy. Pacemakers may be able to replace pharmacologic agents when the medication itself is associated with multiple adverse side-effects or when there are difficulties with patient compliance. In a significant number of cases, pharmacologic therapy reduces but does not eliminate the tachycardia, and the combination of drugs and pacing therapy is proving to be extremely beneficial.[29,30] Used inappropriately, however, pacing may cause a stable arrhythmia, particularly ventricular tachycardia, to degenerate into a more malignant one, such as ventricular fibrillation.[31] At the present time, none of these devices should be employed in the absence of detailed electrophysiologic evaluation. Some investigators have suggested that they should never be used in the ventricle for ventricular tachycardia without the backup protection of an implantable automatic defibrillator.

In the United States, the number of individuals who die suddenly from presumed ventricular fibrillation superimposed on coronary artery disease is estimated to be over 300,000 per year. Studies with the implantable defibrillator began in humans in 1980 and hold exciting promise for the future.[32] Merging the implantable defibrillator with standard antitachycardia pacing systems and merging both techniques with antibradycardia pacing, because protracted asystole may follow the termination of a tachyarrhythmia, are on the medical horizon.

DIAGNOSTIC CAPABILITY

Because pacemakers are capable of pacing and sensing in both chambers of the heart, of being programmed to millions of potential parameter

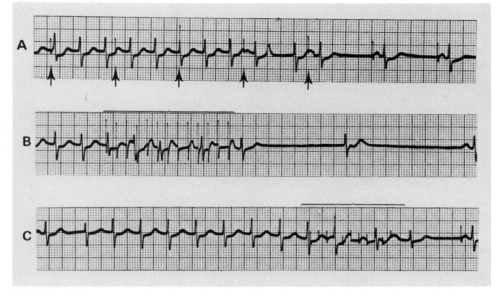

FIG. 20–4. Three examples of termination of a tachyarrhythmia by pacing techniques. **(A)** Underdrive competition. **(B)** Burst pacing without backup support. **(C)** Burst pacing with backup bradycardia support.

combinations, and of responding to pathologic tachyarrhythmias, identification of normal pacing system function is becoming progressively more complicated. The manufacturers are addressing these concerns by providing multiple diagnostic capabilities in present-generation devices, capabilities that can be expected to increase with future units.

Most present-generation dual-chamber pacing systems are capable of being interrogated about their program settings, and, in some cases, actual measurements of lead and battery function can be obtained. One such printout is shown is Figure 20–5. This printout also summarizes the results of capture-and-sensing threshold tests performed as part of the follow-up evaluation.

Because the paced rhythm now entails the interaction between two pacing systems, atrial and ventricular, as well as native events occurring in either the atrium or ventricle, it is not uncommon

for a "normal" rhythm to be misinterpreted as a pacing system malfunction. If this misconception is allowed to persist, a normally functioning device might be inappropriately removed. The reliability of the present-generation devices is so good that if a "malfunction" is encountered, it is usually caused by a lead problem or the inappropriate program settings of the pacemaker, but it is not a true device failure. To aid the physician in interpreting the possible rhythms that may result from even normal function, two capabilities are provided. One is marker pulses, which are signals telemetered directly from the pacemaker that indicate paced and sensed events in each chamber and, in some cases, refractory periods (Fig. 20–6).[33] This can be taken one step further with the programmer actually completing a diagnostic diagram of the pacer system function.[34]

In the early days of cardiac pacing, the physician did not have to concern himself with native

```
                PACESETTER SYSTEMS INC.
                  Version 1 5  - 1277

DATE :    APR 30, 1985 10:20 AM
MODEL :   283  SERIAL :    15876
PATIENT : ......................................
PHYSICIAN : ....................................

----------- PROGRAMMED PARAMETERS ----------

MODE .................................. DDI
RATE ..................................  70 PPM
VENTRICULAR CHANNEL :
   REFRACTORY ......................... 325 MSEC
   PULSE WIDTH ........................ 0.6 MSEC
   PULSE AMPLITUDE .................... 3.0 VOLTS
   SENSITIVITY ........................ 4.0 MVOLT

ATRIAL CHANNEL :
   REFRACTORY ......................... 325 MSEC
   PULSE WIDTH ........................ 0.6 MSEC
   PULSE AMPLITUDE .................... 3.0 VOLTS
   SENSITIVITY ........................ 2.0 MVOLT

AV INTERVAL ........................... 240 MSEC

BLANKING PERIOD .......................  13 MSEC

MAGNET :  ON

--------------- MEASURED DATA ---------------

PACEMAKER RATE ........................ 70.0 PPM

MAGNET RATE ........................... 80.0 PPM

CHANNEL MEASUREMENTS :
                      VENTRICLE    ATRIUM
   PULSE VOLTAGE         3.0         3.0     VOLTS
   PULSE CURRENT         4.1         6.0     MAMPS
   PULSE ENERGY          5           10      µJOULES
   PULSE CHARGE          2           3       µCOULOMBS
   LEAD IMPEDANCE        732         500     OHMS

BATTERY DATA : ( W.G.8074 - NOM.2.3 AHR )
   IMPEDANCE .......................... 1.0 KOHMS
   VOLTAGE ............................ 2.83 VOLTS
   CURRENT ............................ 16 µAMPS

--------------- TEST RESULTS ---------------

FILTERED R-WAVE AMPLITUDE : >14 MVOLTS
          SAFETY MARGIN : > 3 :1

VENTRICULAR CAPTURE THRESHOLD : 0.9 VOLTS
          AT 0.6 MSEC PULSE WIDTH

FILTERED P-WAVE AMPLITUDE : 7.0 MVOLTS
          SAFETY MARGIN : 3.5 :1

ATRIAL CAPTURE THRESHOLD : 0.9 VOLTS
          AT 0.6 MSEC PULSE WIDTH
```

FIG. 20–5. *Printout of the final interrogation after a pacing system evaluation of the Pacesetter AFP Pulse Generator. The top section summarizes the program settings; the middle section details the measurements of rate, lead, and battery function; and the bottom section is a synopsis of the capture and sensing threshold test results.*

atrial arrhythmias in the patient with complete heart block and a ventricular pacemaker. Devices that are now capable of sensing and tracking intrinsic atrial activity to restore rate responsiveness may also respond to abnormal atrial tachyarrhythmias and present a multiplicity of confusing rhythms caused by tracking of these endogenous signals.[35-37] Utilization of marker pulses in this setting merely restates the obvious, particularly if a P wave is not visible, that is, an event is being sensed on the atrial channel and thus triggers a ventricular output. Some devices are capable of telemetering the actual atrial or ventricular electrogram that will not only facilitate evaluation of pacing system function but also will aid in the interpretation of the native rhythms (Fig. 20–7).[38] In the future, marker pulses, diagnostic diagrams, and endocardial electrograms all will be telemetered simultaneously from the pacing system.

Some presently available systems can also act as a mini-Holter monitor in that they are capable of providing the frequency of pacing and sensing in each chamber and even of identifying the incidence of ventricular premature beats (Fig. 20–8). The pacemaker's definition of a ventricular premature beat, however, may differ slightly from that of the clinician.[39]

FUTURE DIRECTIONS

The majority of pacemakers in the not to distant future will be dual-chamber devices that are the size of the present-generation single-chamber units with a similar expected longevity. They will be programmable to either single- or dual-chamber function and will have the programmable features of all of the single-chamber units now available. They will be able to be programmed to a multiplicity of antitachycardia modes and possibly even to automatic defibrillation. Simple patient-activated programmers that will permit the knowledgeable and responsible

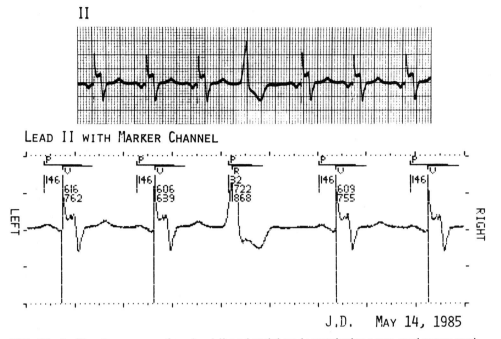

II

LEAD II WITH MARKER CHANNEL

J.D.   MAY 14, 1985

FIG. 20–6. Simultaneous surface lead-II and atrial and ventricular pace, and sense and refractory markers telemetered directly from the pacemaker. The letters *A* and *V* refer to paced events in their respective chambers, and *P* and *R* refer to native depolarizations in the atrium and ventricle, respectively. A lead-II rhythm strip recorded simultaneously with a standard single-channel analogue ECG machine is shown above for comparison. Note that the markers indicate that a P wave was sensed coincident with the leading edge of the ventricular premature beat. Was this really a P wave or was it the R wave first being sensed by the atrial lead?

patient to have some control over his pacemaker after a careful assessment by the physician are being developed. One of the basic parameters that might be programmed by the patient is the rate. He can then increase his paced rate during exercise or decrease it during sleep, depending on which might be better for him. However, a variety of implantable physiologic sensors are under investigation that will permit autoregulation of the pacemaker to maintain optimal physiologic function, eliminating the need for a patient-activated device or frequent reprogramming by the physician.

Transtelephonic monitoring systems will increase in sophistication and capability, and will be able to fully interrogate the pacemaker by telephone and, possibly, to program it as well. Pacemakers will be capable of acquiring and storing a variety of physiologic data, analagous to Holter monitor recordings, and then will be able to transmit this information to the physician on request. Implantable devices will also be able to be used for serial electrophysiologic testing without the need for repeat invasive procedures each time the physician wishes to assess the continued appropriateness of a given pharmacologic or

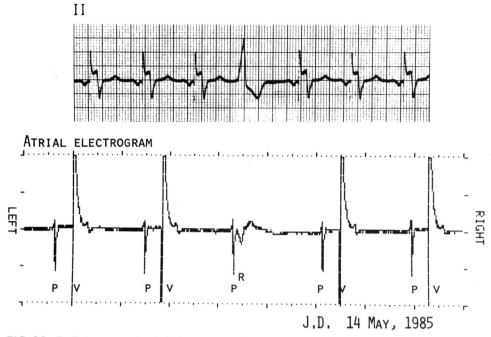

FIG. 20–7. Telemetered atrial electrogram from the same rhythm shown in Figure 20–6. The P wave is large and discrete. The ventricular pacing pulse is seen as a large signal, and although the ventricular premature beat is also visible, it is clear that a P wave coincides with its leading edge to account for the atrial sensing.

```
283-01-008328              SEP 10 '85 03:09 PM    *   I
           DIAGNOSTIC DATA ( CARDIAC CYCLES )          N
                                                       T
EVENT COUNTERS LAST CLEARED.. MAR 26, 11:40 AM        E
NO. OF PREMATURE VENTRICULAR EVENTS..... 2,277        R
NO. OF ATRIAL SENSE EVENTS FOLLOWED                   M
    BY VENTRICULAR SENSE EVENT......11,801,396        E
NO. OF ATRIAL SENSE EVENTS FOLLOWED                   D
    BY VENTRICULAR PACE EVENT....... 7,073,183        I
NO. OF ATRIAL PACE EVENTS FOLLOWED                    C
    BY VENTRICULAR SENSE EVENT........ 301,573        S
NO. OF ATRIAL PACE EVENTS FOLLOWED                    .
    BY VENTRICULAR PACE EVENT......... 185,879
PERCENT PACED - ATRIUM......................... 3%    I
PERCENT PACED - VENTRICLE.................... 37%     N
      DISPLAY MISCELLANEOUS EVENTS                    C
                                                      .
   PRINT      CLEAR EVENT COUNTERS       RETURN       *
```

FIG. 20–8. Printout of the diagnostic data available from an Intermedics Cosmos Pulse Generator.

stimulating regimen for arrhythmia control. Basically, the possible technologic advances are only limited by the extent of our knowledge and imagination. As research in the basic science laboratories continues to expand our understanding of normal and abnormal physiology, the technology is available to refine our therapeutic and diagnostic capabilities.

SUMMARY

Pacemakers today are extremely reliable and complex devices that are capable of lasting 5 to 10 years and possibly longer. They are small and reasonably comfortable for the patient. In many units, parameters can be noninvasively programmed to obtain the maximal therapeutic benefit and safety while aiding in the subsequent diagnostic evaluation and solution of many problems that previously required operative intervention. Dual-chamber pacemakers, which more closely reproduce the normal cardiac physiology, and units specifically designed to control a multiplicity of tachyarrhythmias, including ventricular fibrillation, are currently available and are being further refined. The ICHD code for the presently available pacing systems has been reviewed, but it will be inadequate for future-generation devices and additional revisions can be anticipated. Some of the directions toward which the industry is working have been also summarized briefly.

REFERENCES

1. Elmquist R, Senning A: Implantable pacemaker for the heart. In Smyth CN (ed): Medical Electronics, p 253. Springfield, Illinois, Charles C Thomas, 1960
2. Barold SS, Mujica J (eds): The Third Decade of Cardiac Pacing, Advances in Technology in Clinical Application. Mount Kisco, New York, Futura Publishing, 1982
3. Schaldach M, Furman S (eds): Advances in Pacemaker Technology. New York, Springer-Verlag, 1975
4. Tyers GFO, Brownlee RR: Current status of pacemaker power sources. Ann Thorac Surg 25:571–587, 1978
5. Hauser RG, Klodnycky M: Clinical reliability of programmable pacemakers. In Feruglio GA (ed): Cardiac Pacing, Electrophysiology and Pacemaker Technology, p 763. Padova, Italy, Piccin Medical Books, 1982
6. Stokes K. Stephenson NL: The implantable cardiac pacing lead, just a simple wire? In Barold SS, Mujica J (eds): The Third Decade of Cardiac Pacing, Advances in Technology in Clinical Application, 365–416. Mount Kisco, New York, Futura Publishing, 1982
7. Mujica J, Ripart A: Twelve years experience with cardiac pacing leads, Clinical conclusions from 8004 cases. Clin Prog Pacing Electrophysiol, 2:513–532, 1984
8. Timmis GC, Helland J, Westveer C et al: The evolution of low threshold leads. Clin Prog Pacing Electrophysiol 1:313–334, 1983
9. Irnich W: Engineering concepts in pacemaker electrodes. In Schaldach M, Furman S (eds): Advances in Pacemaker Technology, p 241. New York, Springer-Verlag, 1975
10. Ripart A, Mujica J: Electrode-heart interface: Definition of the ideal electrode. PACE 6:410–431, 1983
11. Levine PA: Why programmability? Indications for and clinical benefits of multiparameter programmable pacemakers. Sylmar, California, Pacesetter Systems Inc, 1981
12. Billhardt RA, Rosenbush SW, Hauser RG: Successful management of pacing systems malfunction without surgery: The role of programmable pulse generators. PACE 5:675–682, 1982
13. Levine PA: Proceedings of the policy conference of the North American Society of Pacing and Electrophysiology on Programmability and Pacemaker Follow-up Programs. Clin Prog Pacing Electrophysiol 2:145–196, 1984
14. Hauser RG: Multiprogrammable cardiac pacemakers: Applications, results and follow-up. Am J Surg 145:740, 1983
15. Levine PA, Belott PH, Bilitch M et al: Recommendations of the NASPE policy conference on pacemaker programmability and follow-up. PACE 6:1221–1222, 1983
16. Sholder J, Levine PA, Mann BM, Mace RC: Bidirectional telemetry and interrogation in cardiac pacing, In Barold SS, Mujica J (eds): The Third Decade of Cardiac Pacing, Advances in Technology in Clinical Application, pp 145–166. Mount Kisco, New York, Futura Publishing, 1982
17. Tyers GFO, Brownlee RR: Telemetry in cardiac pacemakers. In Varriale P, Naclerio E (eds): Cardiac Pacing, A Concise Guide to Clinical Practice, Chap 23. Philadelphia, Lea & Febiger, 1979
18. Levine PA, Mace RC: Pacing Therapy, A Guide to Cardiac Pacing for Optimum Hemodynamic Benefit, pp 3–18. Mount Kisco, New York, Futura Publishing, 1983

19. Ausubel K, Furman S: The pacemaker syndrome. Ann Intern Med 103:420–429, 1985
20. Griffin JC: Pacemaker selection for the individual patient. In Barold SS (ed): Modern Cardiac Pacing, pp 411–420. Mount Kisco, New York, Futura Publishing, 1985
21. Sutton R, Perrins J, Citron P: Physiologic cardiac pacing. PACE 3:207–219, 1980
22. Harthorne JW: Indications for pacemaker insertion. Prog Cardiovasc Dis 23:393–400, 1981
23. Parsonnet V, Furman S, Smyth NPD: Revised code for pacemaker identification. PACE 4:400–403, 1981
24. Bernstein AD, Brownlee RR, Fletcher R et al: Pacing mode code. In Barold SS (ed): Modern Cardiac Pacing, pp 307–322. Mount Kisco, New York, Futura Publishing, 1985
25. Rossi P, Plicchi G, Canducci G et al: Respiratory rate as a determinant of optimal pacing rate. PACE 6:502–507, 1983
26. Griffin J, Jutzy KR, Claude JP et al: Central body temperature as a guide to optimal heart rate. PACE 6:498–501, 1983
27. Goicolea A, Ayza MW, LaLlana RD et al: Rate responsive pacing, clinical experience. PACE 8:322–328, 1985
28. Rickards AF: Rate responsive pacing. In Barold SS (ed): Modern Cardiac Pacing, pp 799–809. Mount Kisco, New York, Futura Publishing, 1985
29. Osborn MJ, Holmes DR: Anti-tachycardia pacing. Clin Prog Electrophysiol Pacing 3:239–267, 1985
30. Camm J, Ward D: Pacing for Tachycardia Control. London, Butler and Tanner Ltd, 1983
31. Fisher JD, Mehra R, Furman S: Termination of ventricular tachycardia with bursts of rapid ventricular pacing. Am J Cardiol 41:94–102, 1978
32. Echt DS, Winkle RA: Management of patients with the automatic implantable cardioverter/defibrillator. Clin Prog Electrophysiol Pacing 3:4–16, 1985
33. Kruse I, Markowitz T, Ryden L: Timing markers showing pacemaker behavior to aid in the follow-up of a physiologic pacemaker. PACE 6:801–805, 1983
34. Olson WH, McConnell MV, Sah RL et al: Pacemaker diagnostic diagrams. PACE 8:691–700, 1985
35. Levine PA, Seltzer JP: Runaway on normal pacing? Two cases of normal rate responsive (VDD) pacing. Clin Prog Pacing Electrophysiol 1:177–183, 1983
36. Levine PA, Seltzer JP: A-V universal (DDD) pacing and atrial fibrillation. Clin Prog Pacing Electrophysiol 1:275–281, 1983
37. Greenspan AM, Greenberg RM, Frankl WS: Tracking of atrial flutter during DDD pacing. PACE 7:955–960, 1984
38. Levine PA, Sholder J, Duncan JL: Clinical benefits of electrogram telemetry in evaluation of DDD function. PACE 7:1170–1177, 1984
39. Sanders R, Martin R, Frumin H et al: Data storage and retrieval by implantable pacemakers for diagnostic purposes. PACE 7:1228–1233, 1984

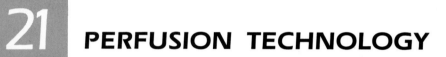

21

PERFUSION TECHNOLOGY

Thomas Hankins
Arthur J. Roberts

COMPUTER CONCEPTS AND APPLICATIONS IN CARDIAC SURGERY

To improve perfusion during cardiopulmonary bypass (CPB) from a condition of "controlled shock" to one as normal as possible, there must be a more precisely controlled method of perfusion. Subjective or empirical criteria used as a basic means of management may place a patient in a compromised condition. Now, sophisticated perfusion management could conceivably avoid such a dilemma. Physiologic events, such as increased vascular resistances, lactic acid production, and calculated oxygen debt might go unnoticed because sufficient data may not be generated or processed during the routine conduct of CPB.

During cardiopulmonary bypass, patients undergo changes in temperature, depth of anesthesia, blood pressure, blood flow, urine output, hemodilution, and biochemical components. The parameters by which most perfusionists determine adequate perfusion are mean arterial pressure, arterial blood gases, blood flow, and urine output. These few parameters have long been the standard for measurement of perfusion adequacy.[1-4] Perfusion may be judged to be adequate by these parameters alone, but is perfusion as optimal as possible under these conditions? Due to patients' ever-changing conditions, other parameters such as venous blood gases, vascular resistances, oxygen consumption, oxygen availability and oxygen extraction might give additional beneficial information if continuously monitored and evaluated.[5-18]

Monitoring of critically ill patients with the aid of a computer has been explored for more than a decade.[19-25] The management of critically ill patients in the postoperative period has also been described.[26-31] Using the computer as a real-time clinical tool, multiple parameters can quickly and efficiently be evaluated and subsequent pharmacologic or mechanical intervention instituted. As perfusion becomes an increasingly complicated technology, the use of computers in this field will probably develop with enthusiastic support. As early as 1975, perfusionists became interested in this new tool.[32-40]

FUNCTIONAL CONCEPTS AND APPLICATIONS

DATA ACQUISITION

The main function of the computer is to acquire data. There are two basic mechanisms through which a computer can acquire data: one is by manual entry at a keyboard and the other is by automated data capture by either analog-to-digital conversion or digital-to-digital processing. Because the use of computers as a clinical tool in the operating room is basically still in its infancy, almost all collection of data is done manually. For a computer to accept and process data, a program must be written that will allow the computer to function. Most programs utilized in the operating room environment use either BASIC or FORTRAN as an operating language. Currently, there is a trend toward the use of PASCAL as an oper-

Cardiac Surgical Procedure Menu

orprocmenu

1. Pressures	2. Temperatures
3. Blood Gases	4. Blood Gas Correction Factors
5. Lab Data	6. Medications
7. Times	8. Initial Bypass Data
9. Vascular Resistance Calc	10. Oxygen Index Calculations
11. Urine Output	12. Cardiac Index Calculations
13. Heparin Response Curve	14. Post Bypass Data
15. Cardiac Dynamics Calculations	16. Reports and Procedure End

Enter Choice: [ ] or use the Softkeys below, and then Press 'Proceed'.

Proceed   Next   Previous   Last   Help   Main
          Choice   Choice   Choice   Menu

FIG. 21–1. Example of user-selectable menu options for use during cardiac surgery.

ating language among those involved in automation.

Programs that will allow multiple selections at various times are called menu-driven programs. A menu in a computer program is similar to a menu in a restaurant in that it allows the user to choose the portion of the program he wishes to utilize. For example, we have collaborated with Hewlett-Packard Company and developed a menu-driven program for cardiopulmonary bypass (Fig. 21–1). In a program of this type, each time an element is selected, a timed entry is used to mark the exact time of data collection. Once the selected element is finished, the program returns to the original menu. The advantage of this methodology is that each element can be used as many times and as frequently as necessary. Examples of these elements can be seen in Figures 21–2 to 21–13.

DATABASE MANAGEMENT

When one starts entering and saving data on the computer, there must be a reasonable and reliable means of retrieving the stored data. To ac-

complish this, one must utilize a database management system when dealing with large arrays of data. A database management system functions by storing data into files, records, and fields. For example, suppose that a patient has coronary artery bypass graft surgery on October 15, 1985. His pump time is 60 minutes and the aortic cross-clamp time is 30 minutes. The vessels bypassed were the left anterior descending (LAD), obtuse marginal, and right coronary arteries. If one wished to store and retrieve this information, how could it be accomplished? First, a file labeled "OPEN HEART" would be created. Next a record would be created with the following fields of information: (1) patient name, (2) data of surgery, (3) number of vessels bypassed, (4) pump time, (5) cross-clamp time, (6) vessel #1 (7) vessel #2, (8) vessel #3. An example of how this record would look can be seen in Table 21–1. Once the data are entered into the appropriate fields in the record, the file is then closed and stored in the computer's memory. One of the benefits of this database system is that similar data can be synthesized and updated over time. For example, if a surgeon wants to know how

(Text continues on p. 284.)

Cardiac Surgery Procedure Record
_____

or_procedure2

ID Number: _____   Procedure Date: / /   at   : :

Hct: _____ vol%   Hgb: _____ g/dl   Barometric Pressure: ___ mmHg

Priming Volume: Plasmalyte A: _____ cc Albumin: ___ cc Hespan: _____ cc

Mannitol: __ cc   Packed Cells: ___ cc

Height: _____ cm   Weight: _____ kg   BSA ___ m2

Final Dilution Hct: _____ Vol%

Electrolytes: Na: ___ mmol/dl   K: ___ mmol/dl

Please Choose a Function from the Softkeys Below:
Accessing the CDMS Cardiac Surgery Database

Find	Add	Update	Delete		Help			OR
Mode	Data	Data	Data					Menu

FIG. 21–2. Example of the prebypass pump prime calculation information. For example, this information allows the calculation of the hematocrit the patient will have as soon as bypass is initiated.

Cardiac Surgery Initial Bypass Record
_____

orinitbyp

ID Number: _____   Date of Procedure: / /   at   : :

BSA: ___ m2

Minimum Pressure of __ mmHg at   \
Optimal Pressure of __ mmHg at   >   Calculated Maximum Flow: _____ cc/min
Maximum Pressure of __ mmHg at   /

Calculated Minimum Flow: _____ cc/min

Please Choose a Function from the Softkeys Below:

Accessing the CDMS Cardiac Surgery Database

Find	Add	Update	Delete		Help			OR
Mode	Data	Data	Data					Menu

FIG. 21–3. Calculated maximum and minimum flow rates as well as the optimal pressure range for an individual patient.

```
                    Cardiac Surgery Pressure Record
                                                                orpress
  ID Number:                  Date of Procedure:   /  /     at   :   :
```

```
  ┌─────────────────────────────────────────────────────────────────────┐
  │ Systolic Arterial:        ___ mmHg    Mean Arterial:        ___ mmHg │
  │ Diastolic Arterial:       ___ mmHg                                   │
  │- - - - - - - - - - - - - - - - - - - - - - - - - - - - - - - - - - - │
  │ Systolic Pulmonary Artery:  ___ mmHg   Mean Pulmonary:      ___ mmHg │
  │ Diastolic Pulmonary Artery: ___ mmHg                                 │
  │- - - - - - - - - - - - - - - - - - - - - - - - - - - - - - - - - - - │
  │ Central Venous:           ___ mmHg    Mean Left Atrial:     ___ mmHg │
  │- - - - - - - - - - - - - - - - - - - - - - - - - - - - - - - - - - - │
  │ Arterial Line:            ___ mmHg    Cardioplegia Line:    ___ mmHg │
  │ Aortic Root:              ___ mmHg                                   │
  ├─────────────────────────────────────────────────────────────────────┤
  │   If Automatic Entry of Date/Time when ADDing is desired, enter "X": _│
  │      Manual Date and Time of Entry:  __/__/____  at  __:__:__ ___     │
  └─────────────────────────────────────────────────────────────────────┘
```

```
              Please Choose a Function from the Softkeys Below:
                 Accessing the CDMS Cardiac Surgery Database

  __Find__  __Add___  _Update_  _Delete_      __Help__  _____ _____  __OR__
  __Mode__  __Data__  __Data__  __Data__      _____  _____ _____  _Menu_
```

FIG. 21–4. Example of the pressure information screen.

```
                 Cardiac Surgery Cardiac Index Record
                                                              orcindx
  ID Number:                 Date of Procedure:   /  /     at   :   :
```

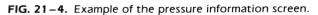

```
           ┌──────────────────────────────────────────────────┐
           │  BSA:        ___ m2      Weight: ___ kg           │
           │- - - - - - - - - - - - - - - - - - - - - - - - - -│
           │  Flows:      ___ L/min            ___ cc/min      │
           │- - - - - - - - - - - - - - - - - - - - - - - - - -│
           │              ___ cc/kg/min        ___ cc/min/m2   │
           └──────────────────────────────────────────────────┘
```

```
  ┌───────────────────────────────────────────────────────────────────┐
  │  If Automatic Entry of Date/Time when ADDing is desired, enter "X": X│
  │     Manual Date and Time of Entry:  __/__/____  at  __:__:__ ___    │
  └───────────────────────────────────────────────────────────────────┘
```

```
           Please Choose a Function from the Softkeys Below:

              Accessing the CDMS Cardiac Surgery Database

  __Find__  __Add___  _Update_  _Delete_    __Help__  _____ _____  __OR__
  __Mode__  __Data__  __Data__  __Data__    _____  _____ _____  _Menu_
```

FIG. 21–5. Example of the cardiac index screen. This is particularly useful for those involved in pediatric surgery.

```
                    Cardiac Surgery Laboratory Data Record
                                                                    orlab
    ID Number:                      Date of Procedure:   /  /    at   :  :
```

```
    ┌─────────────────────────────────────────────────────────────────────┐
    │  Hemoglobin: ____ mg/dL   Hematocrit: ____ vol%   Platelets: ___  mm3 │
    │  - - - - - - - - - - - - - - - - - - - - - - - - - - - - - - - - - -  │
    │  Sodium:                 _____ mmol/dl    Potassium:      ___ mmol/dl │
    │  - - - - - - - - - - - - - - - - - - - - - - - - - - - - - - - - - -  │
    │  Ionized Calcium:    ____ mmol/dL    Glucose:            ___ mmol/dl  │
    │  - - - - - - - - - - - - - - - - - - - - - - - - - - - - - - - - - -  │
    │  Arterial Lactic Acid: ____ mmol/dl   Venous Lactic Acid: ____ mmol/dl│
    └─────────────────────────────────────────────────────────────────────┘
```

```
    ┌─────────────────────────────────────────────────────────────────────┐
    │  If Automatic Entry of Date/Time when ADDing is desired, enter "X": _ │
    │     Manual Date and Time of Entry:  __/__/____  at  __/__/__ __       │
    └─────────────────────────────────────────────────────────────────────┘
```

```
              Please Choose a Function from the Softkeys Below:

              Accessing the CDMS Cardiac Surgery Database

    _Find_  _Add_   _Update_  _Delete_       _Help_ _____ _____  _OR_
    _Data_  _Data_  _Data_    _Data_         _____ _____ _____  _Menu_
```

FIG. 21–6. Example of the laboratory data screen.

```
                    Cardiac Surgery Oxygen Index Record
                                                                   oro2idx
    ID Number:                      Date of Procedure:   /  /    at   :  :
```

```
    ┌─────────────────────────────────────────────────────────────────────┐
    │  Flow: ____ l/min  Arterial PO2:    ___ mmHg   Venous PO2:   ___ mmHg │
    │  - - - - - - - - - - - - - - - - - - - - - - - - - - - - - - - - - -  │
    │  BSA:  ____ m2     Arterial O2 Sat: _____ %    Venous O2 Sat: _____ % │
    │  - - - - - - - - - - - - - - - - - - - - - - - - - - - - - - - - - -  │
    │          Hemoglobin:       ___ g/Dl     Hematocrit:    ___ vol%      │
    │                                                                       │
    │  Arterial O2 Content: ____ ml/100ml  Venous O2 Content: ____ ml/100ml│
    │  A-VdO2:              ____ ml/100ml   VO2:              ___ ml/min    │
    │  O2 Extraction Ratio: ____ O2ex      Red Cell Flow:    ___ ml/min    │
    │  Tissue Oxygen Extraction Index: _____ ml/min/m2                      │
    │                                                                       │
    │  If Automatic Entry of Date/Time when ADDing is desired, enter "X": X │
    │     Manual Date and Time of Entry: __/__/____   at  __:__:__          │
    └─────────────────────────────────────────────────────────────────────┘
```

```
              Please Choose a Function from the Softkeys Below:
              Accessing the CDMS Cardiac Surgery Database

    _Find_  _Add_   _Update_  _Delete_       _Help_ _____ _____  _OR_
    _Mode_  _Data_  _Data_    _Data_         _____ _____ _____  _Menu_
```

FIG. 21–7. Example of the oxygen index screen. With basic blood gas and laboratory data, important calculations such as oxygen consumption, oxygen availability, and oxygen extraction are readily available.

```
                    Cardiac Surgery Medications Record
                                                                  orrxl
ID Number:                    Date of Procedure:   /  /    at   :  :

   Plasmalyte A:        ____ cc    Inderal:          _ mg   Protamine:   ____ mg
   Lactated Ringers: ____ cc       Decadron:         _ mg   Other:
   D5W:                 ____ cc    Solumedral:       _ mg   [          ]  ___ mg
   Hespan:              ____ cc    Pavulon:          ___ mg
   Albumin 5%:          ____ cc    Sublimase:        ___ mg
   Albumin 25%:         ____ cc    Sodium Pentothal: ___ mg
   Mannitol:            ____ cc    Sufenta:          ___ mg
   Lasix:               ____ mg    Morphine:         ___ mg
   Potassium:           __ mEq     Packed Cells:     ___ cc
   Calcium:             _ G        FFP:              ___ cc
   Sodium Bicarb:       __ mEq     Platelets:        ___ cc
   Lidocaine:           ___ mg     Heparin:          ___ mg

   If Automatic Entry of Date/Time when ADDing is desired enter "X": _
        Manual Date and Time of Entry:  __/__/____  at __/__/__ ___

                Accessing the CDMS Cardiac Surgery Database

   Find    Add    Update  Delete       Help  _____  _____  OR
   Mode    Data    Data    Data         _____  _____  _____  Menu
```

FIG. 21–8. Example of the medications screen. This screen offers most of the common drugs used in cardiac surgery. The screen also tracks the total amount of each drug administered.

```
                    Cardiac Surgery Urine Output Record
                                                                orurine
ID Number:                    Date of Procedure:   /  /    at   :  :

          Cumulative Bypass Urine Output: ____ cc
          ------------------------------------------
          Minutes on Bypass: ___ min
          ------------------------------------------
          Average Bypass Urine Output: __ cc/min


   If Automatic Entry of Date/Time when ADDing is desired, enter "X": X
        Manual Date and Time of Entry: __/__/____  at  __:__:__ ___

          Please Choose a Function from the Softkeys Below:

                Accessing the CDMS Cardiac Surgery Database

   Find    Add    Update  Delete       Help  _____  _____  OR
   Mode    Data    Data    Data         _____  _____  _____  Menu
```

FIG. 21–9. Example of the urine output screen. This screen enables one to keep a cumulative record of the urine output throughout the case.

```
                    Cardiac Surgery Cardiac Dynamics Record
                                                                    orcarddx
  ID Number:                  Date of Procedure:    / /     at    :  :
```

```
┌──────────────────────────────────────────────────────────────────────┐
│  Cardiac Output: ▧  L/min  Heart Rate: ▧  B/min                        │
│  - - - - - - - - - - - - - - - - - - - - - - - - - - - - - - - - - -   │
│  Mean Arterial: ▧  mmHg     Mean PA: ▧  mmHg        PA Wedge: ▧  mmHg   │
│                                                                        │
│  Stroke Volume: ▧ cc/beat  Pulmonary Vascular Resistance: ▧ dyne sec/cm5/M2 │
│  - - - - - - - - - - - - - - - - - - - - - - - - - - - - - - - - - -   │
│  Left Cardiac Work: ▧  kg/min/M2  Right Cardiac Work: ▧  Kg/min/M2      │
│  - - - - - - - - - - - - - - - - - - - - - - - - - - - - - - - - - -   │
│  LV Stroke Work:  ▧  G/min/m2     RV Stroke Work:  ▧  G/min/m2          │
└──────────────────────────────────────────────────────────────────────┘
```

```
          Please Choose a Function from the Softkeys Below:
            Accessing the CDMS Cardiac Surgery Database
```

Find	Add	Update	Delete		Help			OR
Mode	Data	Data	Data					Menu

FIG. 21–10. Example of the cardiac dynamics screen. This screen is particularly useful to the anesthesiologist in comparing prebypass data with postbypass cardiac data.

```
                              Valve Data
                                                            orvalve
  ID Number:                  Date of Procedure:   / /    at   :  :
```

```
              ┌────────────────────────────────┐
              │  Location:    _____        │
              │ -----------------------------   │
              │  Type:        _____        │
              │ -----------------------------   │
              │  Manufacturer: [_____]       │
              │ -----------------------------   │
              │  Model Number: _____       │
              │ -----------------------------   │
              │  Date Code:   _____        │
              └────────────────────────────────┘
```

```
     Please Choose a Function from the Softkeys Below:

  Accessing the CDMS Ventricular Angiography Database
```

FIG. 21–11. Example of the valve data screen. This is useful because the valves can be traced if there is a recall or if there is any question about a device installed previously.

```
_____Cardiac Surgery Vascular Resistance Record_____
                                                                      orvasres
ID Number:                       Date of Procedure:   /  /    at   :  :
═══════════════════════════════════════════════════════════════════════════════

┌─────────────────────────────────────────────────────────────────────────────┐
│ Mean Arterial Pressure: ___ mmHg      Central Venous Pressure: __ mmHg        │
│ - - - - - - - - - - - - - - - - - - - - - - - - - - - - - - - - - - - - - -   │
│ Blood Flow: ____ cc/min                                                       │
│ - - - - - - - - - - - - - - - - - - - - - - - - - - - - - - - - - - - - - -   │
│ PRU: ___ mmHg/ml/min                  SVR: ____ dyne-sec/cm-5/m2              │
└─────────────────────────────────────────────────────────────────────────────┘


┌─────────────────────────────────────────────────────────────────────────────┐
│ If Automatic Entry of Date/Time when ADDing is desired, enter "X": X          │
│    Manual Date and Time of Entry: __/__/____  at  __:__:__ __                 │
└─────────────────────────────────────────────────────────────────────────────┘

            Please Choose a Function from the Softkeys Below:

            Accessing the CDMS Cardiac Surgery Database

  Find     Add     Update   Delete        Help   _____  _____   OR
  Mode     Data    Data     Data          _____  _____  _____  Menu
```

FIG. 21–12. Example of the resistance screen. This screen is one of the most frequently used screens.

```
_____Cardiac Surgery Procedure - Time Stamp_____
                                                                   ortimestamp
ID Number:                       Date of Procedure:   /  /    at   :  :
═══════════════════════════════════════════════════════════════════════════════

┌─────────────────────────────────────────────────────────────────────────────┐
│                        Event Code: [_____]                                 │
└─────────────────────────────────────────────────────────────────────────────┘

┌─────────────────────────────────────────────────────────────────────────────┐
│                              For automatic entry of date/time,                │
│                                 enter "X" in box below:                       │
│ - - - - - - - - - - - - - - - - - - - - - - - - - - - - - - - - - - - - - -   │
│ Start Time: __/__/____ at __:__:__ now          X                            │
│ - - - - - - - - - - - - - - - - - - - - - - - - - - - - - - - - - - - - - -   │
│ Stop Time:  __/__/____ at __:__:__ __           _                            │
└─────────────────────────────────────────────────────────────────────────────┘

        Please Choose a Function from the Softkeys Below:

        Accessing the CDMS Ventricular Angiography Database

  _____   _____   _____   _____      _____   _____   _____   _____
  _____   _____   _____   _____      _____   _____   _____   _____
```

FIG. 21–13. Example of the time stamp. This is useful to mark events such as going on bypass, application of the cross-clamp, and so forth.

TABLE 21–1
RECORD FOR CARDIOPULMONARY BYPASS PATIENT

Structure for file: A: OPEN HEART.DBF
Number of records: 01000
Date of last update: 11/20/85
Primary use database

FLD	NAME	TYPE	WIDTH	DEC
001	NAME	C	025	
002	DATE	N	008	
003	NUMVESSL	N	002	
004	PUMPTIME	N	003	
005	CRSCLAMP	N	003	.
006	VESSEL1	C	015	
007	VESSEL2	C	015	
008	VESSEL3	C	015	
TOTAL			00087	

many patients had bypass grafts to the LAD in the previous six months, all that has to be done is to recall the file "OPEN HEART," and the database management program will display all of the patients who had LAD bypass grafts during that period. The same analytical benefit applies for a perfusionist. For example, a search for patients that required sodium bicarbonate administration during CPB for correction of metabolic acidosis might identify perfusion-related problems. The computer allows ready access to information that can help to identify clinical shortcomings.

PERFUSION MANAGEMENT

Several papers have been presented that describe the use of a microcomputer or programmable calculator during CPB.[38-42] The computer can also aid in the utilization of peripheral vascular resistance, oxygen consumption, and arteriovenous oxygen content difference to attain parameters useful in optimizing perfusion. In examining the factors influencing oxygen delivery, the following observations must closely be examined. If the blood flow through a particular tissue becomes increased, either pharmacologically or

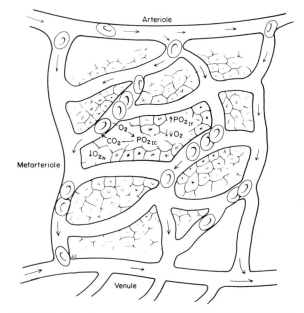

FIG. 21–14. Example of optimal perfusion of tissue with normal red cell flow through the capillary network. Notice the increased interstitial fluid PO_2 and the normal respiration between the tissues and the red cells. ($PO_{2_{IF}}$, interstitial fluid PO_2; O_{2_N}, oxygen need; $PO_{2_{IC}}$ intracellular PO_2; and $\dot{v}O_2$, oxygen consumption)

mechanically, greater quantities of oxygen are transported into the area in a given time (Fig. 21–14). The tissue PO_2 becomes correspondingly increased, reducing A-V_dO_2, and at the same time increasing oxygen availability. As a result, there is optimal perfusion to that area. Optimal perfusion can be diagramed as seen in Figure 21–15.

If there is a decrease in blood flow, which may occur during perfusion utilizing conventional perfusion techniques, there will be a corresponding increase in the oxygen extraction ratio and A-V_dO_2. With a decrease in blood flow, there is a corresponding decrease in oxygen availabil-

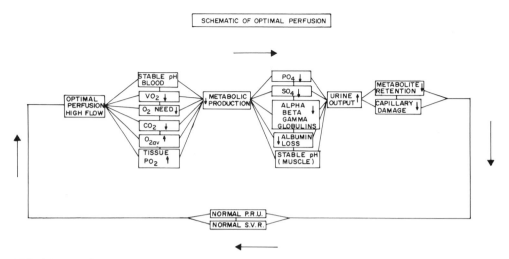

FIG. 21–15. *Schematic example of optimal perfusion and its relational effects on body subsystems. Note the increased oxygen availability (O_{2av}) along with the decreased metabolite production.*

ity and interstitial fluid PO_2. Since oxygen is always being utilized by the tissue cells, even during hypothermia, the intracellular PO_2 remains lower than the surrounding interstitial fluid PO_2. When there is a reduction in the interstitial fluid PO_2 as a result of inadequate perfusion, there is a large reduction in the intracellular PO_2. When the intracellular PO_2 is allowed to decrease significantly, an oxygen debt occurs. When an oxygen debt occurs, tissue metabolites, especially lactic acid, are increased, and the tissue is weakened by a metabolic acidosis.[10,18,41] Muscle pH and PCO_2, unlike muscle PO_2, remain unaltered until the production of lactic acid is increased for certain time periods.[41]

In a state of metabolic acidosis, red cell membrane rigidity increases.[42] The limited flexibility of red cell membranes causes transient slowing or stoppage of flow during their transit through the capillary bed. As a result of sluggish movement of blood through the capillaries and of interstitial fluid through the lymphatic system, an increasing amount of tissue hypoxia occurs, leading to a further increase in the generation of metabolic acidosis. The plasma pH falls because the tissues, in their increased production of acid metabolites, release PO_4 and SO_4. Lactic acid levels continue to rise because of anaerobic glycolysis, in which the conversion of pyruvate to CO_2 and H_2O is impaired and the generation of CO_2 content in the blood is increased.[43] With the continued rise in lactic acid, HCO_3 is used to bind, millimole for millimole, with lactic acid. This process generates a need for exogenous sodium bicarbonate to replace the depleted HCO_3 level and to correct the metabolic disorder.

With inadequate perfusion, the blood levels of excretory products may build up because the flow of bile and urine may be inadequate to remove them. Blood amino acid levels increase because of deficient deamination as well as deficient excretion. Also, because urea synthesis by the liver is impaired, the blood ammonia level will increase. The α, β, and γ globulins

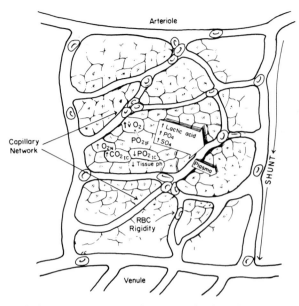

FIG. 21–16. Example of changes in the micro-vasculature in relation to inadequate perfusion. Some deleterious effects that accompany vasoconstriction and its maldistribution of flow are red cell rigidity, increased capillary permeability, edema, decreased tissue *pH*, and increased lactic acid production. Note the increased use of interstitial fluid PO_2 **($PO_{2_{IF}}$)** and the decreased intracellular PO_2 **($PO_{2_{IC}}$)**.

may increase while the albumin level may fall due to increased permeability. This increase in capillary permeability usually generates large losses of plasma into the extravascular spaces (Fig. 21–16). Increased permeability is believed to be due to capillary damage caused by the effect of increased tissue metabolites, in particular lactic acid. Poor perfusion can be diagramed as in Figure 21–17.

The consequences of lactic acidosis are significant. Lactic acidosis has been shown previously to impair the effects of catecholamines, to decrease intraventricular conduction, to decrease myocardial contractility, and to cause the loss of

the digitalis effect.[19–21, 44–46] During the rewarming phase of CPB, when blood flow is being reestablished into areas with no or poor perfusion, a lactic acid washout phenomena occurs. It should be pointed out that one can routinely monitor both arterial and venous blood lactic acid levels during CPB. The venous sample is particularly important in that it assesses the lactic acid washout phenomena very closely. The positive value of routine monitoring of blood lactate during CPB has been suggested.[40]

The information described previously outlines some of the metabolic conditions of the patient during CPB. The following section will present an actual technique to maintain perfusion during bypass. Without the use of the computer to accurately assess all of the associated variables, the goals of this technique, which are to maximize oxygen availability to the tissues and to ensure that no oxygen debt occurs, probably could not be realized.

A computer system quickly derives data using one of the formulas given in Table 21–2. Table 21–3 lists the normal ranges of these variables. Once a maximum calculated flow, utilizing a car-

TABLE 21–2
FORMULAS UTILIZED IN COMPUTER COMPUTATIONS

Arterial oxygen content (O_{2act})
$(1.34 \times HGB \times (AO_{2sat}/100)) + (.0031 \times$ temp corr $PaO_2)$
Venous oxygen content (O_{2vct})
$(1.34 \times HGB \times (AO_{2sat}/100)) + (.0031 \times$ temp corr $PaO_2)$
Arterial–venous oxygen content difference ($A\text{-}V_dO_2$)
$(O_{2act} - O_{2act})$
Oxygen consumption (VO_2)
$((A\text{-}V_dO_2 \times$ flow cc/min)/100)
Oxygen extraction ratio (%) (O_{2ex})
$(A\text{-}V_dO_2/O_{2act}) \times 100$
Oxygen availability (O_{2av})
$((O_{2act} \times$ flow liters/min) $\times 10)$
Peripheral resistance (mm Hg/ml/min)
$((MAP - CVP)/$flow cc/sec)
Body surface area (BSA m²)
$(WT kg^{.425}) \times (HT CM^{.725}) \times (.007184)$

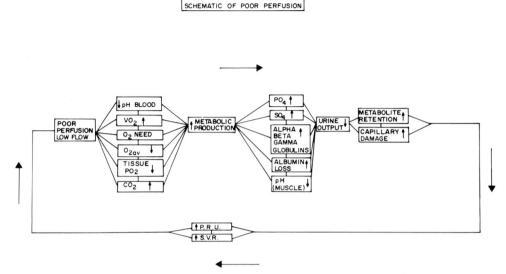

FIG. 21–17. *Schematic example of poor perfusion and its relational effects on body subsystems. Note the decreased oxygen availability (O$_{2av}$), increased oxygen consumption, and metabolite production.*

diac index of 2.4 liter/minute/m², is determined by the computer, calculations using the computer subroutine shown in Table 21–4 are made to determine the optimal mean arterial pressure and the acceptable mean arterial pressure range for the maximum calculated flow to obtain a vascular resistance of 0.9 to 1.1 mm Hg/ml/minute. Unlike conventional perfusion techniques, the bypass flow is held at a constant 2.4 liter/minute/m² even during hypothermia.

Arterial and venous blood gases are drawn 10 minutes after bypass begins and at 20-minute intervals thereafter. Blood gas samples are temperature-corrected to the arterial reservoir and venous return port temperatures, respectively. It is important that paired blood gas samples be evaluated. Without venous blood gas samples, it is impossible to accurately assess the patient's physiologic status. During bypass, A-V$_d$O$_2$, oxygen consumption, and the oxygen extraction ratio are usually lowered. At the same time, oxy-gen availability can be maintained and the systemic vascular resistance kept between 0.9 and 1.1 mm Hg/ml/minute. Because of the small range of tolerance, the resistance is constantly monitored at 10-minute intervals and more frequently if there is any trouble maintaining the resistances within the normal range. The vascular resistance is maintained within the normal range with the use of sodium nitroprusside or with Neo-Synephrine Hydrochloride.[19-22] The vascular resistance is lowered slightly below normal with nitroprusside if the oxygen consumption and A-V$_d$O$_2$ increase too quickly during rewarming. Nitroprusside dosages average 0.5 to 3 μg/kg/minute and are given as needed to adjust the resistances. The continuous computerized management of these variables easily enables the perfusionist to control and optimize the perfusion and delivery of oxygen to the tissues of the patient.

Figure 21–18 illustrates a typical case in which

TABLE 21–3
NORMAL RANGE OF VALUES FOR FORMULAS
LISTED IN TABLE 21–2

$O_{2act} = 18 - 20$ ml/100 ml
$O_{2vct} = 14 - 15$ ml/100 ml
$A-V_dO_2 = 4.25 - 5.25$ ml/100 ml
$VO_2 = 142 \pm 8$ ml/min
$O_{2ex} = 26 \pm 1\%$
$O_{2av} = 560 \pm 43$ ml/min
$PRU = 0.9 - 1.1$ mm Hg/ml/min

TABLE 21–4
COMPUTER SUBROUTINE FOR RESISTANCE
CALCULATIONS

```
1650 Print tab(20); ''=(Initial Bypass Data) = ''
1660 Maxflow = (BSA*2.4)
1670 Minflow = (BSA*2.0)
1680 Print tab(20); "Enter time (hh/mm/ss)": input times$
1690 Print
1700 Print tab(10); "calculated Maximum Flow:"; maxflow;
"L/min"
1710 Print tab(10); "Calculated Minimum Flow:"; minflow;
"L/min"
1712 RPM = (maxflow*1000)
1713 I = RPM
1715 For A = 0 to 110
1716 B = (I/60)
1717 C = (A/B)
1718 IF C < .9 then goto 1720
1719 Print tab(10); "Pressure mmHg = "; A; "Flow
cc/min = "; I; "PRU = ";C
1720 IF C > 1.1 then goto 1722
1721 Next A
1722 Next I
1725 Print
```

this computerized perfusion technique is used. It depicts the precise control of oxygen consumption, $A-V_dO_2$, and vascular resistances in an 89-kg male undergoing CPB for myocardial revascularization. During the procedure, a flow of 4.8 liters/minute was maintained. Vascular resistances were maintained relatively constant and averaged 0.97 mm Hg/ml/minute throughout the surgery. Nitroprusside was administered throughout the majority of the surgery. Initially, oxygen consumption during bypass was 145 ml/minute. During hypothermia, it dropped to 35 ml/minute, and at the end of bypass, it was 147 ml/minute. Initially, $A-V_dO_2$ during bypass was 3.1 ml/100 ml; during hypothermia, it dropped to 0.7 ml/100 ml; and at the end of bypass, it was 3.2 ml/100 ml. Oxygen consumption and $A-V_dO_2$ returned to normal postbypass because of the prevention of vascular bed constriction during CPB. In this process, increased blood flow and optimal oxygen availability and utilization occurred during surgery.

The values of other variables at the end of bypass nearly equaled the initial bypass levels. Lactic acid levels remained stable and never increased above 1.8 mmol/liter (normal 0.5 mmol to 2.5 mmol/liter), either intraoperatively or postoperatively. No sodium bicarbonate was required either intraoperatively or postoperatively. (Arbitrarily, sodium bicarbonate is administered if the base excess falls below −3.) It has been noted previously that a strict method of calculat-

ing an optimal bypass flow rate (*e.g.,* 2.4 liter/minute/m²) does not guarantee that the patient's metabolic requirements will be met.[5] It does, however, provide a constant value from which calculations and decisions, based on the accurately assessed metabolic requirements, can be made intraoperatively. Commonly, perfusionists alter flow rates up or down from the calculated flow during the course of bypass. There are disadvantages to using this technique, particularly when used to counter increasing arterial pressure. It has been shown that even small decreases of flow are reflected by diminished skeletal muscle PO_2 along with associated metabolic acidosis, increased lactic acid levels, and impaired liver function.[41,47–49] Many authors rationalize that during hypothermia, the maximum calculated flow is not required because of reduced metabolic needs. However logical it may seem, this approach may be less than ideal because of a perfusion-related deficiency, which causes defi-

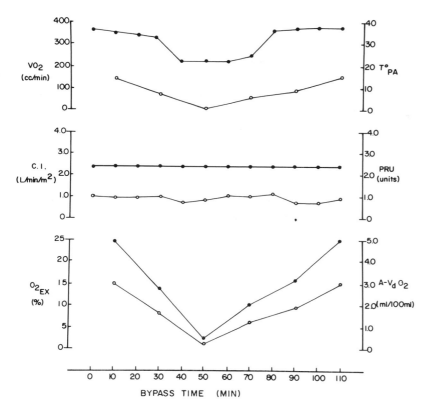

FIG. 21–18. The control of patients utilizing a computer to assess techniques is summarized in this typical bypass case. Filled circles represent pulmonary artery **(PA)** temperature, cardiac index **(C.I.)**, and oxygen extraction ratio **(O$_{2_{EX}}$)**. Open circles represent oxygen consumption **(VO$_2$)**, peripheral resistance **(PRU)**, and arteriovenous oxygen content difference **(A-V$_d$O$_2$)**. This illustration shows the precise control of this patient that resulted from constant assessment of important parameters. Of particular importance is the fact that no oxygen debt occurred, which is evidenced by the fact that these variables returned to initial bypass levels and the arterial and venous lactic acid levels never increased above the normal range.

ciencies in oxidative metabolism.

It may also be incorrect to assume that if there is a reasonable systemic arterial pressure, there is adequate tissue perfusion. As stated previously, when flow is reduced, peripheral vasoconstriction occurs. When vasoconstriction occurs, there is an increase in peripheral vascular resistance. An increase in peripheral resistance will tend to maintain an arterial pressure in the presence of a falling blood flow.[13] When vasoconstriction is present, there is maldistribution of flow and there will be areas that are not being adequately perfused.[50] The cellular components in these underperfused areas utilize all of the available oxygen within the cells and the interstitial fluid, causing oxygen debt, an increase in CO_2, a decrease in tissue pH, an increase in lactic acid pro-

duction, and generally a need for sodium bicarbonate. If sodium bicarbonate is required, either intraoperatively or postoperatively, then optimal perfusion has not been attained.

Utilizing the constant assessment of oxygen consumption, A-V$_d$O$_2$, and vascular resistance, it is possible to avoid oxygen debt, metabolic acidosis, and the need to administer sodium bicarbonate. By routinely computerizing these variables, it is possible to attain optimal perfusion, optimal oxygen delivery, and utilization during CPB.

MATHEMATICAL COMPUTATIONS

One of the most useful elements of support provided by computerization during bypass is the computers' ability to do multiple complex calculations at an incredible rate. Many of today's computers can perform 3 million bits of calculations per second. The routine calculations used during bypass include body surface area (BSA), blood volume, blood flow, blood gas temperature correction, urine output, drug dosages, vascular resistances, and oxygen indices such as oxygen consumption, A-V$_d$O$_2$, oxygen extraction, oxygen availability, oxygen transfer. In a typical 90-minute CPB case, by incorporating all of the complex calculations normally done by hand or pocket calculator, we have found that one can reduce recording and calculation time from 47% to 8% (unpublished observation). This dramatic reduction in the time required for recording and calculation allows the perfusionist to have more time to watch the oxygenator and to make more sound clinical decisions based on more available data.

With the advent of the vast number of calculations now available to the perfusionist, many new and important parameters can be constantly monitored, corrected, and changed accordingly. Because of this ability, a patient can be monitored more closely. In addition, the perfusionist can observe the subtle changes that can and do occur during bypass.

LIMIT DETECTION

Limit detection through use of a computer offers a tremendous monitoring advantage both to the perfusionist practitioner and to students of perfusion technology. Setting limits within the computer program (*e.g.*, a PCO$_2$ value is too high) allows the computer to flash this value repeatedly to the perfusionist, instantly calling attention to it and making sure that an effort is made to return the value to normal. Along with limit-detection mechanisms, normal-range values can be placed on the screen to remind or teach in certain situations.

AUTOMATIC DATA COLLECTION

Automated data collection is probably the ultimate in patient management during cardiopulmonary bypass, and even postoperatively. However, this system is also the most difficult to achieve. Table 21–5 shows a typical flow pattern for data in an automated collection system. One of the major advantages of real-time/on-line data collection is that data are collected, manipulated, and stored at the exact times specified in the programming, unlike manual entry, in which many functions can be occurring at once, and entries can be missed or late in time sequences. A typical configuration of real-time processing is shown in Figure 21–19. One of the most difficult problems in setting up a real-time system is getting appropriate analog or digital information from all of the different vendors of monitoring devices. However, many of the manufacturers are beginning to realize the importance of having an RS-232 access port on their equipment. An RS-232 port is a device that allows the computer to gain access into the monitoring device to sam-

TABLE 21–5
FLOW PATTERN OF DATA IN AN AUTOMATED DATA COLLECTION SYSTEM

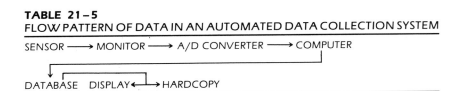

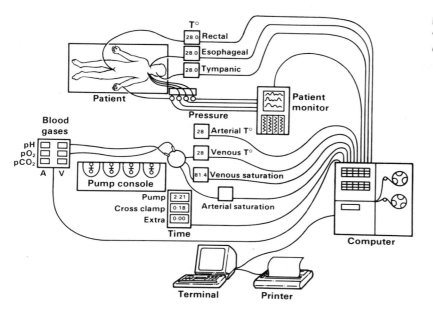

FIG. 21–19. Some of the various data sites utilized in capturing real-time data.

ple data from it. However, data collection without centralization and automation is an absolute nightmare! In any typical open-heart suite, recording, sampling, and informational devices are scattered all over the room. This creates tremendous distractions for the perfusionist and other professionals as well. By centralizing all of the data on one screen located in front of the perfusionist, for example, safety has been increased and risk has been decreased.[51] With the tremendous graphics capabilities of many computers, the display of user-friendly information can be practically unlimited.

CONCLUSION

Computer-assisted bypass management is becoming increasingly accessible. More general applicability occurs, particularly when it is coupled with other computer systems that allow the physician to follow the patient from admission through cardiac catheterization, surgery, intensive care, and floor care with subsequent yearly follow-up. Perfusion technology has grown by bounding leaps in the past few years. Perfusionists should no longer fly by the seats of their pants because the art of perfusion is giving way to a more exacting science. Without the aid of the computer, excellence in the management of patients undergoing cardiac surgery might never be accomplished.

REFERENCES

1. Galletti PM, Brecher GA: Heart Lung Bypass: Principles and Techniques of Extracorporeal Circulation, pp 213–222. New York, Grune & Stratton, 1962
2. Clark LC: Optimal flow rate in perfusion. In Allen JG (ed): Extracorporeal Perfusion, pp 150–163. Springfield, Illinois, Charles C Thomas, 1958
3. Nose Y: Manual on Artificial Organs. Vol II: The Oxygenator, p 237. St. Louis, CV Mosby, 1973
4. Reed CC, Clark DK: Cardiopulmonary Perfusion, p 306. Houston, Texas Medical Press, 1975

5. Mandl JP, Motley JR: Oxygen consumption plateauing: A better method of achieving optimum perfusion. J Extracorp Tech 11(2):69–77, 1979

6. Bagby E: An extracorporeal flow formula for all patients. J Extracorp Tech 11(3):101–106, 1979

7. Stanley TH, Isern–Amaral J: Mixed venous oxygen tension: A simple metabolic monitor of adequacy of perfusion during cardiopulmonary bypass. Amsect Proc 11:41, 1974

8. Vetto RR, Winterschied LC, Merendino KA: Studies in the physiology of oxygen consumption during cardiopulmonary bypass. Surg Forum IX:163, 1958

9. Starr A: Oxygen consumption during cardiopulmonary bypass. J Thorac Cardiovasc Surg 38(1):46, 1959

10. Simmons DH, Alpas AP, Tashkin DP, Coulson A: Hyperlactatemia due to arterial hypoxemia or reduced cardiac output or both. J Appl Physiol 45(2):195–202, August 1978

11. Daniel A, Alan D, Cohen J et al: The relationship among arterial oxygen flow rate, oxygen binding by hemoglobin and oxygen utilization in chronic cardiac decompensation. J Lab Clin Med 91(4):635–649 April 1978

12. Kiecberg J, Gitelson S: A study of blood pyruvic acid levels in patients with congestive heart failure. J Clin Pathol 7:116, 1954

13. Shoemaker WC: Hemodynamics and oxygen transport patterns of common shock syndromes. Proceedings of a Symposium on Recent Research Developments and Current Clinical Practices in Shock. Sponsored by the Upjohn Company, Baltimore, MD, 1974

14. Hickey RF, Hoar PE: Whole-body oxygen consumption during low-flow hypothermic cardiopulmonary bypass. J Thorac Cardiovasc Surg 86:903–906, 1983

15. Shoemaker WC, Reinhard JM: Tissue perfusion defects in shock and trauma states. Surg Gynecol Obstet 137:980–986, 1973

16. Shoemaker WC: Shock in low and high flow states. In Forscher BK, Lillehei RC, Stubbs SS (eds): Exerpta Medica, pp 119–130. Amsterdam. 1972

17. Stainsby WN, Otis AB: Blood flow, blood oxygen tension, oxygen uptake and oxygen transport in skeletal muscle. Am J Physiol 206:858–866, 1964

18. Kasnitz P, Druger GL, Yorra F, Simmons DH: Mixed venous oxygen tension and hyperlactatemia. Survival in severe cardiopulmonary disease. JAMA 236:570–574, 1976

19. Kurusz M, Christman EW, Arens JF, Tyson KR: Sodium nitroprusside as an adjunct to pediatric perfusion. J Extracorp Tech 11(5):189–194, 1979

20. Miller RR, Vismara LA, Zelis R et al: Clinical use of sodium nitroprusside in chronic ischemic heart disease. Circulation 51:328–336, 1975

21. Suzuki M, Penn I: The effect of therapeutic agents upon the microcirculation during general hypothermia. Surgery 60:867–878, 1966

22. Lappas DG, Lowenstein E, Waller J et al: Hemodynamic effects of nitroprusside infusion during coronary operation in man. Circulation (Suppl III) 54:4–10, 1976

23. Weil MH, Shubin H, Rand W: Experience with a digital computer for study and improved management of the critically ill. JAMA 198:1011–1016, 1966

24. Glaeser DH, Thomas LJ: Computer monitoring in patient care. Annual Review of Biophysics and Bioengineering, Vol 1, pp 449–476. California Annual Reviews, Inc, 1972

25. Cox JR, Nolle FM, Fozzard HA, Oliver GC: AZTEC, A preprocessing program for real time ECG rhythm analysis. IEEE Trans Biomed Eng 15:128–129, 1968

26. Osborn JJ, Beaumont JO, Ratson JS, Abbot, RP: Computation for quantitative on line measurements in an intensive care ward. Comp Biomed Res 3:207–237, 1969

27. Russel RP, Rackley CE: Hemodynamic Monitoring in a Coronary Intensive Care Unit. Mount Kisco, New York, Futura Publishing, 1974

28. Tompkins WJ: A portable microcomputer based system for biomedical applications. Biomed Sci Instrum 14:60–66, 1978

29. Bushman JA: The use of computers in the care of the acutely ill, pp 167–170. In Payne JP, Hill DW (eds): Real Time Computing in Patient Management. Steven, G. E., Eng Peregrinus, 1976, WB 141, R228, 1975

30. Sheppard LC, Kouchoukos NT, Kurtts MA, Kirklin JW: Automated treatment of critically ill patients following operation. Ann Surg 168:596–604, 1968

31. Osborn JJ, Beaumont JO: Computerized intensive care: Data processing. Hospitals 44:49, 1970

32. Mollison DR, Streczyn MV: In depth evaluation of arterial line filtration of air emboli in bubbler and membrane oxygenators. Am SECT Proceedings 4:99–112, 1976

33. Riley JB, Snyder JE: A technique for extrapolation of analyzed values of blood pH, PCO_2 and PO_2 to hypothermic states. J Extracorp Tech 9(2):86–95, 1977

34. Davis J: Flow bench for the evaluation of thermal dilution cardiac output computer. J Extracorp Tech 9(4):187–195, 1977

35. Streczyn MV: Gas emboli arterial line filtration efficiencies of the pall and J-J filters under stress conditions. Am SECT Proceedings 5:6–17, 1977

36. Abts LR, Beyer RT, Karlson KE et al: Low heparin levels and microemboli effects on the Johnson and Johnson arterial line filter. Am SECT Proceedings, 5:18–22, 1977

37. Riley JB, O'Kane KC: A computer simulation of maintaining total heart lung bypass for basic education. Am SECT Proceedings 5:42–49, 1977

38. Rose EA, Haubert SM, Spotnitz HM: Programmable pocket calculator and cardiopulmonary bypass. J Extracorp Tech 12(1):19–23, 1980

39. Holdt DW, Mandl JP: A new pumpside aid for decision making: The pocket programmable calculator. J Extracorp Tech 12(1):19–23, 1980

40. Hankins T: Computer Assisted Bypass Management J Extracorp Tech 12(4):95–102, 1980

41. Furuse A, Brawley RK, Struve E, Gott VL: Skeletal muscle gas tension: Indicator of cardiac output and peripheral tissue perfusion. Surgery 74(2):214–222, 1973

42. Berman HJ: Clinical applications of microcirculation research in cardiovascular dynamics. In Baan J, Noordergraaf A, Raines J: Cardiovascular System Dynamics, pp 232–244. Cambridge, Massachusetts, MIT Press, 1978

43. Fine J: Shock and peripheral circulatory insufficiency. Handbook of Physiology, pp 2037–2069. In Dow P, Hamilton WF (eds): Baltimore, Waverly Press, 1965

44. Campbell GS, Houle DB, Crisp NW et al: Depressed response to intravenous sympathicometric amines in humans during acidosis. Chest 33:18, 1958

45. Smith LL, Moore FP: Refractory hypotension in man—Is this irreversible shock? New Engl J Med 267:733, 1962

46. Sutherland GW, Robinson GA: The role of cyclic-3',5'AMP in response to catecholamines and other hormones. Pharmacol Res Commun 18:145, 1966

47. Crafoord C, Norberg B, Senning A: Clinical studies in extracorporeal circulation with a heart-lung machine. Acta Chir Scand 112:220, 1957

48. Wall RA, Warden HE, Gott VL et al: Total body perfusion for open cardiotomy utilizing the bubble oxygenator. J Thorac Cardiovasc Surg, 32:591, 1956

49. Anderson M, Senning A: Studies in oxygen consumption during extracorporeal circulation with a pump oxygenator. Ann Surg 148(1):59–65, 1958

50. Couch NP, Dmochowski JR, Van De Water JM et al: Muscle surface pH as an index of peripheral perfusion in man. Ann Surg 173(2):173–183, 1971

51. Riley JB, Hurdle MB, Winn BA, Wagoner PA: Automation of cardiopulmonary bypass data collection J Extracorp Tech 17(1):7–12, 1985

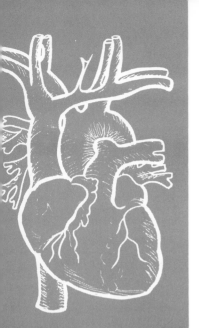

22

CARDIAC ANESTHESIA

Nathaniel Sims

Judy O'Young

Daniel M. Philbin

GOALS FOR THE ANESTHESIOLOGIST

Rapid and profound changes in anesthesia and surgery in the past 40 years have led to the development of cardiac anesthesia as a subspeciality. This has been dictated by the need for the anesthesiologist involved in the care of cardiac patients to synthesize information from pharmacology and physiology, and clinical knowledge of heart diseases and anesthetic techniques. This should allow the anesthesiologist to complete the following:

1. *Assess* the patient preoperatively, with determination of anesthetic considerations for induction and intraoperative and postoperative management.
2. Formulate a *plan of anesthetic management,* anticipating likely problems in view of the particular hemodynamic disorder involved.
3. *Institute monitoring,* in the preinduction period, of sufficient sophistication to enable accurate, continuing assessment of cardiovascular performance. Monitoring must be adequate to permit prompt recognition and treatment of failure or ischemia, which may occur following surgical manipulation in the preoperative or postbypass period.
4. *Induce surgical anesthesia* and maintain it without adversely affecting the patient's hemodynamics.
5. Participate effectively in the *management of cardiopulmonary bypass,* with particular attention to adequacy of venous drainage, myocardial protection, pump flow, perfusion pressure, and renal function at appropriate times.

6. Have *strategies* for the following:
   a. Dealing safely with *changes in sympathetic (particularly vasomotor) tone* related to induction of anesthesia.
   b. Treating episodes of ischemia, arrhythmias, or failure by precise management of heart rate, right and left heart preload, coronary perfusion pressure, and myocardial contractility.
   c. *Protection* of the *brain* and *kidney* during cardiopulmonary bypass, and of the *spinal cord* during cross-clamping for surgery on the thoracic aorta.
   d. Management of rare complications such as drug reactions, lung injury resulting in severe bronchospasm, and pulmonary hypertension.
7. Institute *postoperative management* through the period of rewarming and ventilatory support.

HISTORY

The achievement of the goals described above is made more challenging by changes in the population and preoperative conditions of patients undergoing cardiac surgery.

The population for elective surgery has more severe cardiac disease and is older, with a higher incidence of preoperative renal, carotid, and other systemic disease. Antianginal therapy has improved, percutaneous coronary transluminal angioplasty has a high success rate, and the indications for coronary artery bypass grafting (CABG) are more limited. Thus most patients undergoing operation, at least for CABG, have severe three-vessel disease with compromised left ventricular function and often rest angina with maximal therapy.

There is a large group of patients undergoing operation with acute hemodynamic instability, including a population of patients who required preoperative intra-aortic balloon counterpulsation for treatment of ischemia, and a group of patients undergoing operation for emergent CABG following failed percutaneous transluminal coronary angioplasty.

There are more patients undergoing reoperation after prior CABG or prior valve replacement. These patients often have significant hemodynamic compromise, and yet the interval between the induction of anesthesia and the institution of cardiopulmonary bypass can be long. With the heart inaccessible for pacing or other intervention, far more demand is placed on the anesthesiologist for management.

New operations including transplants, automatic internal defibrillator placement, and arrhythmia surgery have appeared, and in the pediatric area, early total correction of congenital heart disease has taken precedence over palliation.

It is fortunate, then, in view of these new challenges, that the anesthesiologist's armamentarium has been augmented by a variety of new techniques, new medications, and fresh approaches to certain difficult problems. We will describe a few of these below.

PREOPERATIVE EVALUATION

VALVULAR HEART DISEASE

Aortic Stenosis. Patients with critical aortic stenosis and congestive heart failure have abnormalities of contractile function and require an anesthetic that minimizes myocardial depression. This can be achieved with narcotic-oxygen–relaxant techniques. There are many factors that predispose the aortic stenosis patient to ischemic events, including left ventricular hypertrophy, elevated wall tension during systole, shortened time for diastolic coronary perfusion, low coronary perfusion pressure, and occasionally coexistent coronary disease. Because of this, maintenance of systemic blood pressure and precise control of heart rate are essential for preservation of coronary perfusion. Inadvertent sympatholysis during induction of anesthesia must be treated early and aggressively using norepinephrine or phenylephrine infusions. Heart rate should be maintained at the preinduction rate, because tachycardia will cause ischemia and bradycardia will cause systemic hypotension due to the rate-dependence (fixed stroke volume) of cardiac output. Avoidance of tachycardia is challenging because these patients are usually not receiving beta blockers. In addition, sinus rhythm must be maintained, because ventricular filling is highly dependent on left atrial contraction. The facility for rapid direct current cardioversion and for pacing capability must be immediately available. Finally, filling pressures must be maintained, guided by measurement of left-sided filling pressures.

Mitral Stenosis. A mean left atrial pressure of up to 25 mm Hg to 30 mm Hg may be required to maintain an acceptable cardiac output at rest. "Reactive" pulmonary hypertension may be present, with varying degrees of right ventricular enlargement, failure, and tricuspid insufficiency. The most important considerations are maintenance of a slow heart rate, which will maintain left ventricular filling, and avoidance of any factors (hypercarbia, acidosis, vasoconstrictors) that may exacerbate pulmonary hypertension. Thus preoperative continuation of digoxin for rate control in atrial fibrillation, avoidance of vagolytic drugs, and a smooth transition from spontaneous to positive pressure ventilation are essential. It should be recognized that these patients can be extremely sensitive to narcotic premedication.

Aortic Insufficiency. Volume overload of the left ventricle occurs in both acute and chronic aortic insufficiency. In chronic cases, the ventricle has acquired high diastolic compliance and is well adapted to high volumes; in acute cases, the ventricle is operating on the steep noncompliant portion of the pressure–volume curve. The anesthetic priority is to control heart rate and systemic vascular resistance. Increases in heart rate are beneficial, because diastolic time is shortened and the degree of regurgitation per beat decreases. Similarly, the regurgitant fraction will be decreased by careful afterload reduction; this should be done in conjunction with pulmonary artery pressure monitoring for adjustment of preload.

Mitral Insufficiency. Mitral insufficiency may occur on a structural basis (prosthetic-valve failure, rheumatic) or as a consequence of ischemia, leading to left ventricular dilatation and/or papillary muscle dysfunction. Anesthetic considerations will vary depending on the cause and duration in a particular patient, but in general, as for aortic insufficiency, control of heart rate and systemic vascular resistance are essential, using the size of the V wave in the pulmonary capillary wedge (PCW) tracing as an index of the degree of regurgitation. Increases in heart rate and decreases in systemic vascular resistance will reduce the regurgitant fraction. In addition, if ischemia is a factor in causing mitral insufficiency, both preload reduction (to reduce ventricular size) and measures to improve perfusion are useful. It may be difficult to determine the relative hazards and benefits of afterload reduction versus maintenance of perfusion pressure; intra-aortic balloon counterpulsation achieves both during every cardiac cycle and may be required preoperatively.

Coronary Artery Disease. The patient with severe coronary artery disease, with or without prior myocardial infarction or depressed ejection fraction, may manifest ischemia in a variety of ways. The ventricle may be noncompliant and may respond to increases in preload by dilating, with increases in wedge pressure or with the appearance of V waves in the wedge tracing. Alternatively, ischemia, especially if it is due to tachycardia, may manifest as changes on the electrocardiogram (ECG). Because there is ample reason to believe that perioperative ischemic events are associated with infarction, it is essential that the anesthesiologist have the ability to detect them, which usually requires a pulmonary artery catheter. The hemodynamic goals include aggressive control, primarily, of heart rate, and, secondarily, of blood pressure, contractility, and coronary perfusion pressure. Patients with medically refractory angina will require preoperative intra-aortic balloon counterpulsation, provided the aortic valve is competent.

PREOPERATIVE PREPARATION

Appropriate preoperative assessment and management of the patient's psychological, physiologic, and pharmacologic condition is crucial for the best intraoperative management and outcome. It is essential that evaluation be thorough and complete prior to surgery and that qualified consultants be asked to assist in this process. Of equal importance is preoperative patient and family teaching with the use of audiovisual aids and discussion by clinical specialists.

PREMEDICATION

The purpose of preoperative medication is to decrease anxiety, to produce amnesia, and to reduce stress on the cardiovascular system, thus preventing an increase in myocardial oxygen demand. Anxiety and postoperative pain are further reduced by a careful and thorough preoperative discussion with the anesthesiologist. The maximum sedation possible without further cardiorespiratory depression is used. For patients with ischemic heart disease, our approach is to give morphine sulfate (0.1 mg/kg intramuscularly), and scopolamine (0.3 mg to 0.4 mg intramuscularly) 1 hour prior to induction. Occasionally, lorazepam (1 mg to 2 mg PO) is added. Other drug combinations can be equally effective in preventing anxiety and catecholamine-induced increases in afterload and heart rate. For patients with severe heart failure or valvular disease, dosages are reduced or, in some cases, eliminated.

PERIOPERATIVE MEDICATION WITHDRAWAL

Perioperative medications must be reviewed and the effects of their withdrawal evaluated. In general, all antihypertensive medications should be continued up to and including the morning of surgery. Oral nitrates and nitropaste, calcium channel blockers, and beta blockers are continued until the time of surgery. The potential for adverse interactions of these medications with anesthesia exists but such interactions do not commonly occur. It should be noted that patients receiving large doses of beta and calcium channel blockers may require more inotropic support; however, patients maintained on nifedipine are less likely to experience a "rebound" increase in systemic vascular resistance and to require vasodilators. Sudden discontinuation of propranolol may be hazardous in patients with ischemic disease who are receiving chronic therapy. Digitalis is discontinued at least two half-lives before surgery to eliminate digitalis toxicity as a possible cause of perioperative arrhythmias. Exceptions to this include patients with valvular disease and atrial fibrillation, with ventricular responses in excess of 80 beats per minute and severe heart failure. Diuretics result in electrolyte and intravascular volume depletion, which can exacerbate intraoperative hemodynamic instability. We, therefore, if possible, discontinue diuretics 2 days before surgery and administer additional oral potassium as needed, recognizing that the patient may still be totally potassium depleted. Aspirin and other antiplatelet drugs affect platelet function without decreasing their number. Patients should not take any aspirin-containing compounds for at least 10 days prior to surgery to allow for a complete regeneration of the platelet population. Moreover, a normal bleeding time does not necessarily ensure normal platelet function.

MONITORING

Monitors employed in the intraoperative management of cardiac surgical patients provide an indication of variations from the expected and allow immediate feedback after interventions have been made. Primary concerns are the prompt and early recognition of ischemia, the quantitation of volume status, and the ability to gauge organ perfusion. Minimum monitoring includes temperature, two ECG leads, arterial pressure, central venous pressure, and urine output. Pulmonary artery catheters (with pacing capability, when needed) are used in the majority of patients, as are surgically placed left atrial catheters. Pulse oximeters are extremely helpful, particularly in patients with systemic desaturation caused by congenital heart disease. Transesophageal echocardiography is used occasionally.

We favor the use of a multichannel oscilloscope with a strip chart recorder in the operating room. The tracing of arterial, pulmonary artery, central venous (and, when indicated, left atrial) pressures, together with two ECG leads and the output of a heart-rate counter, are recorded on eight-channel paper. The actual values of intravascular pressures are taken from the paper tracing or are estimated from a calibrated screen, rather than read from a digital display. Whenever possible, intravascular tracings are displayed as phasic signals, so that the maximum amount of qualitative information can be derived from observation of A, C, and V waves. The creation of a permanent paper record of each case is done routinely at minimal inconvenience and serves as a guide for intervention, as an indicator of trends, as a permanent record, and as a vehicle for teaching and for "quality control" of anesthetic practice.

Other points with regard to monitoring are as follows:

Electrocardiogram: A multiple-lead system is necessary to detect ischemia, conduction abnormalities, and arrhythmias. Leads II and V_5 should be monitored simultaneously to detect inferior and anterolateral changes. Posterior ischemia will be undetected by this system.

Pulmonary artery catheters: We insert pulmonary artery catheters percutaneously from the internal jugular vein preoperatively in the awake, sedated patient just prior to induction of anesthesia. This allows us to obtain a full hemodynamic profile as a baseline prior to induction and to have full monitoring during induction of anesthesia.

Left atrial catheters: Left atrial catheters permit precise adjustment of filling pressures in critically ill postbypass patients. They serve as a backup in the event that the pulmonary artery catheter fails to wedge postoperatively, and they can be used for infusion of vasoactive agents into the systemic circulation.

INDUCTION OF ANESTHESIA

TECHNIQUES

Once the anesthesiologist has assessed the patient, formulated a list of anesthetic considerations, and established satisfactory monitoring/pacing, anesthesia is induced. Drugs (narcotic and/or inhalational) must be administered incrementally and their adequacy tested with a series of graded stimuli. The transition from spontaneous to positive pressure ventilation is made carefully, especially when tamponade or constrictive pericarditis exists. The graded stimuli indicate the need for either laryngoscopy and endotracheal intubation, and the hemodynamic effect of each maneuver is ascertained. Alterations in sympathetic tone (usually vasodilation) due to the anesthetic are treated, and corrections of heart rate, preload, and contractile state are made. Intermittent high-speed recordings of the pressure tracings and ECG and measurement of cardiac output aid in the assessment of both the stimuli and the treatment.

CHOICE OF ANESTHETIC AGENTS

There are no recipes for anesthetic technique and no mandatory drugs in cardiac anesthesia. Skill and knowledge are the basic requirements. Generally, it is our practice to use narcotic–oxygen relaxants, adding volatile anesthetics when vasodilation or controlled depression of contractility is needed. The use of volatile agents as the sole anesthetic during cardiac surgery is much less common and somewhat controversial. Similarly, the use of nitrous oxide is generally avoided, particularly in the immediate postbypass period. The narcotics fentanyl, sufentanil, alfentanil, and morphine appear to be benign with respect to myocardial metabolism and circulation, and have their advantages and disadvantages in terms of effects on autonomic tone, heart rate, histamine release, and chest wall rigidity. These effects can often be exploited to enhance hemodynamic performance in a particular patient. Similarly, newer muscle relaxants that have minimal hemodynamic effects are available, and others whose effects on heart rate or histamine release can be utilized to advantage also are available.

MANAGEMENT OF CARDIOPULMONARY BYPASS

Although the responsibility for the management of cardiopulmonary bypass is shared, the anesthesiologist has several responsibilities. These include but are not limited to the following:

1. Assessing the adequacy of venous drainage of the head and upper extremities, by examining the patient frequently and transducing the central venous pressure cephalad to the superior vena caval tourniquet.
2. Judging adequacy of myocardial protection by close observation of the ECG for recurrence of fibrillatory waves.
3. Ensuring that adequate heparinization has been achieved prior to and during the period of bypass.
4. Monitoring the early onset of left ventricular distention prior to and after the institution of left ventricular venting. If a left atrial line is not present prior to bypass, mean pulmonary artery pressure may suffice.
5. Ensuring that adequate flow and perfusion pressures are maintained.
6. Monitoring renal function and perfusion by means of urine output and administering osmotic or other diuretics as indicated, or low-dose (1 μg to 3 μg/kg/minute) dopamine.
7. Ensuring that adequate muscle relaxation exists to prevent the increase in oxygen consumption that would be associated with shivering during rewarming.
8. Assisting the perfusionist in interpreting acid–base status during hypothermia. In most centers during the early 1980s, a transition was made to the use of "uncorrected" arterial blood gases, the practical effect of this change is that carbon dioxide is no longer routinely added to the pump during rewarming.

SEPARATION FROM CARDIOPULMONARY BYPASS

Prior to separation from bypass, the anesthesiologist, working together with the surgeon and perfusionist, must anticipate the need for infusion of vasoactive drugs, if any, for modification of contractility and/or vasomotor tone; consider use of a left atrial drug line for catecholamines, if pulmonary hypertension is expected to be a problem; evaluate cardiac rhythm and the ECG and, if necessary, establish atrial or AV sequential pacing with the appropriate rate and intervals; determine that lung compliance changes have not occurred while the patient has been on bypass; and ensure that rewarming is adequate.

The process of separation from bypass involves progressive occlusion of venous return until an appropriate filling pressure is reached for the particular patient. Pump flow into the arterial perfuser is simultaneously reduced, and when the pump is off, visual inspection of the heart, comparison of left- and right-side filling pressures, evaluation of pulmonary arterial and systemic pressures, and measurement of cardiac output, acid–base status, and oxygenation will provide direction for subsequent therapy. If, as occasionally occurs, there is an element of right ventricular failure and/or pulmonary hypertension in association with systemic hypotension, infusion of drugs into the right and left sides of the circulation separately may be of immense benefit.

POSTBYPASS AND POSTOPERATIVE MANAGEMENT

Following separation of the patient from cardiopulmonary bypass, it is important that the following steps be taken:

1. Confirmation of adequate reversal of anticoagulation using quantitative measures such as activated coagulation time (ACT), prothrombin time (PT), partial prothrombin time (PTT), and thrombin time (TT).
2. Assessment of cardiac performance using intermittent determinations of cardiac output, left- and right-side filling pressures, and pulmonary artery pressures. Volume status must be assessed continuously. This is especially important immediately prior to and immediately after chest closure, so that the effect of this maneouver on cardiac performance can be documented, and so that the rate of infusion of vasoactive drugs can be appropriately regulated.
3. Aggressive therapy of atelectasis (often denoted by the appearance of a gradient between the pulmonary artery diastolic pressure and mean PCW pressure) and of bronchospasm and air trapping, because lung dysfunction during this period can adversely affect cardiac filling, and pulmonary hypertension can be detrimental to right ventricular function.

Finally, upon arrival in the intensive care unit, the anesthesiologist should ensure that the following procedures have been implemented:

An adequate dose of narcotic, appropriate to the expected duration of continued rewarming

A minute ventilation that is appropriate to the metabolic activity expected at the patient's temperature

Positive end-expiratory pressure (PEEP) settings that are appropriate to the patient's hemodynamics

Adequate muscle relaxant to prevent the sudden increases in oxygen consumption that may be associated with shivering

Preparation of personnel to manage the changes in vascular tone of both resistance and capacitance vessels that will occur both with rewarming and with return of sympathetic tone

SPECIAL PROBLEMS

TREATMENT OF INTRAOPERATIVE ISCHEMIA/FAILURE

The anesthesiologist has a variety of options available for the treatment of intraoperative ischemia or failure because volatile and intravenous anesthetic agents can be combined with other therapies. In the anesthetized patient, the appearance of ECG changes, elevations of PCW pressure, or V waves in the PCW tracing are sensitive indices. Assessment begins with confirmation that acid–base status, oxygenation, and ventilation are satisfactory. Cardiac output, and pulmonary artery, central venous, and PCW pressures must be measured to identify right or left ventricular dysfunction. The anesthesiologist must then judge whether the problem is due primarily to any of the following conditions:

Tachycardia, in which case the treatment options include beta blockade; narcotics with vagotonic effect, such as fentanyl; or volatile agents, such as halothane, which slow the heart rate.

Left ventricular distention due to low diastolic compliance, in which case preload reduction with nitroglycerin may be indicated.

Inadequate perfusion pressure due to the effect of sympatholysis on the tone of resistance vessels, which may respond to phenylephrine infusion.

Enhanced contractility as a result of intense sympathetic stimulation, causing an imbalance between myocardial oxygen demand and supply. This may be treated best by achieving reversible, controlled depression of contractility, using beta blockers or volatile anesthetics.

Coronary artery spasm, which may respond to intravenous nitroglycerin and/or calcium channel blockers.

Successful therapy of ischemia/failure in a particular patient may sometimes require several simultaneous therapies. Combinations of propranolol, fentanyl, nitroglycerin, phenylephrine, and halothane occasionally are required.

MANAGEMENT OF SEVERE PULMONARY HYPERTENSION FOLLOWING CARDIOPULMONARY BYPASS

Severe pulmonary hypertension leading to life-threatening right ventricular failure may occur occasionally following cardiopulmonary bypass. It most commonly occurs in patients undergoing mitral valve replacement, especially those with preoperative congestive heart failure and/or pulmonary hypertension; and in patients who have had drug reactions or reactions to transfused blood prior to or during bypass, all resulting in alterations in pulmonary vascular resistance. A variety of therapeutic modalities, including inotropic agents, vasodilators, high-dose steroids, and intra-aortic or intrapulmonary artery balloon counterpulsation, have been tried with less than satisfactory results. An alternative therapy has evolved; it is a technique that combines the pulmonary vasodilatory effects of prostoglandin E_1, which is infused into the pulmonary circulation, with support of systemic pressure using norepinephrine, which is given

through a left atrial line. This technique takes advantage of rapid metabolism of prostaglandin E_1 during its first pass through the lungs (thus minimizing the drug's systemic hypotensive effect), avoids a bolus effect of norepinephrine on the pulmonary vasculature, and utilizes the systemic capillary bed's capacity to remove some of the norepinephrine before returning to the right ventricle.

SPINAL CORD PROTECTION

The anesthesiologist dealing with cardiac surgical patients will be involved in the management of patients having potential central nervous system (CNS) ischemic insults. These occur during aortic cross-clamping for repair of coarctation, during repair of traumatic interruptions of the descending thoracic aorta, or when interruption of carotid blood flow is necessary for surgery on the aortic arch. Two traditional roles for the anesthesiologist during such periods are to ensure that at least mild systemic hypothermia is achieved and that perfusion pressure is adequate to maximize collateral blood flow to the CNS. To these has been added a third modality — intravenous administration of magnesium prior to the ischemic event. Studies in rabbits have shown that administration of 5 mmol/kg of $MgCl_2$ (a dose sufficient to produce neuromuscular blockade) in combination with a 3°C reduction in systemic temperature caused a threefold increase in the duration of ischemia, which could be sustained before irreversible damage ocurred in a rabbit spinal cord ischemia model. The potential benefit for this in humans is yet to be determined.

SUMMARY

Anesthetic considerations can and must be formulated for each individual patient based on a sound understanding of pathophysiology. Safe anesthetic techniques can be designed to optimize cardiac performance during the critical pre- and postbypass periods and should be guided by aggressive monitoring of critical hemodynamic parameters. The variety of new pharmacologic interventions and monitoring devices available makes this possible.

SELECTED REFERENCES

Angelini P, Feldman MI, Lufschanowski R et al: Cardiac arrhythmias during and after heart surgery. Prog Cardiovasc Dis 16:469, 1974

Arkins R, Smessaert AA, Hicks RG: Mortality and morbidity in surgical patients with coronary artery disease. JAMA 190:455–458, 1964

Beaupre PN, Kremer PF, Cahalan MK et al: Intraoperative detection of changes in left ventricular segmental wall motion by transesophageal 2D echocardiography. Am Heart J 107:1021–1023, 1984

Cohn PF, Gorlin R, Cohn LH et al: Left ventricular ejection fraction as a prognostic guide in surgical treatment of coronary and valvular heart disease. Am J Cardiol 34:136, 1979

Dalton B: A precordial ECG lead for chest operations. Anesth Analg 55:740–741, 1976

D'Ambra MN, LaRaia PJ, Philbin DM et al: Prostaglandin E_1 (PGE$_1$): A new therapy for refractory right heart failure and pulmonary hypertension after mitral valve replacement. J Thorac Cardiovasc Surg 88:965–971, 1985

Foex P: Postoperative assessment of patients with cardiac disease. Br J Anaesth 50:15–22, 1978

Goldman L, Caldera DL, Nussbaum R et al: Multifactorial index of cardiac risk in noncardiac surgical procedures. N Engl J Med 297:845–850, 1977

Lowenstein E, Foex P, Francis CM et al: Regional ischemic ventricular dysfunction in myocardium supplied by a narrowed coronary artery with increasing halothane concentration in the dog. Anesthesiology 55:349–359, 1981

Nachlan MM, Abrams SJ, Goldberg MM: The influence of arteriosclerotic heart disease on surgical risk. Am Heart J 101:447–455, 1961

Philbin DM, Foex P, Drummond G et al: Postsystolic shortening of canine left ventricle supplied by a stenotic coronary artery when nitrous oxide is added in the presence of narcotics. Anesthesiology 62:166–174, 1985

Prys–Roberts C, Meloche R, Foex P: Studies of anesthesia in relation to hypertension. I. Cardiovascular response of treated and untreated patients. Anaesthesia 43:122–136, 1971

Rao TLK, El-Eltra A: Myocardial reinfarction following anesthesia in patients with recent infarctions. Anesth Analg 60:271, 1981

Rao TLK, Jacobs KH, El-Etra A: Reinfarction following anesthesia in patients with myocardial infarction. Anesthesiology 59:499–505, 1983

Ream AK, Reitz BA, Silverberg GS: Temperature correction of PCO_2 and pH in estimating acid–base balance. Anesthesiology 56:41–44, 1982

Reiz S: Nitrous oxide augments the systemic and coronary hemodynamic effect of isoflurane in patients with ischemic heart disease. Acta Anaesthesiol Scand 27:464–469, 1983

Reiz S, Balfors E, Sorensen MB et al: Isoflurane — A powerful coronary vasodilator in patients with coronary artery disease. Anesthesiology 59:91–97, 1983

Steen PA, Tinker JH, Tarhan S: Myocardial reinfarction after anesthesia and surgery. JAMA 239:2566–2570, 1978

Tarhan S, Moffitt EA, Taylor WF et al: Myocardial infarction after general anesthesia. JAMA 20:1451–1454, 1972

Vacanti FX, Ames A: Mild hypothermia and Mg^{++} protect against irreversible damage during CNS ischemia. Stroke 15:695–697, 1984

Waller JL, Johnson SP, Kaplan JA: Usefulness of pulmonary artery catheters during aortocoronary bypass surgery. Anesth Analg 61:221–222, 1982

Waller JL, Zaidan JR, Kaplan JA et al: Hemodynamic responses to preoperative vascular cannulation in patients with coronary artery disease. Anesthesiology 56:216–221, 1982

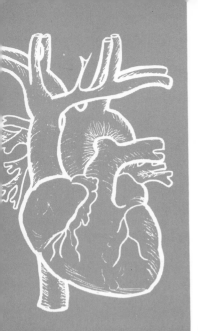

23

PRE- AND POSTINFARCTION UNSTABLE ANGINA: THOUGHTS ON PATHOGENESIS AND THERAPEUTIC STRATEGIES

C. Richard Conti

When a patient seeks medical help, the physician must answer several questions about the patient's condition. What is the diagnosis? What is the best therapy? What is the prognosis? Why did it happen? The answer to the last question often determines the best course of therapy and the prognosis. The purpose of this chapter is to summarize the current understanding of pathogenetic mechanisms that may underlie pre- and post-infarction angina pectoris and influence its management.

UNSTABLE ANGINA: PREINFARCTION

Patients may present with a variable history and different laboratory abnormalities. Most will have severely limited exercise tolerance, with minimal or no effort, because of angina. A few patients will have a normal exercise tolerance and only recurrent rest angina (e.g., classic Prinzmetal's angina). Variable changes on the electrocardiogram (ECG) (*e.g.*, ST-segment depression or elevation, or T-wave peaking or inversion during chest pain) may indicate varying degrees of myocardial ischemia. Coronary angiographic findings are not uniform and range from normal to severely obstructed multiple-vessel disease, including left main coronary artery stenosis. Ventricular function may be normal or abnormal because of regional dysfunction or global dysfunction. These variable clinical and laboratory expressions of the unstable state suggest that different mechanisms may be active in different patients.

POTENTIAL CAUSES OF UNSTABLE ANGINA

Several factors should be considered in each patient who presents with unstable angina both prior to and soon after a myocardial infarction. These include extracardiac factors, rapid progression of atherosclerosis, platelet aggregation in diseased vessels, transient coronary artery thrombosis, hemorrhage into an atheromatous plaque, and abnormal vasoconstriction of a conductive coronary artery.

Extracardiac (Aggravating) Factors. Because unstable angina commonly occurs at rest, it is likely that myocardial ischemia is the result of conditions in which coronary blood flow and oxygen supply are unable to meet the myocardial demand for oxygen under resting conditions. In patients with severe coronary artery stenosis and limited coronary flow reserve, factors such as tachyarrhythmias, systemic hypertension, thyrotoxicosis, and use of sympathomimetic drugs may increase myocardial oxygen demand and may be responsible for this imbalance of supply and demand. Any systemic illness may precipitate an increase in the frequency, duration, or intensity of angina pectoris. Anemia may also result in tachycardia (increased demand) and decreased oxygen supply to the myocardium.

Coronary Atherosclerosis: Rapid Progression. Most patients with unstable angina have atherosclerotic coronary obstructions. The majority have multiple-vessel disease, and about half have angiographic evidence of collateral circulation.[1] In addition, approximately 10% have significant disease of the left main coronary artery.

Moise and colleagues reported on 38 patients with unstable angina who had coronary angiography performed before and shortly after the onset of unstable symptoms.[2] Progressive coronary artery stenosis was found in about 75% of patients with unstable angina, compared to 30% of a similar group of matched patients with stable angina. This report suggests that the anatomical progression of atherosclerosis may be a factor in the development of unstable angina, but it also indicates that 25% of these patients had no evident progression of disease and still had unstable symptoms. A point that must be kept in mind is that "progression of coronary artery stenosis," which is determined by angiography, does not necessarily mean "progression of atherosclerosis."

Coronary angiography reveals normal angiograms in approximately 10% of patients studied, single-vessel disease in 20% to 30% (left anterior descending [LAD] obstruction is common), and multiple-vessel coronary artery disease in 40% to 60%. This latter group will have numerous and severe stenoses. Significant left main coronary artery stenosis will be found in approximately 10% to 15% of these patients. Unfortunately, the majority of these patients were not studied at the time of admission to the hospital or before active treatment was begun, but at some point after stabilization. Thus the precise nature of the coronary artery pathology, at the time of the unstable condition, is not known.

In the individual patient, it is not possible to know whether progressive atherosclerosis is responsible for the acute ischemic syndrome unless one can use serial coronary angiography. In addition, even if serial angiography is performed, it still may be impossible to distinguish between progressive atherosclerosis or incorporated recent thrombus that has formed a plaque.

Platelet Aggregation in Diseased Vessels. In theory, severe coronary artery stenosis will produce turbulent flow and stasis and may increase local platelet aggregation. Several experiments in animals have shown that platelet aggregation can be transient at the site of a stenotic vessel and can produce transient decreases in coronary blood flow. Uchida and associates and Folts and colleagues demonstrated this phenomenon in the dog.[3,4] In their experiments, constrictors were placed on the coronary artery, while coronary blood flow, distal coronary perfusion pressure, and aortic pressure were measured. Transient reductions in coronary blood flow and distal coronary perfusion pressure were noted despite maintenance of normal aortic pressure. These investigators also provided pathologic evidence that platelets accumulate at the site of the severe stenosis in dog coronary arteries at the time of reduction of distal coronary blood flow and pressure. These phenomena can be prevented by the administration of aspirin.

Bolli and colleagues performed similar experiments in dogs and found that reductions in distal coronary flow was not affected in 32 of 34 dogs after heparin administration (1000 units/kg).[5] In contrast, intravenous administration of aspirin (30 mg/kg) suppressed flow reduction in all dogs tested. These authors conclude that platelet aggregation, rather than fibrin deposition, is the cause of the observed cyclic reductions of coronary flow.

More recent evidence suggests that the release of thromboxane and serotonin from aggregating platelets and infiltrating white blood cells is a key factor in promoting platelet aggregation and the cyclic flow alterations in this experimental model.[6-8]

Clinical evidence to support the hypothesis of increased platelet aggregation in diseased coronary arteries is provided by the observations of Hirsh and associates, which indicate an increase in transcardiac thromboxane levels in patients with active unstable angina pectoris, and by the

Veterans Administration Cooperative Trial of 1266 men with unstable angina.[9] In this clinical trial, 625 men received 324 mg of aspirin per day, and 642 received placebo.[10] Nonfatal acute myocardial infarction was 51% lower in the aspirin group (21 patients) compared to that of the placebo group (44 patients). The reduction of mortality in the aspirin group was also 51% (10 patients), compared with that of the group taking placebo (21 patients).

Circumstantial evidence implicating platelet aggregation is provided by the link between cigarette smoking and coronary artery disease. Cigarette smoking is a known risk factor for coronary events. Platelet aggregation may be enhanced by cigarette smoking because nicotine stimulates catecholamine secretion.

Transient Coronary Artery Thrombosis. It is no longer merely a hypothesis that coronary thrombosis occurs in patients with acute evolving myocardial infarction.[11,12] Nor is there any doubt that the majority of patients with an acute myocardial infarction have evidence of severe coronary artery stenosis secondary to atherosclerosis. Because most patients with unstable angina, either prior to or after a myocardial infarction, have severe atherosclerosis, it seems reasonable to suspect that these patients might have similar phenomena occurring on a transient basis.

Vetrovec and colleagues reported on 12 patients with unstable angina who had angiographic findings of intracoronary thrombus in 11 of 13 ischemia-related vessels within 5 days of the onset of the unstable state.[13] Mandelkorn and associates provide additional evidence to support this hypothesis.[14] In nine patients with unstable angina, intracoronary nitroglycerin was administered. Only one totally occluded vessel was opened in response to intracoronary nitroglycerin. However, a major vascular obstruction remained and was eliminated by the administration of streptokinase. In four of these nine

patients, responses to streptokinase infusion included opening of an occluded vessel, a decrease in coronary stenosis, dissolution of a intracoronary filling defect, or a combination of these responses. Most of these patients were studied on the day of their chest-pain episode. In patients studied longer than 1 week after the onset of the rest-pain syndrome, thrombolysis could not be demonstrated.

Capone and associates examined coronary angiograms of 119 consecutive patients who had rest angina occurring within 14 days prior to catheterization.[15] Intracoronary thrombi were found in 37%. In a subset of patients (44) whose most recent pain occurred within 24 hours of angiography, coronary thrombi were found in 52%.

Lawrence and associates reported a clinical trial of fibrinolytic therapy in patients with unstable angina.[16] Forty patients were randomly assigned to receive streptokinase infusion for 24 hours and subsequent treatment with Coumadin, or to receive Coumadin therapy only. At 6 months, 1 of 20 patients treated with streptokinase and Coumadin and 8 of 20 patients treated with Coumadin only, experienced a cardiovascular event (sudden death or myocardial infarction). Although the numbers of patients are small and angiographic evidence for thrombosis was not obtained, it is tempting to attribute the better results to thrombolytic therapy.

Further clinical evidence to support the role of intracoronary thrombus formation in patients with unstable angina comes from a randomized trial comparing intravenous heparin and oral atenolol therapy in 214 patients with the "intermediate coronary syndrome."[17] This was a short-term trial designed to assess which therapy would best prevent myocardial infarction. During the trial period, transmural myocardial infarction developed in 17% of the 54 patients receiving placebo, in 14% of 60 patients receiving atenolol, in 2% of 51 patients receiving heparin, and in 4% of 49 patients receiving heparin and atenolol combined. The results indicate that intravenous heparin therapy helped to prevent infarction in patients with the intermediate coronary syndrome. The investigators speculate that intermediate coronary syndrome could be a result of the gradual development of a thrombus and that heparin treatment may prevent propagation of the thrombus if given early in the clinical course.

Autopsy studies lending support to the concept of gradually developing coronary stenosis secondary to thrombus are provided by Falk.[18] He reported 25 cases of sudden death due to acute coronary artery thrombosis. Eighty-one percent of the thrombi had a "layered structure" with thrombus material of differing age, indicating that the thrombi were formed by repeated mural deposits, causing progressive lumen narowing over time. In addition, 73% of the thrombi were associated with intermittent fragmentation of thrombus-causing microinfarctions.

One can ask the question, "Why should thrombus formation occur in a patient with moderately severe coronary atherosclerosis?" The answer is not known, but Horie and colleagues postulated that an increase of intraplaque pressure resulting from a honeycomblike accumulation of foam cells, cholesterol clefts, and blood infiltration through the injured endothelial cells might produce a break of the atheromatous plaque.[19] They further postulate that rupture into the vessel lumen may proceed and may stimulate platelet aggregation, with the eventual formation of an occluding thrombus and the onset of acute myocardial ischemia.[19]

Hemorrhage into an Atheromatous Plaque. It is impossible to tell, by coronary angiography, whether intramural hemorrhage into a plaque has occurred; autopsy studies are required. However, one can be suspicious if serial angiography reveals rapid progression of a 50% or 60% steno-sis to a near total occlusion. How often this mechanism occurs in patients with ischemic heart disease is unknown. In a series of 6800 consecutive autopsies, only 8% of the total occlusions noted were thought to be due to "intramural hemorrhage" into a plaque.[20]

Recently, Davies and Thomas reported their findings in 100 subjects who died of ischemic heart disease in less than 6 hours.[21] They report the presence of coronary thrombi in 74 of 100 subjects. All thrombi occurred in relation to massive fissuring of lipid-rich atheromatous plaques. These investigators make an important distinction between the terms "plaque hemorrhage" and "plaque fissure." They define the latter term as the formation of an opening from the lumen into the intima (formally called "dissecting hemorrhage"). In contrast, pure plaque hemorrhage is defined as the presence of red cells within a plaque and is derived from small capillaries crossing into the intima from the media. They propose that plaque fissuring is an important process, whereas pure plaque hemorrhage is so universal in both test and control hearts that its importance is ignored. In their 100 patients, intraluminal thrombus was found in 74%, intraintimal thrombus with plaque fissure in 19%, and intraintimal thrombus alone in only 2%. These investigators view the coronary artery lesions in patients who die suddenly of ischemic heart disease as identical to those found in patients with unstable angina. Based on the available information, isolated hemorrhage into a plaque (intraintimal hemorrhage) does not seem to be a common mechanism to produce unstable angina, but intraintimal thrombus with plaque fissuring does.

Abnormal Vasoconstriction of a Conductive Coronary Artery. Coronary artery spasm can be considered an abnormal constriction of the conductive arteries. The "classic" clinical manifestation of coronary spasm is rest angina associated with ST-segment elevation on the ECG. Unfortunately, ST-segment elevation does not define coronary artery spasm because many other factors, which have been previously discussed, can produce total occlusion of a coronary artery and a decrease in coronary blood flow, and can result in ST-segment elevation on the ECG. This transient decrease in blood flow may result from different causes, depending on the state of the coronary arteries. For example, in the case of a patient with "normal coronary arteries," the most likely cause of ST-segment elevation is abnormal vasoconstriction of the conductive arteries. In patients with 50% to 70% stenosis, spasm still may be the cause of the chest pain, especially if the stenosis is due to an eccentric plaque. In patients with higher degrees of coronary artery stenosis, turbulent flow, stasis and platelet aggregation, and associated thromboxane and seratonin release coupled with relatively low prostacyclin concentration at the sites of endothelial injury can account for thrombosis and can result in complete occlusion of the coronary artery and ST-segment elevation on the ECG.

Thus to *prove* the existence of coronary artery spasm, coronary angiography must be performed during the episode of chest pain.

UNSTABLE ANGINA: EARLY POSTINFARCTION

This section will present a strategy for the management of symptomatic patients with recurrent angina immediately (hours or days rather than weeks) following a myocardial infarction. The specific clinical problem of a patient with recurrent angina in the immediate postinfarction state seems to require urgent action to prevent the recurrence of acute myocardial infarction. Unfortunately, there are no long-term clinical trials in these patients that provide guidelines for the clinician; only anecdotal experiences have been reported.

APPROACH TO SPECIFIC CAUSES OF RECURRENT ANGINA

As with unstable preinfarction angina, recurrent angina occurring soon after infarction is due to either a transient increase in myocardial oxygen demand over a fixed coronary reserve or a transient decrease in myocardial oxygen supply.

Increased myocardial oxygen demand can be due to either extracardiac (aggravating) factors or cardiac mechanical problems.[22] Extracardiac factors responsible for recurrent angina include tachyarrhythmias, hypertension, hypotension, anemia, hypermetabolic state, drugs, hypervolemia, and hypovolemia. Mechanical problems such as left ventricular aneurysm, mitral regurgitation, ventricular septal defect (VSD), or severe global left ventricular failure can markedly increase myocardial oxygen demands over a fixed coronary reserve.

Decreased myocardial oxygen supply can be related to either transient thrombosis or platelet aggregation in severely diseased vessels or to abnormal constriction of the conductive arteries at or near the site of the atherosclerotic narrowing.[23-25]

Of course, one must be sure that the recurrent chest discomfort is related to myocardial ischemia. Thus the obsevations of transient ECG changes and/or changing physical signs such as the development of a murmur of mitral regurgitation or the transient appearance of a fourth heart sound are helpful.

It makes no difference how the patient with myocardial infarction was treated initially. The overwhelming majority of patients with acute myocardial infarction will have evidence of severe coronary artery disease in one or more vessels. If the patient has recurrent angina, attempts must be made to understand why angina is recurring. The patient must be evaluated comprehensively by history, physical exam, simple blood and chemical laboratory tests, and hemodynamic assessment (*i.e.*, coronary angiography, ventriculography, and physiologic measurements).

APPROACH TO SPECIFIC TREATMENT OF RECURRENT ANGINA PECTORIS

There is no universal or standard treatment for patients with early postinfarction angina. This should not surprise anyone because there is no universal or standard definition of this symptomatic group of patients. There are numerous variables that must be considered, such as time of onset of recurrent ischemia from the onset of infarction, number of ischemic episodes per hour or day, ischemic manifestations (*i.e.*, only chest pain, only ECG changes, or both ECG changes and chest pain), and mechanism for recurrence of ischemia (*e.g.*, increased myocardial oxygen demand or decreased myocardial oxygen supply).

Conditions That Increase Myocardial Oxygen Demand. *Extracardiac Factors.* If tachycardias occur, they must be controlled with the appropriate therapy (*i.e.*, digitalis, calcium antagonists, beta blockers, or specific antiarrhythmics). If blood pressure is elevated, it should be lowered appropriately by either drugs or diuretics (if hypervolemia is the problem). If blood pressure is low due to hypovolemia, then fluids must be given. If anemia is present, it should be corrected by the transfusion of packed red blood cells. A hypermetabolic state such as hyperthyroidism should be treated appropriately, initially with propranolol but concomitantly with appropriate antithyroid medication. Any drugs that increase myocardial oxygen consumption, such as bronchodilators, nasal decongestants, and so forth, should be discontinued.

Mechanical Cardiac Problems. When these problems arise, surgery may be required in the early stages after myocardial infarction to resect an aneurysm, to replace the mitral valve, or to close a VSD. However, in the patient with heart failure secondary to an aneurysm, mitral regurgitation, VSD, or severe generalized left ventricular dysfunction, in most instances, initial efforts should be made to stabilize the patient, if possible, by using inotropic agents, diuretics, and vasodilators. Afterload-reducing agents of choice are intravenous nitroglycerin or intravenous nitroprusside.[26,27] Intra-aortic balloon counterpulsation can also provide temporary support until the appropriate surgical procedure can be performed.[28] In the patient with severe global left ventricular dysfunction, it must be determined at the time of angiography whether this is related to myocardial ischemia and therefore reversible, or to myocardial infarction and irreversible. Some clues can be obtained by assessing the effects of intravenous nitroglycerin on left ventricular function in this type of patient.[29]

Conditions That Decrease Myocardial Oxygen Supply. *Abnormal Constriction of Conductive Coronary Arteries.* If coronary artery spasm is found at the time of angiography, the treatment of choice is coronary vasodilation. Nitrates and/or calcium antagonists are suitable for this purpose.[30] However, one must be careful to make sure that abnormal vasoconstriction is the mechanism rather than some other cause of transient obstruction of the coronary artery.

Transient Thrombosis and/or Platelet Aggregation. If mechanical obstruction of the coronary artery is determined, at the time of angiography, to be caused by thrombosis, and this spontaneously lyses, intravenous heparin and aspirin should be given to prevent recurrent thrombosis.[17] If medical therapy is selected for long-term management, then the patient should receive aspirin and possibly Coumadin over the long term.[10] In these patients with severe coronary artery disease who are prone to recurrent coronary artery thrombosis, it seems reasonable to perform coronary angioplasty at some time during the initial hospitalization for myocardial infarction. This is especially true in the typical patient, who has a residual high-grade coronary stenosis following spontaneous or drug-related thrombolysis.[31] If the stenosis is 90% or greater, I would recommend percutaneous transluminal coronary angioplasty (PTCA). In contrast, if the stenosis is 50% or less, aggressive therapy with anticoagulants and antiplatelet agents might be acceptable. In the patient who has coronary artery disease of moderate severity (*i.e.*, 70% stenosis), I recommend PTCA if recurrent angina remains a problem despite anticoagulant and antiplatelet therapy.

POTENTIAL PROBLEMS UNIQUE TO THE POSTINFARCTION ANGINA PATIENT

A major question arises when patients develop angina after infarction, that is, is this reinfarction or is the ischemia without infarction? On occasion, initial therapy of the patient will help to answer this important question. For example, if one begins with an intravenous infusion of nitroglycerin and the patient responds crisply, the angina is more likely to be due to ischemia rather than to infarction.

Another issue that needs to be addressed is the safety of performing coronary angioplasty in the immediate postinfarction period. It is possible that angioplasty might make the patient's condition worse. If that happens, it may be necessary to perform urgent coronary bypass surgery because of damage to the coronary artery. The risk of coronary bypass surgery in the immediate postinfarction period is greater than if it is performed weeks or months later when the infarction has healed.

Proponents of PTCA in patients with recent myocardial infarction argue that experience has shown that the risk of complication is not great.[32] Despite this optimistic attitude, most who advocate the procedure would not attempt to completely revascularize a patient and would only perform angioplasty of the vessel responsible for recurrent ischemia.

It is important to point out that there have been no controlled clinical trials performed in which PTCA is used in the immediate postinfarction period in patients with recurrent angina pectoris. However, the logic of performing his procedure in a patient with severe coronary artery stenosis who has already had one episode of thrombosis is reasonable in my view.

Some information can be extrapolated from the National Heart, Lung, and Blood Institute (NHLBI) PTCA registry.[33] Although these were patients with unstable angina, they were not unstable in the immediate postinfarction period. Investigators concluded from this report that PTCA can be performed safely and successfully in patients with unstable angina. Whether these data can be extrapolated to include patients with unstable angina in the immediate postinfarction period is speculative.

SUMMARY AND CONCLUSIONS

The pathophysiology of unstable angina, both pre- and postinfarction, is incompletely understood because the population of patients labeled as having unstable angina is not uniform and the definition of this condition is not precise. One must ask the question, "Why does a patient suddenly become unstable?" Several conditions can be responsible, acting alone or in combination with each other. These conditions include extracardiac (aggravating) factors, rapid progression of coronary atherosclerosis, rapid decrease in coronary lumen size secondary to hemorrhage into an atherosclerotic plaque, transient platelet aggregation in severely diseased vessels, transient coronary artery thrombosis, and abnormal coronary artery vasoconstriction (spasm) in normal or diseased vessels. Figure 23–1 summarizes a hypothetical scheme relating the above conditions to the degree of coronary artery stenosis.

In patients with preinfarction unstable angina, most investigators still believe that severe coronary atherosclerosis and its consequences are the major pathogenic mechanisms in most patients with ischemic heart disease. If spasm is the mechanism, then obviously the use of vasodilators is warranted. However, if thrombosis is clearly defined in these patients, then thrombolytic therapy in the early stages seems reasonable. If severe coronary artery disease is found (with or without thrombosis), one can make a strong argument for therapy with anticoagulants such as intravenous heparin during the acute phase of the illness. A similar argument could be

made for the use of antiplatelet agents during the convalescent phase.

If extracardiac (aggravating) factors are present, they must be corrected appropriately. It may not be possible to identify the appropriate mechanism responsible for unstable angina in every case, but the clinician must attempt to do so, because the selection of appropriate therapy for the individual patient depends on the pathophysiologic mechanism responsible for the symptoms.

The approach to the patient with postinfarction recurrent angina pectoris must also be systematic and logical. Diagnostic and therapeutic principles used in patients with preinfarction unstable angina apply to postinfarction angina patients as well. Coronary angiography is performed principally to determine the extent of coronary artery disease and the presence or absence of thrombosis, abnormal constriction of a

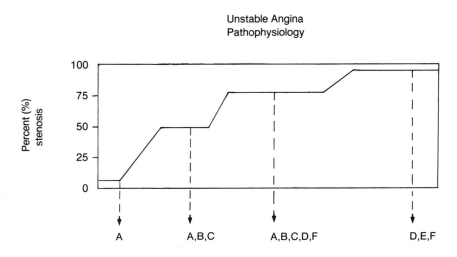

FIG. 23–1. Hypothetical scheme of the pathophysiology of unstable angina. Six conditions or factors responsible for the unstable state are related to the degree of coronary atherosclerosis. (**A**, spasm (epicardial arteries, microvascular); **B**, CAD progression; **C**, plaque hemorrhage; **D**, platelet aggregation; **E**, transient thrombosis; **F**, extracardiac factors)

conductive coronary artery, or mechanical dysfunction of the heart. If recurrent thrombosis is found or a patent vessel with a residual high-grade (90%) stenosis is present, performance of PTCA in the affected artery seems logical to prevent recurrence of myocardial infarction.

Thus each patient with pre- or postinfarction unstable angina becomes a clinical trial. In those in whom ischemia continues despite drug therapy, hemodynamic investigation must be performed to sort out the appropriate therapy for the individual patient. In either group of patients, initial therapy should begin with intravenous nitroglycerin and intravenous heparin as well. However, heparin is only given if there is no contraindication to the use of anticoagulants. In patients who continue to have chest pain, an intravenous beta blocker (preferably ultra–short acting) should be added and, if the chest pain continues, perhaps calcium antagonists. However, calcium antagonists generally have not added much after treatment with intravenous nitroglycerin, intravenous heparin, and intravenous beta blockade. If ischemia persists, intraaortic balloon counterpulsation might provide relief. As all of this is going on, there is some sense of urgency created in the mind of the physician, and because of this, plans are usually made to prepare for hemodynamic investigation on an urgent basis if pain persists and to prepare the patient for either coronary angioplasty or surgery.

REFERENCES

1. Conti CR, Brawley PK, Griffith LSC et al: Unstable angina pectoris: Morbidity and mortality in 57 consecutive patients evaluated angiographically. Am J Cardiol 32:745–750, 1973
2. Moise A, Therous P, Taeymans Y et al: Unstable angina and progression of coronary atherosclerosis. N Engl Med 309:685–689, 1983
3. Uchida Y, Yoshimoto N, Murao S: Cyclic fluctuations in coronary blood pressure and flow induced by coronary artery constriction. Jpn Heart J 16:454–464, 1975
4. Folts JD, Crowell EB, Rowe LL: Platelet aggregation in partially obstructed vessels and its elimination with aspirin. Circulation 54:365–370, 1976
5. Bolli R, Ware JA, Brandon TA et al: Platelet-mediated thrombosis in stenosed canine coronary arteries: Inhibition by nicergoline, a platelet-active alpha-adrenergic antagonist. J Am Coll Cardiol 3:1417–1426, 1984
6. Bush LR, Campbell WB, Buja LM et al: Effects of the selective thromboxane synthetase inhibitor dazoxiben on variations in cyclic blood flow in stenosed canine coronary arteries. Circulation 69:1161–1170, 1984
7. Bush LR, Campbell WB, Kern K et al: The effects of α-adrenergic and serotonergic receptor antagonists on cyclic blood flow alterations in stenosed canine coronary arteries. Circ Res 55:642–652, 1984
8. Willerson JT, Campbell WB, Winniford MD et al: Conversion from chronic to acute coronary artery disease: Speculation regarding mechanisms. Am J Cardiol 54:1349–1354, 1984
9. Hirsh PD, Hillis LD, Campbell WB et al: Release of prostaglandins and thromboxane into the coronary circulation in patients with ischemic heart disease. N Engl J Med 304:685–691, 1981
10. Lewis HD, Davis JW, Archibald DG et al: Protective effects of aspirin against acute myocardial infarction and death in men with unstable angina. New Engl J Med 309:396–403, 1983
11. DeWood MA, Spores J, Notsk ER et al: Prevalence of total coronary occlusion during the early hours of transmural myocardial infarction. New Engl J Med 303:897–902, 1980
12. DeWood MA, Spores J, Hensley GR et al: Coronary arteriographic findings in acute transmural myocardial infarction. Circulation (Suppl I) 68:139–149, 1983
13. Vetrovec GW, Leinbach RC, Gold HK, Cowley MJ: Intracoronary thrombolysis in syndromes of ischemia: Angiographic and clinical results. Am Heart J 104:946–952, 1982
14. Mandelkorn JB, Wolf NM, Singh S et al: Intracoronary thrombus in nontransmural myocardial infarction and in unstable angina pectoris. Am J Cardiol 52:1–6, 1983
15. Capone GJ, Meyer BB, Wolf NM, Meister SG: Incidence of intracoronary thrombi in patients with active unstable angina pectoris. Circulation (Suppl II) 70:II–415, 1984
16. Lawrence JR, Shepherd JT, Bone I et al: Fibrinolytic therapy in unstable angina pectoris, a controlled clinical trial. Thromb Res 17:767–777, 1980
17. Telford AM, Wilson C: Trial of heparin versus atenolol in prevention of myocardial infarction in intermediate coronary syndrome. Lancet I:1225–1228, 1981

18. Falk E: Unstable angina with fatal outcome: Dynamic coronary thrombosis leading to infarction and/or sudden death. Autopsy evidence of recurrent mural thrombosis with peripheral embolization culminating in total vascular occlusion. Circulation 71:699–708, 1985

19. Horie T, Sekiguchi M, Hirosawa K: Coronary thrombosis in pathogenesis of acute myocardial infarction. Histopathological study of coronary arteries in 108 necropsied cases using serial section. Br Heart J 40:153–161, 1978

20. Friedberg CK: Diseases of the heart, 3rd ed, p 781. Philadelphia, WB Saunders, 1966

21. Davies MJ, Thomas MB: Thrombosis and acute coronary artery lesions in sudden cardiac ischemic death. N Engl J Med 310:1127–1140, 1984

22. Conti CR: Unstable angina: Thoughts on pathogenesis in unstable angina: Current concepts in management. In Hugenholtz PG, Goldman BS (eds): Unstable Angina: Current Concepts and Management, pp 55–64. New York, Schattauer, 1985

23. Mandelkorn JB, Wolff NM, Singh S et al: Intracoronary thrombus in non-transmural myocardial infarction and in unstable angina pectoris. Am J Cardiol 52:1–6, 1983

24. Bresnahan DR, Davis JL, Holmes DR, Smith HC: Angiographic occurrence and clinical correlates of intraluminal coronary artey thrombus: Role of unstable angina. J Am Coll Cardiol 6:285–289, 1985

25. Maseri A, L'Abbate A, Chierchia S et al: Significance of spasm in the pathogenesis of ischemic heart disease. Am J Cardiol 44:788–792, 1979

26. Conti CR: Nitrate therapy for ischemic heart disease. Eur Heart J 6:3–11, 1985

27. Franciosa JA, Guiha NH, Limas CJ et al: Improved left ventricular function during nitroprusside infusion in acute myocardial infarction. Lancet I:650, 1972

28. Levine FH, Gold HK, Leinbach RC et al: Management of acute myocardial ischemia with intraaortic balloon pumping in coronary bypass surgery. Circulation (Suppl I) 58:69, 1978

29. Feldman RL, Conti CR: Relief of myocardial ischemia with nitroglycerin: What is the mechanism? Circulation 64:1098–1100, 1981

30. Conti CR, Hill JA, Feldman RL et al: Comparison of nifedipine and nitrates: Clinical and angiographic studies. In Opie LH (ed): Calcium Antagonists and Cardiovascular Disease, pp 269–275. New York, Raven Press, 1984

31. DeFeyter PJ, Serruys PW, Van Denbrand M et al: Percutaneous transluminal coronary angioplasty in unstable angina pectoris: The Rotterdam experience. In Hugenholtz PG, Goldman BS (eds): Unstable Angina: Current Concepts and Management, pp 229–237. New York, Schattauer-Stuttgart, 1985

32. Pepine CJ, Prida X, Hill JA et al: Percutaneous transluminal coronary angioplasty in acute myocardial infarction. Am Heart J 107:820–822, 1984

33. Faxon DP, Detre KM, McCabe CH et al: Role of percutaneous transluminal coronary angioplasty in the treatment of unstable angina. Report from the NHLBI PTCA and CASS Registries. Am J Cardio 53:131C–135C, 1983

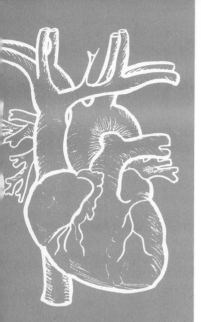

24

HEART TRANSPLANTATION: CURRENT STATUS AND PROSPECTS

G. Arnaud Painvin

Over the past 20 years, cardiac allotransplantation has progressed from an experimental and investigative procedure to a therapeutic modality for the management of end-stage cardiac disease that has been accepted worldwide. In 1984 the 1-year, 2-year, and 5-year survival rates were 85%, 80%, and 60%, respectively.[1-6] The attrition rate per year is now being 5%, as shown by Samuelsson.[7]

Improved and strict selection criteria for potential recipients and donors; optimal perioperative management, including graft preservation and use of frequent endomyocardial biopsies; and, primarily, the introduction of more specific immunosuppression are the major factors contributing to the reestablishment of this procedure worldwide.

This chapter will discuss the history, present status, limitations, and future considerations in isolated cardiac transplantation.

EXPERIMENTAL STUDIES

An excellent review of the experimental background of cardiac transplantation was published recently by Griepp.[8] Briefly, Carrel and Guthrie[9-10] first described the surgical technique of vascular anastomosis, which led to the logical step of the first reported case of cardiac transplantation in 1905. Using a heterotopic model, they transplanted puppy hearts into the neck of larger dogs. None of these grafts survived more than 2 hours. Nevertheless, progress with this heterotopic model was achieved over the next four decades by Mann and Marcus.[11,12] In 1953 Downie and associates were successful in achieving a 10-day survival.[13] Neptune pioneered the techniques of central cooling and circulatory arrest, and Cass and colleagues developed a double atrial anastomosis technique for orthotopic implantation.[14-16] Following these advances, the first successful case of an orthotopic cardiac allograft transplantation was reported by Lower and Shumway.[16-18] In a series of eight cases, there were five patients who survived 6 to 26 days. These reports clearly defined the aspects of the procedure and its feasibility was established. Later, experimental transplantation investigations examined the hemodynamic status of an implanted graft and the diagnosis of acute rejection using the electrocardiogram (ECG).[19]

The first human cardiac transplantation was performed on a 68-year-old male by Hardy and associates in January 1964.[20] The operation consisted of an orthotopic xenograft (chimpanzee), and although technically successful, the patient survived only a few hours. Shortly afterwards, Dr. Barnard in Capetown, South Africa, performed the first allograft transplantation, and this time the patient survived 18 days before dying of pneumonia.[21] Barnard was followed by Cooley and Kantrowitz.[22,23] However, the initial worldwide excitement was premature, and the procedure was almost completely abandoned because of the high failure rate caused by infection. Over the ensuing years, pioneering efforts in the clinical and research arenas were maintained in only a few institutions (Stanford, Richmond, and Paris). Only recently have the results caused a worldwide resurgence of interest in heart transplantation; over 35 institutions in the United States performed more than 300 transplantations in 1984.

INDICATIONS FOR CARDIAC TRANSPLANTATION AND PATIENT SELECTION

In the United States alone, cardiovascular disease affects an estimated 42 million Americans. In 1981 980,000 persons died of cardiovascular disease, and 200,000 of these succumbed before the age of 65.[24] As reported by Evans and associates from the Battelle Human Affairs Research Center, each year up to 300,000 patients from 10 to 54 years of age are hospitalized for significant cardiovascular diseases.[25] Approximately 15,000 die of conditions for which heart transplantation may be indicated. However, the actual number of potential candidates for heart transplantation each year is very difficult to determine because it depends on several factors, specifically, the selection of eligibility criteria. From an extensive review of the literature, the actual number of candidates for heart transplantation varies considerably from 1,000 to 75,000 per year.[26-35] The primary indication for cardiac transplantation is end-stage cardiac disease that is refractory to or unsuitable for treatment by conventional medical or surgical therapies. Strict selection criteria for recipients were defined early in the Stanford program and then were progressively refined over the past decade.[28,36-38] In selecting patients for heart transplantation, four fundamental questions must be answered:

1. Is the patient's illness severe enough to warrant the procedure?
2. Is the disease too advanced, thus minimizing the degree of success?
3. Can the disease be managed with conventional medical and/or surgical therapy?
4. Are there any absolute contraindications to surgery?

Among the clinical conditions considered to be contraindications to orthotopic cardiac allotransplantation is severe (> 8 Wood units) and irreversible pulmonary hypertension. However, some of these patients may be candidates for cardiopulmonary transplantation or heterotopic cardiac transplantation. Other contraindications include recent (< 4 weeks) or unresolved pulmonary infarction, active infection, carcinoma, noncardiac lethal conditions, cardiac cachexia, severe liver and/or renal dysfunction, and insulin-dependent diabetes mellitus. Significant psychological abnormalities or a lack of compliance with chronic medical management on the part of the patient or relatives should also be considered contraindications. The issue of upper age limit is now more controversial because some transplant centers accept patients who are older than 55 years. The mandatory preoperative evaluation and the requirements necessary to organize a transplant program were well described recently by Copeland and Baumgartner.[33,39]

The initial evaluation should include recent right and left cardiac catheterization and respiratory, liver, and kidney function studies. Psychosocial profile, nutritional assessment, immunologic workup, and gastrointestinal tests are also necessary. At least six different departments are involved during this evaluation, under the coordination of the transplant team. A formal in-depth "teaching course" is required for the candidate as well as for family members.[40] At the completion of this evaluation, those candidates who are accepted are placed on the active waiting list. Most patients are then discharged until a suitable donor is identified. The average length of time until the transplantation is usually 5 weeks, although it is highly dependent on the location of the transplant center, the available donor pool, and the effectiveness of the different organ bank networks. The primary cause of cardiac disease in the majority of patients is ischemic heart disease or idiopathic cardiomyopathy. The patient's ages range from 8 months to 63 years (mean of 42 years).

DONOR SELECTION AND CARDIAC PROCUREMENT

The supply of donor hearts remains the single most important factor limiting the clinical expansion of cardiac and cardiopulmonary allotransplantation. As outlined by Evans and coworkers, Bart, Stuart, and Carpenter, some 18,000 persons who die every year in the United States could be considered potential candidates for organ donation.[25,41-43] However, the strict criteria used for cardiac donation, the significant psychological barriers that exist, and the high level of motivation required from the referring physician limits the number of available cardiac donors to 10% to 20% of the total, or between 1000 to 2000 per year.[33] Therefore, the donor-to-recipient ratio in cardiac transplantation is one donor for every nine recipients. As a result of this significant lack of "supply," more than 500 patients die every year awaiting cardiac donors.[43,44] As defined by Bart, the donor for transplantation of the heart is a patient with irreversible brain death from either trauma (60%) or cerebrovascular disease (40%).[41] The guidelines for declaring brain death are clearly defined both medically and legally.[45-48] Adequate assessment and optimal management of potential donors are essential. The selection criteria, contraindications, and "preparation" of donor organs have been outlined by Griepp and colleagues, Cooper, and others.[49-52] The donor must be young (< 35 years for a man and < 40 years for a woman) because the prevalence of coronary artery disease increases beyond this age. Contraindications to

cardiac donation also include active infection, previous cardiopulmonary resuscitation, abnormal ECG, history of cardiac trauma or cardiac disease, and hemodynamic instability requiring significant inotropic support. Hypothermia, diabetes insipidus, and peripheral vascular collapse accompanying brain death must be treated promptly during the stabilization period before transplantation. Size matching in cardiac transplantation is not as important as in cardiopulmonary transplantation; however, a weight discrepancy of more than 20 kg between the recipient and the donor may be of concern. The reasons for adequate matching of ABO blood-group types are obvious, and a search for recipient antibodies against donor cells should be performed routinely by directly cross-matching recipient serum and donor lymphocytes. A positive test is an absolute contraindication for transplantation.

Histocompatibility at the HLA-A2 and HLA-DR (*HLA,* human leukocyte antigen) has not been shown to be as important in cardiac transplantation as it has been in renal transplantation. However, the incidence of late graft atherosclerosis appears to be increased with a HLA-A2 mismatch between the donor and the recipient.[53]

Once the decision for surgery is made, cardiectomy, nephrectomy, and often hepatectomy are performed simultaneously, and close cooperation between surgical teams is mandatory. Because of the significant lack of donors, multiple-organ procurement from a single donor is becoming the rule. The technical and logistic aspects of this difficult procedure were defined recently by Shaw, Goldman, Margreiter, and others.[54-60]

Under full heparinization (300 units/kg) and hemodynamic stabilization, all intra-abdominal dissections are completed prior to cardiac removal. The heart is exposed through a median sternotomy and is then arrested using conventional cold crystalloid-type potassium cardioplegia. The cardiectomy is then carried out within a few minutes by dividing the vena cavae, followed by transection of the pulmonary artery at its bifurcation and of the aorta as far distally as possible. The heart is then elevated and each pulmonary vein is separated. The heart is trimmed by incising the posterior wall of the left atrium between the pulmonary venous orifices. The superior vena cava is ligated at least 2 cm above the sinus node. The right atrium is then opened from the inferior vena cava toward the right appendage, far from the right coronary artery. Viability of the graft is maintained by submersion in iced-saline bags (4°C) until time of the implantation. Distal procurement and jet transportation of the heart have increased the available donor pool and are used routinely by all persons involved in cardiac transplantation.[61–63] Under hypothermic storage, a total ischemic time of up to 4 hours (maximum radius of flight = 1100 miles) is considered to be the maximum allowable ischemic duration for safe transplantation.[61] However, using a portable hypothermic perfusion system, Cooper and associates reported successful clinical implantations after more than 12 hours of ischemic time.[64]

During the cardiectomy and the transplantation, the recipient is brought to the operating room. The general anesthesia is the same as that used for any open-heart surgery; however, these end-stage cardiac patients tend to be more unstable, especially during induction.[65] The technique of graft implantation has been described extensively and was recently detailed by Cabrol and coworkers.[66–68]

POSTOPERATIVE MANAGEMENT OF THE CARDIAC TRANSPLANTATION PATIENT

Apart from immunotherapy, diagnosis, and treatment of rejections, postoperative management of patients following cardiac transplantation is similar to the conventional postoperative care given after cardiac surgery, and it has been simplified since the introduction of cyclosporine. The value of routinely using reverse isolation (sterile isolation of the hospital staff from the recipient) is now questionable for the following reasons: (1) there are no comparative clinical data showing the beneficial long-term effect of this technique, (2) its high cost and psychological impact minimize its use, and (3) the natural defense mechanisms of the recipients are maintained with cyclosporine treatment.[69] Prolonged ischemic time, absence of sympathetic neurogenic stimulation (the graft is denervated), and mild myocardial edema can induce temporary cardiac dysfunction. Therefore, mild inotropic support is recommended during the first 48 hours, and isoprenaline is of particular value during this period. The recipient must be evaluated daily, including clinical examination, chest film, and ECG. A right ventricular endocardial biopsy for histologic assessment of the graft is obtained regularly on a weekly basis during the initial 5 weeks, and more often if a clinical suspicion of possible rejection is present. Using the technique described by Caves and colleagues, a bioptome is introduced by way of the right internal jugular and six to eight 2-mm pieces of right ventricular septal tissue are removed under fluoroscopic guidance.[70] The histologic findings are examined and then graded as mild, moderate, or severe according to the Billingham classification.[71,72] This scoring system is based on the extent of the lesions involving the blood vessels, interstitium, endocardium, and myocytes. Since the introduction of cyclosporine, histologic assessment of the graft is currently the only accurate and predictive method to diagnose rejection in the early phase and to assess the effectiveness of subsequent antirejection therapy.

IMMUNOSUPPRESSION

Optimal immunosuppression, early diagnosis of acute rejection, and adequate assessment of the antirejection therapy are the essential features of the postoperative management. Immunosuppression protocols vary from one center to another. However, since 1980, cyclosporine has been the drug of choice in concert with corticosteroid therapy for most programs. Concern about the long-term use of cyclosporine and its side-effects will probably modify its association with corticosteroid therapy. The recent addition of cyclosporine as a necessary agent for immunosuppression in the transplanted patient has caused renewed worldwide interest in cardiac transplantation, especially in the United States (> 35 centers), Canada (7 centers), United Kingdom (4 centers), France (6 centers), and elsewhere.

Cyclosporine, an endocapeptide extracted from fungi, appears to induce potent reversible and preferential suppression of the recipient's T-helper lymphocytes. Briefly, its mechanism of action can be summarized as follows: cyclosporine blocks the transformation of resting T cells to activated T cells by interfering with the main stimulators; antigens (class I and II) and interleukines I. Cyclosporine probably also interferes with the production of interleukine II from the activated T-helper lymphocytes. However, cyclosporine does not interfere with the nonspecific immune system or bone marrow activities. Cyclosporine's properties, pharmacokinetic studies, metabolism, and mechanism of action have been previously described in detail.[73-80]

A loading dose of cyclosporine is given orally (10 mg to 14 mg/kg) 4 hours prior to transplantation and then is maintained with a single or divided daily dose for an indefinite period. During the initial hospitalization, several serum trough levels of cyclosporine are obtained every other day. The cyclosporine trough levels are maintained between 200 ng and 400 ng/ml by adjusting the daily dose to minimize the risk of toxicity-related side-effects. The addition of steroids to cyclosporine therapy is believed to optimize immunosuppression. Each recipient should receive 0.5 g methylprednisolone at the time of the cardiectomy, followed by 125 mg administered intravenously three times the next day. Prednisone is given daily on a tapering schedule, decreasing to 30 mg daily by day 60 and to 20 mg daily by day 120. Once again, several different immunosuppressive protocols are used clinically at the present time. Other agents used for the purpose of minimizing the side-effects of cyclosporine include azathioprine and antilymphocyte globulin.

DIAGNOSIS AND MANAGEMENT OF REJECTION

Since the introduction of cyclosporine as the immunosuppressive agent of choice, the diagnosis and management of acute rejection are diagnosed according to the histologic findings. In most programs, acute rejections are managed with intravenous methylprednisolone in a 3-day pulse dose of 1000 mg daily, followed by oral prednisone 200 mg on day 4, tapering to 40 mg daily at day 30. The lack of histologic improvement 48 hours after completion of the steroid pulse therapy or the presence of severe myocardial cytolysis are, for most physicians, an indication to add human antilymphocyte globulin.[71,81-83]

INFECTIONS: DIAGNOSIS AND MANAGEMENT

The susceptibility to infection, especially while the patient receives antirejection therapy, has been reduced with the introduction of cyclosporine but remains significant. Therefore, the clinical involvement of the infectious-disease specialist as an integral part of the transplant team is mandatory. Prompt and, if necessary, invasive diagnosis to enable appropriate treatment with specific antibiotics is the basis for management of infected, immunosuppressed patients. Serial cultures (blood, sputum, urine), immunoelectrophoresis, antibody titers, and other screening tests should be ordered according to the clinical status and immunosuppression levels of compromised patients.

IMMUNOMONITORING

Since the introduction of cyclosporine, the clinical value of immunomonitoring has become less critical. The quantitative tests measuring the blood levels of different types of lymphocytes and the qualitative tests using different types of lymphocyte cultures are very sophisticated but yield, in our experience, poor specificity and sensitivity. There is an obvious need for a simple, reproducible, inexpensive test to accurately assess the immune status of the patient treated with cyclosporine.

FOLLOW-UP

Patients are discharged when their cyclosporine serum trough level stabilizes at approximately 250 ng/ml. This usually occurs by the fourth week after transplantation. The patients are followed up at the outpatient clinic once or twice weekly during the first postoperative month, then every 2 weeks during the subsequent 2 months. Thereafter, stable patients return to the care of their referring physicians. The protocols for outpatient cardiac biopsy vary from center to center. After discharge, endomyocardial biopsy is recommended every 2 weeks during the first 2 months, then every month during the following 6 months. Biopsies may be performed by the local cardiologist and the specimens mailed to the transplant center, or they may be obtained at the transplant center. Patients are readmitted annually for complete evaluation of the graft, including coronary angiography and cyclosporine pharmacokinetic studies.

OVERALL RESULTS

As mentioned previously, current medical reports from Stanford, Houston, Pittsburgh, the United Kingdom, Paris, or from one collective review clearly indicated that cyclosporine has contributed to improved survival rates and rehabilitation for cardiac recipients, with a 5-year survival rate beyond 60%.[1,3-6,84-91] These results are remarkable and cannot be matched with other therapeutic modalities involving terminal cardiac or noncardiac diseases. The quality of life of the survivors is of equal importance. Over 95% of the discharged recipients achieve New York Heart Association functional class I. As shown by Lough and others, over 80% of these patients have enjoyed active rehabilitation returning to full-time employment and complete social adaptation.[7,53,92,93]

COMPLICATIONS

REJECTION

The most notable features of acute rejection with cyclosporine-treated patients can be described as follows:

1. The overall incidence of rejection is slightly lower than with conventional immunosuppression. Through the Texas Heart Institute, a cooperative analysis between a similar group of patients who underwent transplantation 14 years ago and a current population revealed that the overall incidence of acute rejection during the first year was 23 episodes per 100 patient-months in 1970 versus 11 per 100 patient-months in 1983.[85] At 18 months, the percentages of those who did not suffer any rejection of the graft and those who did not die of graft rejection were 19% and 34%, respectively, in 1970, versus 40% and 79%, respectively, at the present time.
2. A subacute rather than acute onset of graft rejection is often observed.
3. A high incidence of asymptomatic episodes is observed (up to 40%) despite significant abnormal histologic findings.[91]
4. The clinical signs and symptoms are inconsistent, nonspecific, and nonsensitive. Abnormal hemodynamic parameters such as low blood

pressure and low output syndrome occur late in the clinical picture, when the rejection process itself is irreversible.

5. However, a significant reduction in mortality has been achieved despite the inability to diagnose rejection without biopsy.
6. The difficult reversal of severe rejection with pulse therapy alone may require the addition of human antilymphocyte globulin, as emphasized by Hardesty and colleagues.[86,87]
7. A mild degree of myocardial cellular infiltration may occur regardless of the degree of rejection and has been attributed to the use of cyclosporine.[4,71,94,95]

INFECTION

Perhaps the most striking impact of the addition of cyclosporine to steroid therapy has been a significant reduction in the incidence of fatal infection, resulting in a reduced overall incidence of opportunistic organisms as shown by Reece and colleagues and others.[96-98] From the Texas Heart Institute comparative analysis, the overall incidence of infection in 1970 was 64 episodes per 100 patient-months during the first year versus 34 episodes per 100 patient-months at present.[85] At 18 months, rates for freedom from infection and freedom from total infection were 6% and 42%, respectively, in 1970, versus 24% and 100% currently. We agree with Oyer and colleagues that the superior survival rate obtained with cyclosporine is not directly related to the moderate reduction in the incidence of rejection and infection, but rather to a significant reduction in the mortality of these two frequent complications.[4]

SIDE-EFFECTS AND OTHER COMPLICATIONS OF CYCLOSPORINE

Numerous adverse reactions and complications related to cyclosporine have been reported extensively. Some are minor, but others are significant in terms of frequency or severity.

Nephrotoxicity. Renal dysfunction is diagnosed consistently among cardiac transplantation patients, with an incidence reaching 75% to 80%.[99-103] High blood urea nitrogen levels (> 50 mg/ml) and serum creatinine levels of approximately 2.5 mg to 3 mg/ml are common. Hyperkalemia and mild metabolic alkalosis usually occur.[99,104] The mechanism of this nephrotoxicity is not yet known and seems to persist chronically. The risk of acute renal failure and subsequent hemodialysis for patients with severe pretransplant cardiogenic renal and hepatic dysfunctions is significant during the immediate posttransplantation course, especially when cyclosporine is given intravenously. Strict selection criteria, avoidance of intravenous administration of cyclosporine, and adequate control of cyclosporine serum levels are the major preventive measures currently available to prevent liver and kidney injuries. To minimize the incidence and the severity of the nephrotoxicity, several authors reduce the daily dose of cyclosporine and add other immunosuppressive agents such as azathioprine and/or antilymphocyte globulin.[105-108]

Hypertension. As a consequence of cyclosporine-induced nephrotoxicity, diastolic blood pressure above 90 mm Hg is frequently diagnosed (up to 90% of cases) among cardiac transplantation patients.[4,81,109-111] Adequate control is difficult to achieve and usually requires a combination of diuretic and antihypertensive therapy. Its pathogenesis is unknown, but most likely it involves the renin–angiotensin system as shown by Siegl.[112] Its long-term effect on myocardial function remains unknown, however.

Interstitial Myocardial Fibrosis. Interstitial myocardial fibrosis is reported by nearly all cardiac transplant centers.[4,94,95,109,113,114] The fibrotic histologic pattern may appear as early as 2 to 4 weeks postoperatively and was not originally reported in cardiac recipients treated with conventional immunosuppression. The risk of subsequent restrictive cardiomyopathy remains ill-defined. Preliminary data indicate that fibrosis does not seem to be progressive.[4]

Lymphoproliferative Disease. The overall incidence of lymphoproliferative disease in cyclosporine-treated patients has been reduced to less than 2% and is directly related to the amount and type of immunosuppression added to cyclosporine, as defined by Penn and Thiru.[73,115,116] However, the incidence can reach 10% to 15% when human antilymphocyte globulin is used routinely in conjunction with cyclosporine. Further long-term analyses are needed to assess accurately the actual incidence of malignancies in cyclosporine-treated patients. The tendency to reduce the conventional doses of cyclosporine to minimize its side-effects and to add other agents will probably increase the incidence of malignancies.

Allograft Coronary Atherosclerosis. This well-recognized complication with azathioprine steroid-treated patients has also been observed in patients treated with cyclosporine. The incidence of graft atherosclerosis (up to 10%) has been reported by Jamieson and associates.[110] Chronic rejection, inducing immunologic damage to the vascular endothelium and secondary intimal hyperplasia, could be the initial insult.[117,118] However, whatever the initial mechanism is, this pathologic process may lead to severe atherosclerosis. The exact pathogenesis of atherosclerosis remains unknown, and, therefore, its prevention is not possible. The effects of an antiplatelet regimen in combination with cyclosporine have not yet proven to be effective in preventing this significant complication.[119,120]

Other Complications and Cyclosporine Side-Effects. Several other cyclosporine-related complications have been described. Hepatotoxicity with mild cholestasis, convulsions, hirsutism, tremor, headaches, diarrhea, and pancreatitis,

among others, are the most frequently diagnosed.[121–123,125] A review of cyclosporine side-effects and complications was written recently by Calne.[78] Most of these complications are dose related, transient, and subject to significant individual variation. As mentioned earlier, the long-term effects caused by hypertension, nephrotoxicity, and myocardial fibrosis are of concern but still remain to be defined.

COST

Despite the clinical results obtained in cardiac transplantation, its costs and socioeconomic impacts are debated. Several articles were published that attempted to estimate the overall cost of the procedures. From Knox, Copeland, Centerwall, Pluth, Pennock, and Austen, the average total cost of a single cardiac transplantation, including expenses incurred during the first postoperative year, varies widely from $30,000 to $150,000 depending on the type of analysis and the inclusion of the research expenses related to transplantation.[53,126–129] An excellent review of economic and social costs of cardiac transplantation has been written by Evans.[131] This article provides an extensive analysis of the effectiveness of the procedure from which costs, benefits, and social impacts are assessed. The average cost of the procedure including follow-up and cyclosporine therapy during the first year is $56,000. However, as pointed out by Evans, calculating the cost of a heart transplant without taking into consideration the cost of conventional management (medical and/or surgical) of an end-stage cardiac disease with failure to achieve patient rehabilitation would not provide a realistic and adequate cost-benefit–effectiveness analysis. Therefore, the cost of a transplant procedure should be compared with the expenses incurred during the conventional therapy required for a similar end-stage cardiac patient, including its almost constant failure to provide social and professional rehabilitation. The cost to society of an occupationally incapacitated individual who previously earned a U.S. median wage of $13,000/year was estimated by Thomas and Lower.[132] This cost is about $32,000 per year in support money and loss of occupational contributions. It seems that although transplantation carries a slightly higher economic cost, its social impact may be a highly positive one.

THE FUTURE

The short- and middle-term results of cardiac transplantation clearly indicate its clinical value for end-stage cardiac disease. This achievement cannot be matched with any conventional therapeutic alternative, and the cost-benefit effectiveness and social impact seem favorable. However, the long-term effects caused by cyclosporine, mainly nephrotoxicity, hypertension, and graft fibrosis, remain unclear. Biochemical improvements of the cyclosporine molecule or adequate therapeutic balance among different immunosuppressive agents should minimize these effects. In future years, we predict that total control of the recipient immune system by means of specific or nonspecific immunotolerance techniques may include the option of using mammalian heterografts. If this were to occur, the present lack of human donors would become history. The artificial heart remains in its infancy and, therefore, cannot be used as an indefinite support but rather as a temporarizing modality. Blood-related complications (*i.e.*, thrombosis, hemorrhage, and significant hemolysis) have yet to be solved before use of the artificial heart can be increased despite its good mechanical performance.

REFERENCES

1. Cabrol C, Gandjbakhch I, Pavie A et al: Heart transplantation at Lapitie Hospital, Paris 1968–1984. Journal of Heart Transplantation 4:27, 984

2. Austen WG, Cosimi AB: Heart transplantation after 16 years. N Engl J Med 311:1437, 1984

3. McGregor CGA, Jamieson SW, Oyer PE et al: Heart transplantation at Stanford University. Journal of Heart Transplantation 4:31, 1984

4. Oyer PE, Stinson EB, Jamieson SW et al: Cyclosporine in cardiac transplantation: A 2½ year follow-up. Transplant Proc XV:2546, 1983

5. Shumway NE: Recent advances in cardiac transplantation. Transplant Proc 15:1223, 1983

6. Painvin GA, Reece IJ, Cooley DA, Frazier OM: Cardiopulmonary allotransplantation, a collective review: Experimental process and current clinical status. Texas Heart Institute Journal 10:372, 1983

7. Samuelsson RG, Hunt SA, Schroeder JS: Functional and social rehabilitation of heart transplantation recipients under age thirty. Scand J Thorac Cardiovasc Surg 18:97, 1984

8. Griepp RB, Elrisan Ergin M: The history of experimental heart transplantation. Heart Transplantation III:145, 1984

9. Carrel A: The surgery of blood vessels. Bull J Hopkins 18:190, 1907

10. Carrel A, Guthrie CC: The transplantation of veins and organs. Am J Med 10:1101, 1905

11. Mann FC, Priestley JT, Markowitz J: Transplantation of the intact mammalian heart. Arch Surg 26:219, 1933

12. Marcus E, Wong SM, Luisada AA: Homologous heart grafts: Transplantation of the heart in dogs. Surg Forum 2:212, 1951

13. Downie HG: Homotransplantation of the dog heart. Arch Surg 66:624, 1953

14. Neptune WB, Cookson BA, Bailey CP: Complete homologous heart transplantation. Arch Surg 66:174, 1953

15. Cass MH, Brock R: Heart excision and replacement. Guy Hosp Rep 108:285, 1959

16. Lower RR, Shumway NE: Studies on the orthotopic homotransplantation of the canine heart. Surg Forum 11:18, 1960

17. Lower RR, Stofer RC, Shumway NE: Homovital transplantation of the heart. J Thorac Cardiovasc Surg 41:196, 1961

18. Shumway NE, Lower RR, Stofer RC: Transplantation of the heart. Surg Forum 2:265, 1966

19. Lower RR, Dong E, Shumway NE: Long-term survival of cardiac homografts. Surgery 58:110, 1965

20. Hardy JD, Chavez CM: The first heart transplantation in man: Developmental animal investigation with analysis of the 1964 case in light of current clinical experience. Am J Cardiol 22:772, 1968

21. Barnard CN: The operation: A human cardiac trans-

plantation. An interim report of the successful operation performed at Groote Schuur Hospital, Capetown. S Afr Med J 41:1271, 1967

22. Cooley DA, Bloodwell RD, Hallman GL et al: Cardiac transplantation: Several considerations and results. Ann Surg 169:892, 1969

23. Kantrowitz A, Haller JD, Joos H: Transplantation of the heart in an infant and an adult. Am J Cardiol 22:782, 1968

24. American Heart Association: Heart Facts, 1984. Dallas, American Heart Association National Center, 1984

25. Evans RW, Manninen DL, Gersh BJ et al: The need for and supply of donor hearts for transplantation. Heart Transplantation 3:57, 1984

26. Pennock JL, Oyer PE, Reitz BA et al: Cardiac transplantation in perspective for the future: Survival, complication, rehabilitation and cost. J Thorac Cardiovasc Surg 83:168, 1982

27. Lubeck DP, Bunder JP: The artificial heart: Cost, risks and benefits. Washington, DC, Office of Technology Assessment, 1982

28. Thompson ME: Selection of candidates for cardiac transplantation. Heart Transplantation III:67, 1983

29. Evans RW, Manninen DL et al: The organ procurement program survey. National Heart Transplantation Study, update report No 1 and No 5. Seattle, WA, Battelle Herrian Affairs Research Centers, 1982

30. Ad Hoc Task Force on Cardiac Replacement: Cardiac replacement: Medical, ethical, psychological and economic implications. Bethesda, MD, National Heart, Lung, and Blood Institute, 1969

31. Cooley DA, Frazier OH, Painvin GA et al: Cardiac and cardiopulmonary transplantation using cyclosporine for immunosuppression: Recent Texas Heart Institute Experience. Transplant Proc XV:2567, 1983

32. Jarvik RK: The total artificial heart. Sci Am 244:74, 1981

33. Copeland JG: Facts to be considered prior to undertaking a heart transplantation program. Heart Transplantation III:275, 1984

34. Russel PS, Cosmimi AB: Transplantation. N Engl J Med 301:470, 1979

35. Schroeder JS: Current status of cardiac transplantation. JAMA 241:2069, 1979

36. Cooper DK, Boyd ST, Lanza RP, Barnard CN: Factors influencing survival following heart transplantation. Heart Transplantation 3:88, 1983

37. Griepp RB, Stinson EB, Clark DA, Shumway NE: Determinants of oprative risk in human heart transplantation. Am J Surg 122:192, 1971

38. Lower RR, Szentpetery S, Quinn J et al: Selection of patients for cardiac transplantation. Transplant Proc 11:293, 1979

39. Baumgartner WA, Borkon AM, Achuff SC et al: Heart and heart lung transplantation: Program development, organization, and initiation. Heart Transplantation 4:197, 1985

40. Gunderson L: Teaching the transplant recipient. Heart Transplantation 4:227, 1985

41. Bart KJ, Macon EJ, Humphries Al et al: Increasing the supply of cadaver kidneys for transplantation. Transplantation 31:384, 1981

42. Stuart FP: Need, supply, and legal issues related to organ transplantation in the United States. Transplant Proc XVI:88, 1984

43. Carpenter CB, Ettenger RB, Strom TB: "Free-market" approach to organ donation. N Engl J Med 310:395, 1984

44. Richenbacher WE, Pierce WS: The artificial heart: A progress report. J Cardio Med 36:1057, 1983

45. A definition of irreversible coma: Report of the Ad Hoc Committee of the Harvard Medical School to examine the definition of brain death. JAMA 205:85, 1968

46. Black PM: Brain death. N Engl J Med 299:338, 1978

47. Stuart FT, Veith FJ, Crawford RE: Brain death laws and patterns of current to remove organs for transplantation from cadavers in the U.S. and 28 other countries. Transplantation 31:238, 1981

48. Angstwurm H, Einhaupl K: Organ donors and brain death diagnosis: Experiences in the diagnosis and documentation of brain death. Transplant Proc XVI:95, 1984

49. Griepp RD, Stinson EB, Shumway NE: The cardiac donor. SGO 133:792, 1971

50. Cooper DKC: The donor heart. J Surg Res 21:363, 1976

51. Hardesty RL, Griffith BP, Deeb GM, Starzl TE: Improved cardiac function using cardioplegia during procurement and transplantation. Transplant Proc 15:1253, 1983

52. Cabrol C, Lienhart A, Gandjbakhch I et al: Choice and handling of donors for cardiac transplantation. Transplant Proc XVI:55, 1984

53. Pennock JL, Oyer PE, Reitz BA, Shumway NE: Cardiac transplantation in perspective for the future. J Thorac Cardiovasc Surg 83:168, 1982

54. Shaw BW, Rosenthal JT, Griffith BP et al: Early function of heart, liver, and kidney allografts following combined procurement. Transplant Proc XVI:238, 1984

55. Shaw BW, Rosenthal JT, Griffith BFD et al: Techniques for combined procurement of hearts and kidneys with satisfactory early function of renal allografts. Surg Gynecol Obstet 157:262, 1983

56. Goldman MH, Shapiro R, Capehart J et al: Cardiac procurement in the multiple organ disease. Transplant Proc XVI:231, 1984

57. Margreiter R: Multiple organ procurement. Transplant Proc XVI:261, 1984

58. Rosenthal FT, Shaw BN, Hardesty RL et al: Principles of multiple organ procurement from cadaver donors. Ann Surg 198:618, 1983

59. Brodman RF, Veith FJ, Goldsmith J et al: Multiple organ procurement from one donor. Heart Transplantation 4:254, 1985

60. Cederna J, Toledo–Paaereyra LH: Multiple organ harvesting: Selection, maintenance, surgical techniques. Contemporary Surgery 25:15, 1984

61. Reece IJ, Painvin GA, Okereke J et al: Evaluation of the Texas Heart Institute Distant Organ Procurement Program. Texas Heart Institute Journal 11:38, 1984

62. Mendez–Picon GJ, Goldman MH, Lower RR: Long distance procurement and transportation of human hearts for transplantation. Heart Transplantation 1:63, 1981

63. Watson DC, Reitz Ba, Stinson EB, Shumway NE: Distant heart procurement for transplantation. Surgery 86:56, 1979

64. Cooper DKC, Wicomb WN, Barnard CN: Storage of the donor heart by a portable hypothermic perfusion system: Experimental development and clinical experience. Heart Transplantation II:105, 1983

65. Fernando NA, Keenan RL, Boyan CP: Anesthetic experience with cardiac transplantation. J Thorac Cardiovasc Surg 75:531, 1978

66. Cooley DA: Cardiac transplantation. In Cooley DA (ed): Techniques in Cardiac Surgery, 2nd ed, pp 369–385. Philadelphia, WB Saunders, 1984

67. Cooley DA, Frazier OM, Painvin GA, Kahan BD: Cardiac transplantation with the use of CyA for immunosuppression. Texas Heart Institute Journal 9:247, 1982

68. Cabrol C, Pavie A, Laskar MJ, Mattei MF: Heart and heart lung transplantation: Techniques and safeguards. Heart Transplantation 3:110, 1984

69. Hess N, Brook–Brunn JA, Joy K: Complete isolation: Is it necessary? (abstr) Heart Transplantation 4:112, 1985

70. Caves PK, Stinson EB, Shumway NE: Percutaneous transvenous endomyocardial biopsy in human heart recipient. Ann Thorac Surg 16:325, 1973

71. Billingham ME: Diagnosis of cadiac rejection by endocardial biopsy. Heart Transplantation 1:25, 1981

72. Billingham ME: The role of endomyocardial biopsy in diagnosis and treatment of heart disease in cardiovascular pathology. In Silver MD (ed): Cardiac Pathology, Vol II New York, Churchill Livingstone, 1983

73. Starzl TE: Clinical aspects of cyclosporine therapy: A summation. Transplant Proc XV:3103, 1983

74. Cyclosporine A: A new outlook for immunosuppression in clinical transplantation. Blut 39:81–87, 1979

75. White DJG: Cyclosporine A: Clinical pharmacology and therapeutic potential. Drugs 24:322, 1982

76. Bandlien KO, Toledo–Pereyra LH, MacKenzie GH, Cortez JA: Immunosuppression with cyclosporine. Immunosuppression 118:829, 1983

77. Borel JF: Cyclosporin A. Present experimental status. Transplant Proc XIII:344, 1981

78. Calne RY: Organ transplantation and cyclosporine. Can J Surg 27:12, 1984

79. Bore JF, Laferty KJ: Cyclosporine: Basic science summations. Transplant Proc XV:3097, 1983

80. Borel JF, Lafferty KJ: Cyclosporine: Speculation about its mechanism of action. Transplant Proc XV:1881, 1983

81. Hardesty RL, Griffity BP, Debski RF, Bahnson HT: Experience with cyclosporine in cardiac transplantation. Transplant Proc XV:2553, 1983

82. Reece IJ, Frazier OH, Painvin GA et al: Early results of cardiac transplantation of the Texas Heart Institute. Thorax 39:676, 1984

83. Painvin GA, Reece IJ, Okereke J, Frazier OH: Cardiac transplantation: Indications, procurements, operation, and management. Heart Lung (in press)

84. Painvin GA, Okereke OU, Frazier OH et al: Cardiac transplantation: Current results of cyclosporine treated patients at the Texas Heart Institute. Transplant Proc 17:223, 1985

85. Frazier OH, Cooley DA, Painvin GA et al: Cardiac transplantation at the Texas Heart Institute: Comparative analysis of two groups of patients (1968–1969) and (1982–1983). Ann Thorac Surg 39:304, 1985

86. Griffith BP, Hardesty RL, Thomson ME: Cardiac transplantation CyA: The Pittsburgh Experience. Heart TX II:251, 1983

87. Hardesty RL, Griffith BP, Debski RF et al: Experience with cyclosporine in cardiac transplantation. Transplant Proc 15:2553, 1983

88. Wallwork J, Cory–Pearce R, English TAH: Cyclosporine for cardiac transplantation: U.K. trial. Transplant Proc XV:2559, 1983

89. English TAH, Cory–Pearce R, McGregor C: Cardiac transplantation: 3.5 year experience of Papworth Hospital. Transplant Proc 15:1238, 1983

90. Cabrol C, Pavie A, Cabrol A: Current management of heart transplantation patients to LaPitie Hospital in Paris. Heart Transplantation I:275, 1982

91. Painvin GA, McCormick MC, Roberts AJ: Cardiac and cardiopulmonary transplantation: Current status. Cardiovasc Reviews & Reports 6:178, 1985

92. Greenberg ML, Uretsky BF, Reddy PS et al: Long-term hemodynamic follow-up of cardiac transplant patients treated with cyclosporine and prednisone. Circulation 71:487, 1985

93. Lough ME: Life satisfaction following heart transplantation (abstr). Heart Transplantation 4:111, 1985

94. Griffith BP, Hardesty RL, Bahnson HT: Powerful but limited immunosuppression for cardiac transplantation with cyclosporine and low dose of steroids. J Thorac Cardiovasc Surg 35:87, 1984

95. Griffith BP, Hardesty RL, Bahnson HT et al: Cardiac transplants with cyclosporine A and low dose prednisone: Histologic graduation of rejection. Transplant Proc XV:1241, 1983

96. Reece IJ, Painvin Ga, Gentry BL et al: Infection after cardiac transplantation: Treatment and prognosis. Texas Heart Institute Journal 11:32, 1984

97. Reece IJ, Painvin GA, Zeluff B et al: Infection in cyclosporine immunosuppressed cardiac allograft recipients. Heart Transplantation 3:239, 1984

98. Baumgartner WA: Infection in cardiac transplantation. Heart Transplantation III:75, 1983

99. Egel J, Greenberg A, Thompson ME et al: Renal failure in heart transplant patients receiving cyclosporine. Transplant Proc XV:2706, 1983

100. Nelson PW: Cyclosporine. Surg Gynecol Obstet 159:297, 1984

101. Myers BD, Ross J, Newton OL et al: Cyclosporine associated chronic nephropathy. N Engl J Med 311:699, 1984

102. Devineni R, McKenzie N, Duplan J et al: Renal effects of cyclosporine: Clinical and experimental observation. Transplant Proc XV:2695, 1983

103. Keown PA, Stiller CR, Laupacis AL: Effects and side-effects of cyclosporine: Relationship to drug pharmacokinetics. Transplant Proc 14:659, 1981

104. Foley RJ, VanBuren CT, Hammer R, Weinmann EJ: Cyclosporine associated hyperkalemia. Transplant Proc XV:2726, 1983

105. Griffith B, Hardesty RL, Lee A et al: The response of cyclosporine toxicity to azathioprine and reduced cyclosporine dose (abstr). Heart Transplantation 4:148, 1985

106. Scott WC, Haverich A, Dawkins KD et al: Study of optional cyclosporine immunosuppression in primate orthotopic cardiac transplantation (abstr). Heart Transplantation 4:124, 1985

107. Bolman RM, Elick B, Olivari MT: Improved immunosuppression for cardiac transplantation (abstr). Heart Transplantation 4:123, 1985

108. Canafax DM, Martel EJ, Ascher NL et al: Two methods of managing cyclosporine nephrotoxicity: Conversion to azathioprine, prednisone, or cyslosporine, azathioprine and prednisone. Transplant Proc 27:1176, 1985

109. Hunt SA: Complications of heart transplantation. Heart Transplantation 3:70, 1983

110. Jamieson SW: Recent developments in heart and heart lung transplantation. Transplant Proc 7:199, 1985

111. Thompson ME, Shapiro AP, Griffith BL: New onset of hypertension following cardiac transplantation: A preliminary report and analysis. Transplantation Proc XV:2573, 1983

112. Siegl H, Ryffel B, Petric R, Muller A: Cyclosporine, the renin–angiotensive aldosterone system and renal adverse reactions. Transplant Proc XV:2719, 1983

113. Cohen RG, Hoyt EG, Billingham ME et al: Myocardial fibrosis due to cyclosporine in rat heteroptic heart transplant. Heart Transplantation III:182, 1984

114. Karch SB, Billingham ME: Cyclosporine induced myocardial fibrosis. A unique controlled case report. Heart Transplantation 4:211, 1985

115. Penn I: Lymphomas complicating organ transplantation. Transplant Proc XV:2790, 1983

116. Thiru S, Calne RY, Nagington J: Lymphoma in renal allograft patients treated with cyclosporine as one of the immunosuppressive agents. Transplant Proc 13:359, 1981

117. Kosek JVC, Bieber C, Lower RR: Heart graft atherosclerosis. Transplant Proc 3:512, 1971

118. Hess ML, Hastillo A, Lower RR: Accelerated atherosclerosis in cardiac transplantation: Role of cytotoxic antibodies and hyperlipidemia. Circulation 68:97, 1983

119. Hoyt EG, Gollin G, Billingham M et al: Vessel disease in cardiac allografts: The effect of anti-platelet regimens in combination with cyclosporine. Heart Transplantation (III)195:1984

120. Hoyt G, Gollin G, Billingham M et al: Effects on anti-platelet regimens in combination with cyclosporine on heart allograft vessel disease. Journal of Heart Transplantation 4:54, 1984

121. Loertscher R, Thiel G, Hardee F: Persistent elevation of alkaline phosphotase in cyclosporine treated renal transplant recipients. Transplantation 36:115, 1983

122. Schade RR, Guglielmi A, Vanthiel DH et al: Cholestasis in heart transplant recipients treated with cyclosporine. Transplant Proc XV:2557, 1983

123. Durrant S, Chipping P, Palmers S: Cyclosporine methylprednisolone and convulsions. Lancet 2:829–830, 1982

124. Human DP, McKenzie FN, Kostuk NJ: Restricted myocardial compliance one year following cardiac transplantation. Heart Transplantation III:341, 1984

125. Okereke OJ, Frazier OH, Colley DA, Waldenberger F: Cardiac transplantation: Current results at the Texas Heart Institute. Texas Heart Institute Journal 11:228, 1984

126. Knox RA: Heart transplantation: To pay or not to pay. Science 209:570, 1980

127. Copeland JG, Stinson EB: Human heart transplantation: Current problems in cardiology. (IV)8:45, 1979

128. Centerwall BS: Cost-benefit analysis and heart transplantation. N Engl J Med 304:901, 1981

129. Pluth JR, Kaye MP: Cardiac transplantation: Foolhardy or farsighted. Mayo Clin Proc 56:202, 1981

130. Austen WG, Cosimi AB: Heart transplantation after 16 years. N Engl J Med 311:1437, 1984

131. Evans R: Economic and social costs of heart transplantation. Heart Transplantation 1:243, 1982

132. Thomas FT, Lower RR: Heart transplantation 1978. Surg Clin North Am 58:325, 1978

INDEX

Numbers followed by "t" denote tables; numbers followed by "f" denote figures.